TCM Study Guide Series

Herbology

VOLUME I

by Shi Cun Wu

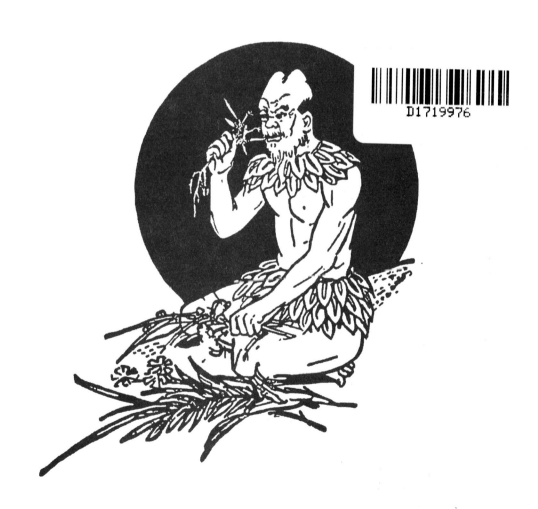

KANG TAI PRESS ☯ CHICAGO

Copyright © 2000 by Kang Tai Press, Inc.

All rights reserved. This book or any part thereof may not be reproduced, stored in a retrieval system, or transmitted, in any form or by any means, electronic, mechanical, photocopying, recording, or otherwise, without the prior written permission of the publisher.

This publication is designed to provide accurate and authoritative information in regard to the subject matter covered. It is sold with the understanding that the publisher is not engaged in rendering medical, legal, or any other advice. If medical advice or other expert assistance is required, the services of a competent, licensed professional should be sought.

Printed in the United States of America

ISBN 1-928537-03-0

2 3 4 5 6 7 8 9 10 Printing / Year 08 07 06 05 04 03 02

TABLE OF CONTENTS

Table of Contents i
Preface iii
Acknowledgments v
About the Author vii
Recommended Reference Texts ix
Terminology Equivalencies xi
Storehouse of Questions (see topical breakdown below)
    Section A *(questions 1–1800)* 1
    Section B *(questions 1801–2500)* 203
    Section C *(questions 2501–3500)* 253
Answers to the Questions 309

TOPICAL BREAKDOWN OF QUESTIONS

Topic or Function	Section A	Section B	Section C
Foundations of TCM	1-39	1801-1809	2501-2537
Release the Exterior	40-104	1810-1856	2538-2585
Clear Heat	105-254	1857-1922	2386-2722
Drain Downward	255-300	1923-1944	2723-2753
Drain Damp, Drain Wind-Damp and Transform Damp	301-436	1945-2004	2754-2864
Transform Phlegm	437-536	2005-2045	2865-2925
Relieve Food Stagnation	537-567	2046-2067	2926-2937
Regulate the Qi	568-650	2068-2113	2938-2969
Regulate the Blood	651-797	2114-2147	2969-3023
Warm the Interior	798-860	2148-2179	3024-3051
Tonify	861-990	2180-2218	3052-3109
Stabilize and Bind	991-1053	2219-2233	3110-3150
Calm the Spirit	1053-1086	2234-2267	3151-3119
Open the Orifices	1087-1113	2268-2269	3168-3179
Extinguish Wind	1114-1177	2270-2301	3180-3210
Expel Parasites *(ext. application)*	1178-1265	2302-2316	3211-3225
Combination Formulas	1266-1800	2317-2500	3226-3500

PREFACE

Traditional Chinese Medicine (TCM) is the legacy of many thousands of years of accumulated experience. The value of this ancient, holistic, health care system is now widely recognized, and well-trained practitioners of Traditional Chinese Medicine have established themselves in many Western health care facilities.

Shi Cun Wu developed the TCM Study Guide Series in order to help fulfill the quest for better English-language learning tools devoted to TCM principles and practice. Through his TCM Study Guide Series, he hopes to provide students and practitioners alike with new means for developing their knowledge and preparing to demonstrate its capacity on board examinations.

The questions in the TCM Study Guide Series have been designed to improve the reader's ability to analyze health problems and make sound judgments within the framework of Traditional Chinese Medicine. They are presented in a multiple-choice format because that represents the most popular method in the United States.

TCM Study Guide Series: Herbology is comprised of two volumes. Volume one contains the Storehouse of Questions—3,500 multiple-choice questions relating to Traditional Chinese Herbal Medicine and Herbal Formulas. These questions are grouped by function and are further grouped by syndrome using Traditional Chinese Herbs or Traditional Chinese Formulas (see Table of Contents). The answers to the Storehouse of Questions in Volume One are found at the back of this book.

Volume Two will contain case studies, practice tests, final examinations, and resource material.

ACKNOWLEDGMENTS

This volume would not have been possible without the help of a number of people, who devoted great time and effort to ensuring it met or exceeded its objectives. Vicki Jarossek, Yosef Pollack, Bill Siegel, Tammy Siegel, Mari Stecker, and Barry Thorne were instrumental in the careful evaluation and revision of its contents. Bill Burck was responsible for the book's overall editing, design, production, and publishing. Of course, the father of the TCM Study Guide Series is Shi Cun Wu, who developed these books as a means of spreading the knowledge and benefits of Traditional Chinese Medicine

Author
SHI CUN WU

Editor/Designer/Publisher
BILL BURCK

Editorial Board
VICKI JAROSSEK
YOSEF POLLACK, L. AC.
BILL SIEGEL
TAMMY SIEGEL
MARI STECKER, L. AC.
BARRY THORNE
AMY YEOSTROS, L. AC.

ABOUT THE AUTHOR

Shi Cun Wu began his formal education in Traditional Chinese Medicine at Jilin Medical University in Jilin, China, where he graduated in the 1950s. His understanding of TCM began much earlier than this, however, under the tutelage of his father, who was himself a TCM physician.

After graduation, Shi Cun Wu engaged in 20 years of TCM clinical practice and research in Chinese hospitals and herbal research bureaus. He authored articles on herbal research for the *Journal of Chinese Herbal Medicine* and presented his findings at academic conferences. He participated in the project to compile the 1977 edition of the *People's Republic of China Pharmacopoeia*, helping to define quality standards for the sections on Traditional Herbal Medicine and Herbal-Based Patent Medicine. In addition, he helped write the *Guangdong Provincial Traditional Herbal Medicine Preparation Handbook* as well as the Traditional Herbal Medicine section of the 1978 edition of the *Guangdong Provincial Medicine Standards Manual*.

After this work, Shi Cun Wu emigrated to the United States, where he has operated an herbal store and taught classes on all aspects of TCM for two decades. He is an NCCA Diplomate in Herbology and Acupuncture.

RECOMMENDED REFERENCE TEXTS

Bensky, Dan and Gamble, Andrew. *Chinese Herbal Medicine Materia Medica*. Seattle: Eastland Press, 1993.

Bensky, Dan and Barolet, Randall. *Formulas and Strategies*. Seattle: Eastland Press, 1990.

Zhang Enqin, et al. *The Chinese Materia Medica*. Shanghai: Shanghai College of Traditional Chinese Medicine, 1990.

Zhang Enqin, et al. *Prescriptions of Traditional Chinese Medicine*. Shanghai: Shanghai College of Traditional Chinese Medicine, 1990.

TERMINOLOGY EQUIVALENCIES

As you use this study guide, you will most likely reference one or more texts on TCM theory and practice. The terminology used can vary widely from text to text. The following list of equivalencies is provided to help bridge some of the terminology differences you may encounter. Each term can be found in alphabetical order, with equivalencies listed to the right. This list is far from comprehensive. Nevertheless, we hope you find it useful.

Ancestral vessels = Eight meridians = Eight extra meridians = Eight extraordinary vessels
Asthenia = Deficiency (or Deficient) = Emptiness = Xu
Backward on the Ko cycle = Counteracting cycle = Insult cycle
Body fluids = Ching ye = Jin-ye
Bowel = Fu = Yang organ
Bu = Supplement = Tonify
Channel = Mai = Meridian = Mo (for instance: Yinweimo = Yinweimai; Du Mo = Du Mai)
Ching Ye = Body fluids = Jin-ye
Chong Mai = Chong meridian = Penetrating meridian
Coating = Moss = Tongue fur
Conception Vessel = Ren meridian = Ren Mo
Control cycle = Interacting cycle = Overacting cycle = Ko cycle
Dai Mai = Dai meridian = Belt meridian
Defensive Qi = Protective energy = Wei Qi
Deficiency (or deficient) = Asthenia = Emptiness = Xu
Disorder stemming from external factors = Exogenous = Externally generated
Disorder stemming from internal factors = Endogenous = Internally generated
Disperse = Reduce = Sedate = Xie
Du meridian = Du Mai = Du Mo = Governing Vessel
Eight meridians = Ancestral vessels = Eight extra meridians = Eight extraordinary vessels
Emptiness = Asthenia = Deficiency (or Deficient) = Xu
Endogenous = Disorder stemming from internal factors = Internally generated

Enlarged tongue = Fat tongue = Flabby tongue = Swollen tongue
Excess = Fullness = Shi = Sthenia
Exogenous = Disorder stemming from external factors = Externally generated
Externally generated = Disorder stemming from external factors = Exogenous
External pathogenic factor (or influence) = Outside evil = Pernicious influence = Perverse energy
Fat tongue = Enlarged tongue = Flabby tongue = Swollen tongue
Five Elements = Five Phases = Wu Xing
Fu = Yang organ = Bowel
Fullness = Excess = Shi = Sthenia
Generation cycle = Interpromoting cycle = Sheng cycle
Governing Vessel = Du meridian = Du Mai = Du Mo
Horary cycle = Mid-day/midnight cycle = Organ clock
Insult cycle = Backward on the Ko cycle = Counteracting cycle
Interacting cycle = Control cycle = Overacting cycle = Ko cycle
Internally generated = Endogenous = Disorder stemming from internal factors
Interpromoting cycle = Generation cycle = Sheng cycle
Ko cycle = Control cycle = Interacting cycle = Overacting cycle
Mai = Channel = Meridian = Mo
Main meridians = Primary meridians = Principal meridians = Regular meridians
Meridian = Channel = Mai = Mo
Mid-day/midnight cycle = Horary cycle = Organ clock
Mo = Channel = Mai = Meridian

Moss = Coating = Tongue fur
Nourishing energy = Nutritive Qi = Ying Qi
Officials = Organs and Bowels = Viscera = Yin and Yang organs = Zang/fu
Organ clock = Horary cycle = Mid-day/midnight cycle
Organs and Bowels = Officials = Viscera = Yin and Yang organs = Zang/fu
Original Qi = Prenatal Qi = Yuan Qi
Outside evil = External pathogenic factor (or influence) = Pernicious influence = Perverse energy
Pectoral Qi = Zhong Qi
Penetrating meridian = Chong Mai = Chong meridian
Pernicious influence = External pathogenic factor (or influence) = Outside evil = Perverse energy
Perverse energy = External pathogenic factor (or influence) = Outside evil = Pernicious influence
Prenatal Qi = Original Qi = Yuan Qi
Primary meridians = Main meridians = Principal meridians = Regular meridians
Principal meridians = Main meridians = Primary meridians = Regular meridians
Protective energy = Defensive Qi = Wei Qi
Reduce = Disperse = Sedate = Xie
Regular meridians = Main meridians = Primary meridians = Principal meridians
Ren meridian = Conception Vessel = Ren Mo
Sanjiao = Three Heaters = Tri-Heater = Triple Burner = Triple Burning Space = Triple Energizer = Triple Heater = Triple Warmer**Sedate** = Disperse = Reduce = Xie

Sheng cycle = Generation cycle = Interpromoting cycle
Shi = Excess = Fullness = Sthenia
Sthenia = Excess = Fullness = Shi
Supplement = Bu = Tonify
Swollen tongue = Enlarged tongue = Fat tongue = Flabby tongue
Tongue fur = Coating = Moss
Tongue proper = Tongue material or tissues
Tonify = Bu = Supplement
Triple Burner = Sanjiao = Three Heaters = Tri-Heater = Triple Burning Space = Triple Energizer = Triple Heater = Triple Warmer
Viscera = Officials = Organs and Bowels = Yin and Yang organs = Zang/fu
Wei Qi = Defensive Qi = Protective energy
Wu Xing = Five Elements = Five Phases
Xie = Disperse = Reduce = Sedate
Xu = Asthenia = Deficiency (or deficient) = Emptiness
YangQiao meridian = Yang Heel meridian
Yang organ = Bowel = Fu
Yangwei meridian = Yang Linking meridian
Yin and Yang organs = Officials = Organs and Bowels = Viscera = Zang/fu
Yin organ = Zang
Ying Qi = Nourishing energy = Nutritive Qi
YinQiao meridian = Yin Heel meridian
Yinwei meridian = Yin Linking meridian
Yuan Qi = Original Qi = Prenatal Qi
Zhong Qi = Pectoral Qi
Yuan Qi = Original Qi = Prenatal Qi
Zang = Yin organ
Zang/fu = Officials = Organs and Bowels = Viscera = Yin and Yang organs

Storehouse of Questions

STOREHOUSE OF QUESTIONS

A. In this section (questions 1–1800), select the one best answer to each question.

1. Who wrote the treatise entitled *Ben Cao Gang Mu* (Compendium of Materia Medica)?
   a. Tao Hong Jing
   b. Sun Si Miao
   c. Li Shi Zhen
   d. Zhang Zhongjing

2. How many kinds of herbs are listed in the *Ben Cao Gang Mu* (Compendium of Materia Medica)?
   a. 844
   b. 921
   c. 1,746
   d. 1,892

3. The *Shen Nong Ben Cao Jing* (Divine Husbandman's Classic of the Materia Medica) is:
   a. The first Chinese pharmacopoeia
   b. The first Chinese materia medica specialty book
   c. The first Chinese diet therapy book
   d. The most famous Chinese biology book

4. How many herbs are covered in the *Xin Xiu Ben Cao* (Newly Revised Materia Medica)?
   a. 730
   b. 1,746
   c. 844
   d. 1,892

5. Which materia medica book was the first official Chinese pharmacopoeia?
   a. *Ben Cao Gang Mu* (Compendium of Materia Medica)
   b. *Shen Nong Ben Cao Jing* (Divine Husbandman's Classic of Materia Medica)
   c. *Xin Xiu Ben Cao* (Newly Revised Materia Medica)
   d. *Qian Jin Yao Fang* (Thousand Ducat Formulas)

6. Who wrote the treatise entitled *Qian Jin Yao Fang* (Thousand Ducat Formulas)?
   a. Sun Si Miao
   b. Huato
   c. Huang Pu Mi
   d. Li Shih Chen

7. Who wrote the treatise on the preparation and broiling of medicinal substances?
   a. Tao Hung Ching
   b. Lei Xiao
   c. Li Ting
   d. Wu Qi Qian

8. Which term is used to describe the process of heating minerals and then immediately immersing them in cold water or vinegar?
   a. Steaming
   b. Boiling
   c. Quenching
   d. Simmering

9. What is the goal when preparing fresh He Shou Wu?
    a. To decrease or remove poisonous side effects
    b. To alter its function
    c. To enhance the ease with which it is prepared and stored
    d. To remove the ineffective portion

10. Preparing herbs by frying with wine fulfills which purpose?
    a. It enhances the function of strengthening the Middle Energizer and benefiting the Qi.
    b. It enhances the function of invigorating the Kidney
    c. It enhances the function of strengthening the Spleen
    d. It enhances the function of promoting Blood circulation

11. Which herb is often prepared by frying with honey?
    a. Bai Zhu
    b. Shan Yao
    c. Bai Shao
    d. Huang Qi

12. Which frying method is used to enhance the dispersal of depressed Liver Qi and the alleviation of pain?
    a. Fry with honey
    b. Fry with wine
    c. Fry with vinegar
    d. Fry with ginger juice

13. Which preparation helps to decrease an herb's poisonous effect?
    a. Fry Yan Hu Suo with vinegar
    b. Fry Yuan Hua with vinegar
    c. Grind Hua Shi to a fine powder while adding water
    d. Fry Xiang Fu with vinegar

14. Which of the five flavors is considered bland?
    a. Acrid
    b. Bitter
    c. Sour
    d. Sweet
    e. Salty

15. Which of the five flavors is categorized as softening?
    a. Acrid
    b. Bitter
    c. Sour
    d. Sweet
    e. Salty

16. What is a function of sour-flavored herbs?
    a. Promote Blood circulation
    b. Harmonize
    c. Astringent
    d. Relieve stranguria by diuresis

17. Bitter-flavored herbs performs which of the following functions?
    a. Promote Qi and Blood circulation
    b. Regulate the Middle Energizer
    c. Drain Damp and relax the bowels in order to eliminate internal Heat
    d. Soften hard lumps, dispel nodules, and purge

18. Acrid-flavored herbs performs which of the following functions?
    a. Drain Damp
    b. Soften hard lumps and purge
    c. Invigorate and regulate the Middle Energizer
    d. Dispel exogenous evils and promote Qi and Blood circulation

19. Salty-flavored herbs are used to treat which of the following?
    a. Night sweats
    b. Blurry vision or dizziness
    c. Coughing caused by Lung Damp-Heat
    d. Scrofula, phlegm nodules, and masses in the abdomen

20. Which flavor has the function of draining Damp?
    a. Sweet
    b. Sour
    c. Bitter
    d. Bland

21. Cold-bitter herbs performs which of the following functions?
    a. Aromatically transform Damp
    b. Expel Wind-Damp and activate the meridians
    c. Clear Heat and eliminating Damp
    d. Drain Damp

22. Which of the following is characterized as lifting and floating?
    a. Sweet, acrid, cool
    b. Acrid, bitter, hot
    c. Acrid, sweet, warm
    d. Bland, sweet, cold

23. The Theory of Meridian Tropism belongs to which of the following?
    a. The doctrine of Yin and Yang
    b. The doctrine of the viscera and Jing Luo (meridians and collaterals)
    c. The characteristics of the four natures of Chinese medicine (cold, cool, warm, hot)
    d. None of the above

24. What are the normal functions of lift and float, and lower and sink?
    a. Lift and float move up and out; lower and sink move up and in
    b. Lift and float move down and out; lower and sink move up and in
    c. Lift and float move up and out; lower and sink move down and in
    d. Lift and float move up and in; lower and sink move down and out

25. In the clinical use of medica, what is the main principle of compatible application?
    a. Mutual restraint and mutual detoxification
    b. Mutual restraint and mutual assistance
    c. Mutual reinforcement and mutual assistance
    d. Mutual restraint and mutual incompatibility

26. Which two herbs belong to the eighteen incompatible herbs?
    a. Ba Dou and Quan Nu Zi
    b. Mang Xiao and San Leng
    c. Gan Cao and Yuan Hua
    d. Li Lu and Ban Xia

27. Which two herbs belong to the nineteen antagonistic medicinal herbs?
    a. Fu Zi and Ban Xia
    b. Ding Xiang and Chuan Wu Tou
    c. Rou Gui and Chi Shi Zhi
    d. Ren Shen and Quan Nu Zi

28. Which herb is incompatible with Ren Shen?
    a. Wu Tou
    b. Li Lu
    c. Gan Cao
    d. San Leng

29. Which two herbs decrease each other's effect?
    a. Fu Zi and Gan Cao
    b. Lai Fu Zi and Ren Shen
    c. Wu Ling Zi and Ren Shen
    d. Sha Shen and Ren Shen

30. Which answer contains an herb that counteracts the toxicity of the other herb?
    a. Fu Zi and Gan Cao
    b. Ban Xia and Ze Xie
    c. Da Ji and Gan Cao
    d. Gan Sui and Sheng Jiang

31. What should be avoided if one has a pyogenic infection and an ulcerous disease of the skin?
    a. Salt
    b. Sugar
    c. Pork
    d. Shrimp

32. Which of the following should be added after the rest of the herbs in a formula have been decocted?
    a. Jin Yin Hua
    b. Sang Ye
    c. Pi Pa Ye
    d. Bai Dou Kou

33. When should tonifying medicine be taken?
    a. After eating
    b. Before eating
    c. Before going to sleep
    d. None of the above

34. Which herb does *not* have to be ground into pills or powder before it is taken?
    a. Lei Wan
    b. Hu Po
    c. Ji Nei Jin
    d. Hua Shi
    e. Niu Huang

35. What was the first government formula pharmacopoeia?
    a. *Tai Ping Sheng Hui Fang* (Hoy Peaceful Benevolent Prescriptions)
    b. *Tai Ping Hui Min He Ji Ju Fang* (Prescriptions of Peaceful Benevolent Dispensary)
    c. *Sheng Ji Zong Lu* (The Complete Record of Holy Benevolence)
    d. *Pu Ji Fang* (Prescriptions for Curing All People)

36. Which treatise contains the most formulas?
    a. *Qian Jin Yao Fang* (Thousand Ducat Formulas)
    b. *Shang Han Lun* (Discussion of Cold-induced Disorders)
    c. *Pu Ji Fang* (Prescription for Curing All People)
    d. *Tai Ping Sheng Hui Fang* (Hoy Peaceful Benevolent Prescriptions)

37. Which treatise contains the eight methods of treatment?
    a. *Jin Gui Yao Lue* (Essentials From the Golden Cabinet)
    b. *Yi Zong Jin Jian* (Golden Mirror for Original Medicine)
    c. *Yi Xue Xin Wu* (A Summary on Medicine from Clinical Practice)
    d. *Huang Ti Nei Jing Su Wen* (The Yellow Emperor's Canon of Internal Medicine)

38. How does the *chen* component function in medicinal recipes?
    a. It is the conductant, which directs action to the affected meridian or site
    b. It is the adjutant, which helps strengthen the principal action
    c. It is the principal ingredient, which provides the principal curative action
    d. It is the correctant, which relieves secondary symptoms or tempers the action of the principal ingredient when the latter is too potent

39. Which statement is *not* true of an herbal formula decoction?
    a. It is quickly absorbed
    b. Some herbs can be added early or removed early
    c. Its effect has a very long duration
    d. It treats all manifestations of a disease

40. Herbs that release the Exterior are important for which of the following conditions?
    a. Coughing caused by Heat-Phlegm
    b. Acrodynia caused by Wind-Damp
    c. Exterior Syndrome caused by Wind-Heat or Wind-Cold
    d. Accumulation of Wind-Phlegm

41. Ma Huang would be the chief herb in treating which of the following?
    a. Exterior Syndrome caused by Wind-Heat
    b. Exterior Syndrome caused by Wind-Cold
    c. Exterior Excess Syndrome caused by Wind-Cold
    d. Exterior Deficiency Syndrome caused by Wind-Cold

42. Which herb is especially useful for treating edema that accompanies an Exterior pathogenic influence?
    a. Ma Huang
    b. Mu Tong
    c. Jin Qian Cao
    d. Tong Cao

43. Which herb promotes diaphoresis, stops asthma, and promotes urination?
    a. Gui Zhi
    b. Sang Bai Pi
    c. Che Qian Zi
    d. Ma Huang

44. What are the characteristics and tastes of Gui Zhi?
    a. Acrid, sweet, cool
    b. Acrid, sour, warm
    c. Acrid, aromatic, warm
    d. Acrid, sweet, warm

45. Gui Zhi performs which of the following functions?
    a. Open the inhibited Lung Qi; anti-asthmatic
    b. Regulate sweat, expel exogenous evils, warm the meridians, and penetrate the Yang
    c. Induce sweat, dispel exogenous evils, and warm the Spleen and Kidney
    d. Circulate the Qi and harmonize the Middle Energizer

46. Which herb treats dysmenorrhea and amenorrhea caused by Cold gathering in the meridians and Cold obstructing the Blood?
    a. Yin Mu Cao
    b. Gui Zhi
    c. Dan Shen
    d. Chi Shao

47. Which herb treats externally contracted Wind-Cold accompanied by a feeling of fullness in the chest or abdomen?
    a. Fang Feng
    b. Sheng Jiang
    c. Jing Jie
    d. Zi Su Ye

48. Zi Su Ye performs which of the following functions?
    a. Diaphoretic and anti-asthmatic
    b. Diaphoretic and promote urination
    c. Release the Exterior and circulate Qi
    d. Release the Exterior and penetrate the Yang

49. Which herb treats Summer Heat (Damp, fever, aversion to cold, vomiting, diarrhea)?
    a. Zi Su Ye
    b. Jing Jie
    c. Fang Feng
    d. Xiang Ru

50. Which of the following functions does Xi Xin *not* perform?
    a. Expel Wind and release the Exterior
    b. Disperse Cold and alleviate pain
    c. Warm the Lungs and transform Phlegm
    d. Dispel congealed Blood and alleviate pain

51. Which herb treats Exterior Syndrome caused by Wind-Cold or Wind-Heat?
    a. Huang Qin
    b. Zi Su Ye
    c. Jing Jie
    d. Fang Feng

52. Which herb treats joint pain (particularly in the upper portion of the body) caused by Wind-Cold-Damp?
    a. Qiang Huo
    b. Fang Feng
    c. Xi Xin
    d. Ge Gen

53. Which herb expels Cold, releases the Exterior, and relieves parietal headache?
    a. Qiang Huo
    b. Xiang Ru
    c. Cang Er Zi
    d. Gao Ben

54. Which herb expels Wind, alleviates pain, and is especially effective at relieving Yangming headache?
    a. Bai Zhi
    b. Qiang Huo
    c. Chai Hu
    d. Cang Zhu

55. Which herb expels Damp, alleviates discharge, reduces swelling, and expels pus?
    a. Cang Er Zi
    b. Fang Feng
    c. Bai Zhi
    d. Pu Gong Ying

56. Which herb treats Wind-Cold common cold where there is vomiting caused by Stomach Cold?
    a. Bai Zhi
    b. Xiang Ru
    c. Sheng Jiang
    d. Fu Zi

57. Which herb disperses Wind, expels Damp, and opens the nasal passages?
    a. Xin Yi Hua
    b. Cang Er Zi
    c. Du Huo
    d. Qin Jiao

58. Which herb expels Wind-Cold and opens the nasal passages?
    a. Fang Feng
    b. Cong Bai
    c. Xin Yi Hua
    d. Xiang Ru

59. Which herb induces sweat, releases the Exterior, regulates the Middle Energizer, and transforms Damp?
    a. Niu Bang Zi
    b. Xiang Ru
    c. Sang Ye
    d. Chai Hu

60. Cool-acrid herbs that release Exterior conditions perform which main function(s)?
    a. Detoxify Fire Poison
    b. Benefit the throat
    c. Pacify the Liver and extinguish Wind
    d. Expel Wind and Heat

61. Bo He performs which of the following functions?
    a. Disperse Wind-Heat and stop spasms
    b. Disperse Wind-Heat and release the muscles
    c. Disperse Wind-Heat, benefit the throat, and encourage rashes to surface
    d. Disperse Wind-Heat and raise the Yang Qi

62. Which herb clears the Liver and the eyes?
    a. Sang Ye
    b. Niu Bang Zi
    c. Sang Bai Pi
    d. Dan Dou Chi

63. Which herb expels Wind-Heat, pacifies the Liver, and extinguishes Wind?
    a. Bo He
    b. Dan Dou Chi
    c. Man Jing Zi
    d. Ju Hua

64. Which herb disperses Wind, stops spasms, clears the eyes, and removes superficial visual obstruction?
    a. Fang Feng
    b. Chai Hu
    c. Chan Tui
    d. Sang Ye

65. Which herb clears Liver meridian Wind-Heat, clears red eyes, and treats children's nightmares?
    a. Ju Hua
    b. Sang Ye
    c. Ge Gen
    d. Chan Tui

66. Which herb disperses Wind-Heat, clears Heat, and detoxifies Fire Poison?
    a. Niu Bang Zi
    b. Bo He
    c. Chan Tui
    d. Sang Ye

67. Which herb provides the best treatment for both of the following: stiffness, numbness, cramping, and heaviness in the limbs caused by Wind-Damp; headache caused by Wind-Heat?
    a. Fang Feng
    b. Ge Gen
    c. Sang Ye
    d. Man Jing Zi

68. Which herb clears Heat, detoxifies Poison, and encourages the rash of measles to surface?
    a. Chai Hu
    b. Sheng Ma
    c. Bo He
    d. Chan Tui

69. Chai Hu is *not* indicated for which of the following?
    a. Disharmonies between the Liver and Spleen
    b. Constrained Liver Qi
    c. Collapse of Spleen Qi
    d. Hyperactivity of Liver Yang

70. Which herb is particularly effective for resolving Half-Exterior/Half-Interior syndromes?
    a. Ge Gen
    b. Niu Bang Zi
    c. Gui Zhi
    d. Chai Hu

71. Which herb clears Heat, nourishes the fluids, and raises the Yang Qi?
    a. Chai Hu
    b. Ge Gen
    c. Sheng Ma
    d. Bo He

72. Which herb treats red eyes and excessive tearing caused by Wind-Heat?
    a. Mu Zei
    b. Fu Ping
    c. Ye Ju Hua
    d. Dan Dou Chi

73. Which herb raises the Yang Qi and treats diarrhea caused by Damp-Heat and Deficient Spleen?
    a. Chai Hu
    b. Sheng Ma
    c. Ge Gen
    d. None of the above

74. Sheng Jiang is specific for treating vomiting caused by which of the following?
    a. Stomach Heat
    b. Deficiency
    c. Cold
    d. Stagnation of Qi

75. Xiang Ru and Ma Huang each perform which of the following functions?
    a. Open inhibited Lung Qi and anti-asthmatic
    b. Promote urination and reduce edema
    c. Expel Summer Heat and transform Damp
    d. Move the Yang and transform Qi

76. Which two herbs each release the Exterior and raise the Yang Qi?
    a. Sheng Ma and Bo He
    b. Chai Hu and Man Jing Zi
    c. Ge Gen and Niu Bang Zi
    d. Chai Hu and Ge Gen

77. Which two herbs each release the Exterior and detoxify Poisons?
    a. Sheng Ma and Niu Bang Zi
    b. Sheng Ma and Bo He
    c. Jin Yin Hua and Sang Ye
    d. Ye Ju Hua and Gui Zhi

78. Which two herbs each treat red, painful, swollen eyes caused by Heat in the Liver meridian?
    a. Mu Zei and Dan Dou Chi
    b. Chan Tui and Sheng Ma
    c. Man Jing Zi and Mu Zei
    d. Fu Ping and Chai Hu

79. Which two herbs each treat Exterior Syndrome and edema?
    a. Sang Ye and Fang Feng
    b. Ma Huang and Gui Zhi
    c. Ma Huang and Fu Ping
    d. Bai Zhi and Xiang Ru

80. Dan Dou Chi performs which of the following functions?
    a. Release the Exterior and alleviate irritability
    b. Release the Exterior and nourish the fluids
    c. Release the Exterior and detoxify Poisons
    d. Release the Exterior and encourage rashes to surface

81. Ge Gen is especially known for treating which of the following syndromes?
    a. Wind-Cold-Exterior Syndrome
    b. Wind-Heat-Exterior Syndrome
    c. Alternating chills and fever
    d. Exterior Syndrome with fever, especially where stiffness or tightness exists in the upper back or neck

82. Which two herbs each expel Wind, clear Heat, and clear the Liver and eyes?
    a. Sang Ye and Chan Tui
    b. Ju Hua and Fang Feng
    c. Sang Ye and Ju Hua
    d. Chai Hu and Bo He

83. Which function does Fang Feng *not* perform?
    a. Promote sweating to expel exogenous evils
    b. Expel Exterior Wind-Damp painful obstruction
    c. Relax muscular spasms
    d. Strengthen energy

84. Which formula induces sweat, dispels exogenous evils, opens inhibited Lung Qi, and is an anti-asthmatic?
    a. Ma Huang Lian Qiao Chi Xiao Dou Tang
    b. Ma Huang Tang
    c. Gui Zhi Tang
    d. Jing Fang Bai Du San

85. Which formula treats Wind-Cold Exterior Excess Syndrome that involves fever, aversion to cold, headache, absence of perspiration, asthma, thin white tongue fur, and a floating-tense pulse?
    a. Gui Zhi Tang
    b. Xiao Qing Long Tong
    c. Ma Huang Tang
    d. Ren Shen Bai Du San

86. In addition to diaphoresis, Gui Zhi Tang performs which of the following functions?
    a. Regulate the Ying and Wei systems
    b. Regulate the Qi and Middle Energizer
    c. Nourish the Blood and expel Wind
    d. Regulate the Stomach Qi

87. Which formula does *not* contain Sheng Jiang?
    a. Xiao Qing Long Tang
    b. Gui Zhi Tang
    c. Da Qing Long Tang
    d. Zhi Gan Cao Tang

88. Which herb is an ingredient of Xiang Su San?
    a. Xiang Fu
    b. Xiang Ru
    c. Chen Xiang
    d. Tan Xiang

89. Sang Ju Yin performs which of the following functions?
    a. In combination with acrid herbs that are cool in nature, expel evil factors from the Exterior, clear Lung Heat, and stop coughing
    b. Expel Wind and clear Heat, open inhibited Lung Qi, stop cough
    c. Expel Wind-Heat, clear Heat and Poisons
    d. Drain because of its acrid flavor and cool nature, clear Lung Heat, calm asthma

90. Which formula releases the Exterior, promotes expectoration, and stops coughing and asthma?
    a. Xiao Qing Long Tang
    b. Ding Chuan Tang
    c. Ling Gui Zhu Gan Tang
    d. Xing Su San

91. Which formula consists of Sang Ye, Ju Hua, Xing Ren, Lian Qiao, Bo He, Jie Geng, Lu Gen, and Gan Cao?
    a. Xing Su San
    b. Sang Ju Yin
    c. Sang Xing Tang
    d. Jing Fang Bai Du San

92. Yin Qiao San and Sang Ju Yin each contain which of the following ingredients?
    a. Sang Jin, Ju Hua, Xing Ren, Lian Qiao, Jie Geng
    b. Bo He, Lian Qiao, Jie Geng, Jin Yin Hua, Gua Lou
    c. Lian Qiao, Bo He, Gan Cao, Jie Geng, Lu Gen
    d. Lian Qiao, Bo He, Gan Cao, Dan Zhu Ye, Niu Bang Zi

93. Yin Qiao San does *not* include which of the following?
    a. Lian Qiao and Jin Yin Hua
    b. Jie Geng and Jing Jie
    c. Bo He and Dan Zhu Ye
    d. Sang Ye and Xing Ren

94. Which formula treats the initial stage of a febrile disease, where the evil is located in the Qi-fen layer with the following symptoms: fever, slight aversion to wind and cold, headache, coughing, sore throat, thirst, redness at tip of tongue, thin white or yellow tongue fur, floating-rapid pulse?
    a. Ma Xing Shi Gan Tang
    b. Sang Ju Yin
    c. Yin Qiao San
    d. Sheng Ma Ge Gen Tang

95. What are the main symptoms indicated for Ma Xing Shi Gan Tang?
    a. Fever, asthma, thirst, rapid pulse
    b. Fever, dry cough, dry tongue, rapid pulse
    c. Fever, intolerance of cold, itching throat, cough, white tongue fur, floating pulse
    d. Fever, cough, yellow phlegm, fullness in the chest, red tongue with greasy fur, slippery-rapid pulse

96. Sheng Ma Ge Gen Tang performs which of the following functions?
    a. Expel Wind, clear Heat
    b. Relieve fever with its acrid flavor and cool nature
    c. Diaphoretic, promote the eruption of measles
    d. Clear Lung Heat

97. Sheng Ma Ge Gen Tang contains which of the following ingredients?
    a. Sheng Ma, Ge Gen, Chi Shao Yao, Gan Cao
    b. Sheng Ma, Ge Gen, Dan Dou Chi, Chai Hu
    c. Sheng Ma, Ge Gen, Niu Bang Zi, Chan Tui
    d. Sheng Ma, Ge Gen, Bo He, Shi Gao

98. Bai Du San contains which of the following ingredients?
    a. Qing Huo, Du Huo, Chai Hu, Qian Hu, Jie Geng, Fu Ling
    b. Qing Huo, Jing Jie, Fang Feng, Qian Hu, Jie Geng, Fu Ling
    c. Ren Shen, Zi Su Yi, Ge Gen, Qian Hu, Jie Geng, Fu Ling
    d. Ren Shen, Chuan Xiong, Fang Feng, Xi Xin, Sheng Jing, Gan Cao

99. Bai Du San performs which of the following functions?
    a. Induce sweat, dispel exogenous evil, expel Wind and Damp
    b. Induce sweat, dispel exogenous evil, expel Wind-Cold
    c. Induce sweat, dispel exogenous evil, expel Wind, clear Poison
    d. Induce sweat, dispel exogenous evil, clear Interior Heat

100. Jia Jian Wei Rui Tang does *not* include which of the following?
    a. Yu Zhu, Cong Bai, Dan Dou Chi
    b. Bo He, Bai Wei, Gan Cao
    c. Da Zao, Jie Geng
    d. Qian Hu, Sheng Jiang

101. Jia Jian Wei Rui Tang performs which of the following functions?
    a. Nourish Blood and expel the evil factors from the Exterior
    b. Nourish Yin, clear Heat, induce sweat, and dispel exogenous evil
    c. Encourage measles to surface and dispel exogenous evil
    d. None of the above

102. Jiu Wei Qiang Huo Tang does *not* include which of the following?
    a. Qiang Huo, Fang Feng, Cang Zhu
    b. Du Huo, Chai Hu, Gan Cao
    c. Xi Xin, Chuan Xiong, Bai Zhi
    d. Sheng Di Huang, Huang Qin, Gan Cao

103. Jiu Wei Qiang Huo Tang is *not* indicated for which of the following symptoms?
    a. Aversion to cold, fever
    b. Hidrosis, headache
    c. Anhidrosis, headache
    d. White tongue fur, floating pulse

104. Zai Zao San performs which of the following functions?
    a. Restore Yang and expel the evil factors in an Exterior Syndrome
    b. Restore Yang, supplement Qi, induce sweat, and promote urination
    c. Supplement Qi, dispel exogenous evil, eliminate Phlegm, and stop coughing
    d. Restore Yang, supplement Qi, induce sweat, and dispel exogenous evil

105. Which herb quells Fire, nourishes Yin, and moisturizes dryness?
    a. Shi Gao
    b. Zhi Zi
    c. Dan Zhu Ye
    d. Zhi Mu

106. Which herb treats toothache caused by Stomach Heat?
    a. Sheng Di Huang
    b. Xuan Shen
    c. Huang Qin
    d. Shi Gao

107. Which herb clears Excess-Heat and Deficiency-Fire?
    a. Huang Lian
    b. Zhi Mu
    c. Zhi Zi
    d. Shi Gao

108. Which herb quells Fire, alleviates irritability, cools Blood, and stops bleeding?
    a. Zhi Zi
    b. Dan Zhu Ye
    c. Mu Dan Pi
    d. Dan Dou Chi

109. Which herb clears Heat, generates fluids, stops vomiting, and expels vexation?
    a. Zhi Mu
    b. Lu Gen
    c. Xia Ku Cao
    d. Tian Hua Fen

110. Which herb clears Heat, promotes urination, and treats pulmonary abscess?
    a. Dan Zhu Ye
    b. Lu Gen
    c. Che Qian Zi
    d. Gua Lou

111. Which herb expels pus, clears Heat, and generates fluid?
    a. Tian Hua Fen
    b. Lu Gen
    c. Dan Zhu Ye
    d. Chuan Shan Jia

112. Which herb clears Liver Fire and treats scrofula goiter caused by Stagnant Phlegm-Fire?
    a. Qing Xiang Zi
    b. Xia Ku Cao
    c. Zhi Zi
    d. Bei Mu

113. Which of the following *best* describes the properties and functions of Dan Zhu Ye?
    a. Sweet, cold, clears Heat, promote urination, stop vomiting
    b. Sweet, bland, cold, clear Heat, nurture Yin
    c. Sweet, bland, cold, clear Heat, alleviate irritability, promote urination
    d. Sweet, bland, cold, clear Heat, stop vomiting and bleeding

114. Which herb does *not* clear Heat and dry Damp?
    a. Huang Lian
    b. Long Dan Cao
    c. Ku Shen
    d. Dan Zhu Ye

115. Which herb *best* treats irritability, thirst, and scanty painful urination caused by Heat?
    a. Lu Gen
    b. Tian Hua Fen
    c. Dan Zhu Ye
    d. Huang Qin

116. Which herb does *not* clear Heat and alleviate irritability?
    a. Zhi Zi
    b. Dan Zhu Ye
    c. Xia Ku Cao
    d. Huang Lian

117. Which herb clears Heat and cools the Blood?
    a. Huang Qin
    b. Zhi Zi
    c. Dan Zhu Ye
    d. Qing Xiang Zi

118. Han Shui Shi performs which of the following functions?
    a. Clear Heat and cool the Blood
    b. Clear Heat and Poisons
    c. Clear Heat and Summer Heat
    d. Clear Heat and dry Damp

119. Which herb is *not* used to treat Liver Heat, superficial visual obstruction, and red, painful, swollen eyes?
    a. Mi Meng Hua
    b. Qing Xiang Zi
    c. Xia Ku Cao
    d. Gu Jing Cao

120. Which herb clears Heat, dries Damp, and is particularly effective at stopping vomiting?
    a. Zhu Ru
    b. Ban Xia
    c. Huang Lian
    d. Long Dan Cao

121. What is the strongest herb for clearing Heart Heat?
    a. Dan Zhu Ye
    b. Huang Lian
    c. Huang Qin
    d. Zi Cao

122. Which herb clears Heat and calms the fetus?
    a. Huang Qin
    b. Huang Lian
    c. Long Dan Cao
    d. Ku Shen

123. Which herb treats diarrhea, dysentery, and vomiting caused by Damp-Heat in the Stomach and Intestines?
    a. Huang Qin
    b. Huang Lian
    c. Da Huang
    d. Huang Bai

124. Huang Qin performs which of the following functions?
    a. Clear Heat, dry Damp, and alleviate irritability
    b. Clear Heat, dry Damp, and clear Liver Fire
    c. Clear Heat, dry Damp, and stop bleeding
    d. Clear Heat, dry Damp, and promote urination

125. Huang Qin is most notable for clearing which of the following?
    a. Heart Fire
    b. Bladder Fire
    c. Lung Fire
    d. Liver Fire

126. Huang Qin is particularly effective in treating which kind of bleeding?
    a. Bleeding caused by an incised wound
    b. Bleeding caused by Heat in the Bladder
    c. Hemoptysis caused by deficiency of Yin or cough caused by deficiency of viscera
    d. Hemoptysis caused by Lung Heat

127. Which herb dries Damp and clears Deficiency-Heat?
    a. Huang Bai
    b. Zhi Mu
    c. Yin Chai Hu
    d. Bai Wei

128. Which herb treats redness, swelling, and pain in the knees and lower extremities that are caused by Damp-Heat pouring down?
    a. Yin Chai Hu
    b. Huang Bai
    c. Huang Lian
    d. Zi Cao

129. Which herb clears Excess-Fire of the Liver and Gallbladder, and drains Damp-Heat from the Lower Energizer?
    a. Xia Ku Cao
    b. Huang Qin
    c. Ku Shen
    d. Long Dan Cao

130. Which herb clears Heat, dries Damp, disperses Wind, and stops itching?
    a. Huang Lian
    b. Huang Qin
    c. Jin Yin Hua
    d. Ku Shen

131. Which herb treats genital itching, eczema, furuncles, scabies, and leprosy?
    a. Ku Shen
    b. Huang Bai
    c. Bai Jiang Cao
    d. Huang Qin

132. Which herb treats Damp-Heat jaundice, fever, convulsions, swelling, genital itching, and eczema?
    a. Long Dan Cao
    b. Huang Lian
    c. Qin Pi
    d. Dan Zhu Ye

133. Which herb clears Heat, cools the Blood, and detoxifies Fire Poison?
    a. Xuan Shen
    b. Sheng Di Huang
    c. Huang Lian
    d. Pu Gong Ying

134. Which herb treats Heat entering the Ying-fen and Xue-fen manifesting as irritability and insomnia?
    a. Sheng Di Huang
    b. Huang Lian
    c. Huang Qin
    d. Ku Shen

135. Which herb clears Heat, cools the Blood, nourishes Yin, and generates fluids?
    a. Sha Shen
    b. Shu Di Huang
    c. Sheng Di Huang
    d. Lu Gen

136. Which herb clears Heat, cools the Blood, and promotes Blood circulation to remove Blood Stasis?
    a. Mu Dan Pi
    b. Xuan Shen
    c. Sheng Di Huang
    d. Xi Jiao

137. Which herb cools the Blood, stops bleeding, and promotes circulation to remove Blood Stasis?
    a. Sheng Di Huang
    b. Bai Mao Gen
    c. Chi Shao
    d. San Qi

138. Which herb promotes Blood circulation to remove Blood Stasis and reduces fever caused by Deficient viscera?
    a. Di Gu Pi
    b. Yin Chai Hu
    c. Lian Qiao
    d. Mu Dan Pi

139. Xuan Shen performs which of the following functions?
    a. Cool the Blood, nourish the Yin, and promote urination
    b. Promote Blood circulation to remove Blood Stasis
    c. Detoxify Fire Poison and reduce abscesses
    d. Quell Fire, detoxify Fire Poison, and nourish the Yin

140. Xuan Shen is *not* indicated for which of the following conditions?
    a. Erythema caused by Blood-Heat
    b. Phlegm nodules, swelling and soreness in the throat
    c. Gangrene
    d. Qi-fen Heat Syndrome, high fever, extreme thirst, and a big pulse

141. Which herb treats sore and swollen throat caused by Deficiency-Fire?
    a. Shan Dou Gen
    b. She Gan
    c. Ban Lan Gen
    d. Xuan Shen

142. Which herb cools the Blood, detoxifies Fire Poison, and draws out rashes?
    a. Bo He
    b. Chai Hu
    c. Chan Tui
    d. Zi Cao

143. What are the characteristics of Jin Yin Hua?
    a. Sweet, cold
    b. Bitter, cold
    c. Acrid, cold
    d. Acrid, bitter, cold

144. Which herb expels externally contracted Wind-Heat, clears Heat, and detoxifies Fire Poison?
    a. Sang Ye
    b. Mu Zei
    c. Jin Yin Hua
    d. Chuan Xin Lian

145. Which of the following provides the *best* therapy for hot sores, carbuncles, and neck nodules caused by Heat accumulation?
    a. Bai Zhi
    b. Lian Qiao
    c. Zhe Bei Mu
    d. Huang Qi

146. Which herb expels externally contracted Wind-Heat, cools the Blood, and stops dysentery?
    a. Jin Yin Hua
    b. Pu Gong Ying
    c. Zi Hua Di Ding
    d. Da Qing Ye

147. Which herb clears Heart Heat and dissipates nodules?
    a. Xia Ku Cao
    b. Lian Qiao
    c. Long Dan Cao
    d. Jin Yin Hua

148. Which herb clears Heat, detoxifies Fire Poison, and reduces abscesses?
    a. Chuan Xin Lian
    b. Bai Tou Weng
    c. Lou Lu
    d. Pu Gong Ying

149. Which symptom is caused by an overdose of Pu Gong Ying?
    a. Constipation
    b. Pain in abdomen
    c. Threatened abortion
    d. Mild diarrhea

150. Which herb treats serious cases of furuncles and mumps?
    a. Pu Gong Ying
    b. Zi Hua Di Ding
    c. Ban Bian Lian
    d. Lian Qiao

151. Which herb clears Heat, detoxifies Fire Poison, stops Wind, relieves infantile convulsions, and awakens a patient from unconsciousness by eliminating Phlegm?
    a. Xi Jiao
    b. She Xiang
    c. Niu Huang
    d. Shi Chang Pu

152. Which herb treats coma, delirium, and lockjaw caused by Hot Phlegm obstructing the Pericardium?
    a. Niu Huang
    b. Xi Jiao
    c. She Xiang
    d. Su He Xiang

153. Which herb clears Heat, detoxifies Fire Poison, and treats lung abscesses and coughing caused by Lung Heat?
    a. Bai Tou Weng
    b. Bai Jiang Cao
    c. Jie Geng
    d. Yu Xing Cao

154. Which herb treats lung abscesses where there is pus and thick, yellow-green sputum is coughed up?
    a. Shan Dou Gen
    b. She Gan
    c. Da Qing Ye
    d. Yu Xing Cao

155. Which of the following is an indication for Bai Jiang Cao?
    a. Stomach pain caused by Deficiency-Cold
    b. Hematemesis caused by Blood-Heat
    c. Headache caused by Blood Deficiency
    d. Pain in abdomen caused by intestinal abscess

156. Which is the most important herb for treating pain in the abdomen caused by intestinal abscesses?
    a. Ma Chi Xian
    b. Hong Teng
    c. Jin Yin Hua
    d. Dong Gua Ren

157. Which herb treats pestilence, mumps, viral pneumonia, and red blotches or skin eruptions caused by Heat Poison in the Blood?
    a. Pu Gong Ying
    b. Jin Yin Hua
    c. Sheng Di Huang
    d. Da Qing Ye

158. Which herb clears Heat, expels Damp, and is especially used for treating syphilis?
    a. Fu Ling
    b. Zhu Ling
    c. Tu Fu Ling
    d. Zi Hua Di Ding

159. Which herb quells Heat, detoxifies Fire Poison, and causes milk to descend?
    a. Mai Ya
    b. Lou Lu
    c. Long Dan Cao
    d. Wang Bu Liu Xing

160. Which herb quells Heat, detoxifies Fire Poison, cools the Blood, and reduces swelling?
    a. Da Qing Ye
    b. Pu Gong Ying
    c. Qing Dai
    d. Jin Yin Hua

161. Bai Hua She She Cao performs which of the following functions?
    a. Clear Heat, detoxify Fire Poison, promote Blood, and cool Blood
    b. Clear Heat, detoxify Fire Poison, expel pus, and dissipate abscess
    c. Clear Heat, detoxify Fire Poison, expel pus, and stop pain
    d. Clear Heat, dissipate abscesses, promote diuresis to drain Damp from the Lower Energizer

162. Which herb clears Heat, detoxifies Poison, promotes urination, and eliminates swelling?
    a. Zi Hua Di Ding
    b. Chuan Xin Lian
    c. Ban Bian Lian
    d. Zhu Ling

163. Which herb treats poisonous snake bites, Fire-Poison patterns (such as carbuncles), and skin disease?
    a. Jin Yin Hua
    b. Bai Jiang Cao
    c. Ye Ju Hua
    d. Ban Bian Lian

164. Which herb clears Heat, detoxifies Fire Poison, expels Phlegm, and benefits the throat?
    a. Ban Bian Lian
    b. Jie Geng
    c. Pi Pa Ye
    d. She Gan

165. Which herb is *not* used to treat dysentery?
    a. Qin Pi
    b. Huang Lian
    c. Huang Qin
    d. She Gan

166. Which herb is particularly effective for treating dysentery?
    a. Bai Tou Weng
    b. Huang Qin
    c. Lian Qiao
    d. Qin Pi

167. Which herb clears Lung Heat, benefits the throat, detoxifies Fire Poison, and stops bleeding?
    a. She Gan
    b. Shan Dou Gen
    c. Ma Bo
    d. Ma Chi Xian

168. Which herb treats painful, swollen throat caused by Hot Phlegm obstruction?
    a. Ma Bo
    b. She Gan
    c. Shan Dou Gen
    d. Yu Xing Cao

169. Which herb treats dysentery caused by Heat-Damp?
    a. Lian Qiao
    b. Zhi Zi
    c. Chuan Xin Lian
    d. Chi Shi Zhi

170. Which herb clears Heat, Damp-Heat, and Liver Fire to treat eye disease?
    a. Sang Ye
    b. Xia Ku Cao
    c. Qin Pi
    d. Yu Xing Cao

171. Which herb treats malaria, dysentery, corns, and warts?
    a. Chang Shan
    b. Ya Dan Zi
    c. Tu Niu Xi
    d. Shan Ci Gu

172. Which herb treats Damp-Heat dysentery which includes tenesmus and stool containing blood and pus?
    a. Lian Qiao
    b. Ge Gen
    c. Jin Yin Hua
    d. Ma Chi Xian

173. Which herb is known especially for treating carbuncles, rashes, and dermal itching due to Damp-Heat?
    a. Huang Qin
    b. Shan Dou Gen
    c. Bai Xian Pi
    d. Da Qing Ye

174. Which herb taken orally or topically clears Heat, detoxifies Fire Poison, and dissipates nodules?
    a. Lu Gan Shi
    b. Ming Fan
    c. Lei Wan
    d. Shan Ci Gu

175. Which herb clears Summer Heat, Excess-Heat, Deficiency fever, and malaria?
    a. Hu Huang Lian
    b. Chang Shan
    c. Xiang Ru
    d. Qing Hao

176. Which herb treats Ying-fen evil that causes a feeling of heat at night and cold in the morning?
    a. Hu Huang Lian
    b. Yin Chai Hu
    c. Qing Hao
    d. Di Gu Pi

177. Which herb cools the Blood, quells Deficiency-Fire, and clears Lung Heat?
    a. Di Gu Pi
    b. Huang Qin
    c. Sang Bai Pi
    d. Qian Hu

178. Which herb drains Damp-Heat and clears Deficiency-Heat?
    a. Huang Lian
    b. Qin Jiao
    c. Zhi Mu
    d. Hu Huang Lian

179. Which herb quells Deficiency-Fire and also treats dysentery?
    a. Qing Hao
    b. Yin Chai Hu
    c. Hu Huang Lian
    d. Bai Wei

180. Huang Lian is especially effective at clearing which of the following?
    a. Lung Heat
    b. Deficiency-Heat
    c. Shao-Yang Heat
    d. Heart Heat

181. Huang Qin is especially effective at clearing which of the following?
    a. Lung Heat
    b. Deficiency-Heat
    c. Shao-Yang Heat
    d. Heart Heat

182. Pu Gong Ying and Zi Hua Di Ding each perform which of the following functions?
    a. Clear Heat and quell Fire
    b. Clear Heat and detoxify Fire Poison
    c. Quell Fire and drain Damp-Heat
    d. Clear Deficiency-Heat

183. Zhu Ye and Dan Zhu Ye each perform which of the following functions?
    a. Clear Heat and detoxify Fire Poison
    b. Clear Heat, alleviate irritability, and promote diuresis
    c. Quell Fire and drain Damp-Heat
    d. Clear Heat and generate fluids

184. Xuan Shen and Sheng Di Huang are both indicated for which of the following conditions?
    a. Heat entering the Ying-fen and Xue-fen with fever, thirst, and a red tongue
    b. Damp-Heat jaundice
    c. Heat in the Qi-fen with excess thirst and irritability
    d. Conjunctivitis, ulcerous disease of the skin, and scrofula

185. Bai Tou Weng and Qin Pi each perform which of the following functions?
    a. Clear Heat to treat eye disease
    b. Clear Heat and generate fluids
    c. Clear Heat and stop dysentery
    d. Clear Heat and promote diuresis

186. Dan Zhu Ye, Huang Lian, and Zhi Zi are all associated with which indication?
    a. Constipation caused by Heat Stagnation
    b. Heat patterns with irritability
    c. Dysentery caused by Damp-Heat
    d. Irregular menstruation from Liver Fire

187. Huang Lian and Hu Huang Lian each perform which of the following functions?
    a. Clear Deficiency-Fire
    b. Clear Heat and drain Damp
    c. Clear Heat and stop cough
    d. Expel Wind-Damp

188. Which of the following is associated with cases of hectic fever caused by Deficient Yin and treated with Di Gu Pi?
    a. Anhidrosis
    b. Hidrosis
    c. Summer Heat
    d. Damp

189. Which of the following is associated with cases of hectic fever caused by Deficient Yin and treated with Mu Dan Pi?
    a. Anhidrosis
    b. Hidrosis
    c. Summer Heat
    d. Damp

190. Huang Bai and Zhi Mu each perform which of the following functions?
    a. Clear Heat and drain Damp
    b. Quell Fire and detoxify Fire Poison
    c. Clear Heat from Yin deficiency
    d. Moisten the Intestines to treat constipation

191. Huang Bai and Zhi Mu each perform which of the following functions?
    a. Clear Heat and drain Damp
    b. Quell Fire and detoxify Fire Poison
    c. Clear Heat and cool the Blood
    d. Clear both Excess-Heat and Deficiency-Heat

192. Ma Bo and She Gan each perform which of the following functions?
    a. Clear Heat to treat eye disease
    b. Clear Heat, detoxify Fire Poison; used to treat intestinal abscesses
    c. Clear Heat, detoxify Fire Poison, and benefit the throat
    d. None of the above

193. Long Dan Cao and Ku Shen each perform which of the following functions?
    a. Clear Heat and detoxify Fire Poison
    b. Clear Heat and quell Fire
    c. Clear Heat and cool the Blood
    d. Clear Heat and drain Damp

194. Which two herbs each clear Heat, cool the Blood, and promote Blood circulation to remove Blood Stasis?
    a. Jin Yin Hua and Lian Qiao
    b. Sheng Di Huang and Xuan Shen
    c. Mu Dan Pi and Chi Shao
    d. E Zhu and San Leng

195. Which three herbs each clear Heat and cool the Blood?
    a. Sheng Di Huang, Zhi Mu, and Mu Dan Pi
    b. Sheng Di Huang, Xuan Shen, and Huang Lian
    c. Chi Shao, Bai Shao, and Chi Xiao Dou
    d. Sheng Di Huang, Xuan Shen, and Zi Cao

196. Which two herbs each clear Deficiency-Fire and cool the Blood?
    a. Sheng Di Huang and Zhi Mu
    b. Mu Dan Pi and Zhi Zi
    c. Di Gu Pi and Hu Huang Lian
    d. Qing Hao and Bai Wei

197. Which two herbs each enter the Liver and Kidney meridians and clear Deficiency-Fire?
    a. Zhi Mu and Di Gu Pi
    b. Di Gu Pi and Chi Shao
    c. Sheng Di Huang and Mu Dan Pi
    d. Huang Lian and Huang Bai

198. Which two herbs each treat infantile malnutrition caused by Fire and clear Deficiency-Fire?
    a. Sheng Di Huang and Di Gu Pi
    b. Hu Huang Lian and Yin Chen Hao
    c. Yin Chai Hu and Hu Huang Lian
    d. Mu Dan Pi and Di Gu Pi

199. Da Qing Ye, Qing Dai, and Ban Lan Gen each perform which of the following functions?
    a. Clear Heat, detoxify Fire Poison, and cool the Blood
    b. Clear Heat, detoxify Fire Poison, and benefit the throat
    c. Clear Heat, detoxify Fire Poison, and alleviate spasms
    d. None of the above

200. Which two herbs each treat the following: Steaming-Bone Syndrome accompanied by afternoon fever; night sweats; irritability caused by deficient Yin with Heat signs; severely Deficient Lungs and Kidneys?
    a. Shi Gao and Zhi Mu
    b. Huang Qin and Huang Bai
    c. Huang Lian and Mu Dan Pi
    d. Zhi Mu and Huang Bai

201. Hong Teng and Bai Jiang Cao each perform which of the following functions?
    a. Clear Heat, detoxify Fire Poison, treat lung abscesses
    b. Clear Heat, detoxify Fire Poison, treat intestinal abscesses
    c. Clear Heat, detoxify Fire Poison, benefit the throat
    d. None of the above

202. Mu Dan Pi and Chi Shao each perform which of the following functions?
    a. Clear Heat, cool the Blood, clear Heat, dry Damp
    b. Clear Excess-Heat and Deficiency-Heat, cool the Blood
    c. Clear Heat, cool the Blood, promote Blood circulation to remove Blood Stasis
    d. Clear Deficiency-Heat, promote Blood circulation to remove Blood Stasis

203. Which two herbs are especially effective at treating breast abscesses?
    a. Bai Jiang Cao and Yu Xing Cao
    b. Pu Gong Ying and Lou Lu
    c. Lian Qiao and Jin Yin Hua
    d. Zi Hua Di Ding and Chuan Xin Lian

204. Which two herbs treat Heat in the Pericardium that causes coma or delirium?
    a. Xi Jiao and Lian Qiao Xin
    b. Huang Lian and Zi Cao
    c. Jin Yin Hua and Zi Hua Di Ding
    d. Mu Dan Pi and Chi Shao

205. Xia Ku Cao and Lian Qiao are both indicated for which of the following conditions?
    a. Rashes and measles or chicken pox
    b. Heat in the Blood with constipation
    c. Red, painful, swollen and ulcerated throat
    d. Scrofula and phlegm nodules

206. Xia Ku Cao and Long Dan Cao each perform which of the following functions?
    a. Clear Heart Heat
    b. Clear Lung Heat
    c. Clear Liver Heat
    d. Clear Stomach Heat

207. How is Ya Dan Zi prepared for oral use?
    a. As a draft
    b. Mixed with water
    c. Wrapped during decocting
    d. As encapsulated powder

208. Which herb clears Heat, stops dysentery, quells Liver Fire, and benefits the eyes?
    a. Qin Pi
    b. Ma Chi Xian
    c. Bai Tou Weng
    d. Hong Teng

209. Which herb clears Lung Heat, benefits the throat, detoxifies Poisons, and stops bleeding?
    a. She Gan
    b. Shan Dou Gen
    c. Ma Bo
    d. Tu Niu Xi

210. Which herb treats internal and external abscesses, and promotes diuresis to drain Damp from the Lower Energizer?
    a. Zi Hua Di Ding
    b. Pu Gong Ying
    c. Da Qing Ye
    d. Chuan Xin Lian

211. Qing Hao is *not* indicated for which of the following conditions?
    a. Summer-Heat patterns
    b. Malaria
    c. Deficiency of Yin
    d. Dysuria

212. Which pattern is *not* an indication for antifebrile formulas?
    a. Heat entering the Qi-fen with high fever and strong thirst
    b. Heat entering the Ying-fen and Xue-fen with delirium and macules
    c. Excess-Heat of the Triple Energizer with fidgetiness
    d. Excess-Heat in the Interior with constipation and delirium

213. Which of the following is a caution for the use of antifebrile formulas?
    a. Deficiency-Heat syndromes
    b. Contraindicated during pregnancy
    c. Old and weak patients
    d. Cold syndromes where there are pseudo-Heat symptoms

214. Bai Hu Tang contains which of the following?
    a. Shi Gao, Zhi Mu, Dan Zhu Ye, and Rice
    b. Shi Gao, Zhi Mu, Lu Gen, and Gan Cao
    c. Shi Gao, Zhi Mu, Zhi Zi, and Gan Cao
    d. Shi Gao, Zhi Mu, Gan Cao, and Rice

215. Which of the following is *not* a caution for the use of Bai Hu Tang?
    a. Lingering Exterior Syndrome
    b. Anhidrosis, fever, and lack of thirst
    c. False Heat Syndrome in appearance which is True Cold Syndrome in nature
    d. Slippery-rapid pulse

216. Zhu Ye Shi Gao Tang can be created by subtracting Zhi Mu from Bai Hu Tang and adding which of the following?
    a. Zhu Ye, Ban Xia, Mai Men Dong, and Ren Shen
    b. Ren Shen, Mai Men Dong, Zhu Ye, and Lian Qiao
    c. Mai Men Dong, Xuan Shen, Zhu Ye, and Huang Lian
    d. Zhu Ye, Mai Men Dong, Ren Shen, and Tian Nan Xing

217. Which formula clears Heat, promotes the production of body fluids, supplements the Qi, and regulates the Stomach?
    a. Bai Hu Tang
    b. Qing Shu Yi Qi Tang
    c. Zhu Ye Shi Gao Tang
    d. Qing Ying Tang

218. Which of the following would you expect to find in a patient who will be treated with Qing Ying Tang?
    a. Red tongue coated with yellow fur
    b. Crimson tongue coated with yellow fur
    c. Crimson, dry tongue
    d. Red tongue coated with greasy yellow fur

219. Qing Ying Tang is *not* indicated for which of the following symptoms?
    a. Fever that is heavy at night
    b. Delirium
    c. Upset temperament and sleeplessness
    d. Violet-black macules

220. What is the main indication for the use of Xi Jiao Di Huang Tang?
    a. High fever that worsens at night
    b. Bleeding from the eyes, ears, nose, mouth, or subcutaneous tissues
    c. Scarlet, dry tongue
    d. Erosion of the mucous membranes of the oral cavity

221. Huang Lian Jie Du Tang contains Huang Lian and which of the following?
    a. Huang Qin, Huang Bai, and Zhi Zi
    b. Huang Qin, Huang Bai, and Zi Hua Di Ding
    c. Huang Qin, Huang Bai, and Long Dan Cao
    d. Huang Qin, Huang Bai, and Zhi Mu

222. Which formula would you select to treat this pattern of symptoms: high fever, fidgetiness, delirium, dry mouth and throat, red tongue with yellow fur, and an Excess, rapid pulse?
    a. Xi Jiao Di Huang Tang
    b. Qing Yin Tang
    c. Huang Lian Jie Du Tang
    d. Bai Hu Tang

223. Bu Ji Xiao Du Yin performs which of the following functions?
    a. Clear Heat, detoxify Fire Poison, and promote Blood circulation to stop pain
    b. Expel Wind, disperse swelling, clear Heat, and detoxify Fire Poison
    c. Clear Heat, detoxify Fire Poison, and promote Blood circulation to remove Blood Stasis
    d. Clear Heat, detoxify Fire Poison, and eliminate tumors

224. What is the main indication for Bu Ji Xiao Du Yin?
    a. Dryness in the mouth without thirst
    b. Redness, swelling and pain in the head and face
    c. Red tongue with greasy yellow fur
    d. Thin-rapid pulse

225. What is the main formula contained in Qing Wen Bai Du Yin and what does it do?
    a. Xi Jiao Di Huang Tang to clear Heat, detoxify Fire Poison, and cool Blood to stop bleeding
    b. Huang Lian Jie Du Tang to quell Excess-Heat of the Triple Energizer
    c. Bai Hu Tang to clear Yangming meridian Heat
    d. None of the above

226. Dao Chi San contains which of the following herbs?
    a. Zhi Zi
    b. Zhu Ye
    c. Hua Shi
    d. Ze Xie

227. Dao Chi San performs which of the following functions?
    a. Clear Heart Fire, nourish the Yin, and promote diuresis
    b. Clear Liver Heat, nourish the Yin, and promote diuresis
    c. Clear Heat, quell Fire, and promote diuresis
    d. Clear Heat, detoxify Fire Poison, and promote diuresis

228. Which formula clears Heat from the Heart and Small Intestine?
    a. Xie Huang San
    b. Bai Tou Wang Tang
    c. Dao Chi San
    d. Yu Ni Jian

229. Which herbs in Long Dan Xie Gan Tang drain Damp and nourish the Yin?
    a. Mu Tong, Che Qian Zi, Ze Xie, Dang Gui, and Sheng Di Huang
    b. Mu Tong, Che Qian Zi, Fu Ling, Bai Shao, and Sheng Di Huang
    c. Mu Tong, Che Qian Zi, Hua Shi, E Jiao, and Sheng Di Huang
    d. Mu Tong, Che Qian Zi, Yi Yi Ren, Sang Jing Sheng, and Sheng Di Huang

230. Long Dan Xie Gan Tang is *not* indicated for which of the following symptoms?
    a. Headache and hypochondriac pain
    b. Bitter taste in the mouth and red eyes
    c. Pruritus or swelling of female pudendum and leukorrhea
    d. Erosion of the mucous membrane in the oral cavity

231. What is the ratio of Huang Lian to Wu Zhu Yu in Zuo Jin Wan?
    a. 3 to 1
    b. 4 to 1
    c. 5 to 1
    d. 6 to 1

232. Zuo Jin Wan is *not* indicated for which of the following symptoms?
    a. Pain in the left hypochondria and distention of the stomach
    b. Vomiting of acid fluid and eructation
    c. Hot, foul breath
    d. Bitter taste in the mouth and a red tongue with yellow fur

233. Xie Bai San contains Chao Sang Bai Pi, Di Gu Pi, and which of the following?
    a. Zhi Gan Cao and rice
    b. Ting Li Zi and rice
    c. Huang Qin and rice
    d. Chuan Bei Mu and Gan Cao

234. Which formula clears Lung Heat and stops cough and asthma?
    a. Bei Mu Gua Lou San
    b. Xie Bai San
    c. Qing Qi Hua Tan Tang
    d. Wei Jing Tang

235. Ting Li Da Zao Xie Fei Tang performs which of the following functions?
    a. Clear Lung Heat, moisturize Dry, stop cough and asthma
    b. Clear Lung Heat, stop cough and asthma
    c. Eliminate water and Phlegm in the lung, relieve cough and asthma
    d. Moisturize the Lung to dissipate Phlegm, clear Heat, and nourish the Yin

236. Qing Wei San contains which of the following herb pairs?
    a. Huang Lian and Sheng Ma
    b. Huang Lian and Zhi Mu
    c. Huang Qin and Sheng Ma
    d. Huang Qin and Zhi Mu

237. Qing Wei San performs the following main functions?
    a. Clear Stomach Heat and detoxify Fire Poison
    b. Clear Stomach Heat and nourish the Blood
    c. Clear Stomach Heat and cool the Blood
    d. Clear Stomach Heat and tonify the Qi

238. Sheng Ma performs which function in Qing Wei San?
    a. Raise the Lung Qi
    b. Release the Exterior
    c. Detoxify Fire-Poison
    d. Encourage the rash of measles to surface

239. Xie Huang San is *not* indicated for which of the following symptoms?
    a. Aphtha and foul breath
    b. Bleeding from the gums
    c. Dry mouth and lips
    d. Fever accompanied by restlessness and polyrexia

240. Which formula contains Shi Gao and Shu Di?
    a. Xie Huang San
    b. Bai He Gu Jin Tang
    c. Yu Nu Jian
    d. Xie Xin Tang

241. Which formula would you select to treat this pattern: headache, teeth pain, fever accompanied by restlessness, excessive thirst, bleeding gums, red tongue with yellow and dry fur?
    a. Qing Wei San
    b. Xie Huang San
    c. Huang Lian Jie Du Tang
    d. Yu Nu Jian

242. Niu Xi performs which of the following functions in Yu Nu Jian?
    a. Induce the downward movement of Heat and invigorate the Kidney
    b. Invigorate the Kidney and Liver
    c. Clear Damp-Heat from the Lower Energizer
    d. None of the above

243. Shao Yao Tang contains which of the following herb pairs?
    a. Chuan Lian Zi and Huang Bai
    b. Sheng Jiang and Da Zao
    c. Zhi Zi and Chen Pi
    d. None of the above

244. Which formula treats this pattern: abdominal pain, bloody stool with red and white mucous, tenesmus, burning feeling in the anus, urination that is brief and dark-colored, diarrhea, greasy yellow tongue fur?
    a. Bai Tou Weng Tang
    b. Shao Yao Tang
    c. Ge Gen Huang Qin Huang Lian Tang
    d. Xiang Lian Wan

245. Rou Gui performs which of the following functions in Shao Yao Tang?
    a. Warm the Interior, expel Cold, and stop pain
    b. Warms the Kidney and fortify the Yang
    c. Warm the meridians, promote menstruation, and alleviate pain
    d. Prevent the bitter-cold herbs from injuring the Yang, strengthen movement of the Blood

246. Which formula treats this pattern: abdominal pain with tenesmus, diarrhea with blood and pus, a burning sensation in the anus, thirst for water, red tongue with yellow fur, wiry-rapid pulse?
    a. Xiang Liang Wan
    b. Bai Tou Weng Tang
    c. Huang Qin Tang
    d. Shao Yao Tang

247. Qing Hao Bie Jia Tang contains which of the following herb pairs?
    a. Zhi Mu and Mu Dan Pi
    b. Zhi Mu and Bai Shao
    c. Zhi Mu and Huang Bai
    d. Mu Dan Pi and Xuan Shen

248. Qing Hao Bie Jia Tang performs which of the following functions?
    a. Nourish the Yin, clear Heat
    b. Nourish the Yin, promote fluids
    c. Nourish the Yin, cool the Blood
    d. Nourish the Yin, dispel Heat

249. Which formula treats this pattern: Heat at night, Cold in morning, when the Heat clears there is anhidrosis, red tongue with little fur, thin-rapid pulse?
    a. Xiao Chai Hu Tang
    b. Qing Hao Bie Jia Tang
    c. Qin Jiao Bie Jia San
    d. None of the above

250. Qing Gu San can be created by removing Sheng Di Huang and Mu Dan Pi from Qing Hao Bie Jia Tang and adding:
    a. Di Gu Pi, Yin Chai Hu, and Hu Huang Lian
    b. Di Gu Pi, Yin Chai Hu, Hu Huang Lian, Qin Jiao, and Gan Cao
    c. Sang Bai Pi, Hu Huang Lian, and Gan Cao
    d. Hu Huang Lian, Di Gu Pi, and Gan Cao

251. Which formula treats this pattern: afternoon fever with steaming bone sensation, upset temperament, dryness of the pharynx, malaise, red lips, night sweats, red tongue with thin fur, thin-rapid pulse?
    a. Qin Jiao Bie Jiu Tang
    b. Qing Hao Bie Jie Tang
    c. Qing Qu San
    d. Qing Ying Tang

252. What are the six Huang in Dang Gui Liu Huang Tang?
    a. Huang Lian, Huang Qin, Huang Bai, Da Huang, Huang Qi, and Di Huang
    b. Huang Lian, Huang Qin, Huang Bai, Da Huang, Huang Qi, and Mu Huang
    c. Huang Lian, Huang Qin, Huang Bai, Huang Qi, Shu Di, and Sheng Di Huang
    d. Huang Lian, Huang Qin, Huang Bai, Huang Qi, Shu Di, and Ma Huang

253. In which formula does Huang Qi function as a deputy (zuo) ingredient?
    a. Bu Zhong Yi Qi Tang
    b. Dang Gui Liu Huang Tang
    c. Bu Yang Huan Wu Tang
    d. Gui Pi Tang

254. Which formula treats this pattern: fever, night sweats, dry mouth, vexation, constipation with dry stool, oliguria with reddish urine?
    a. Qing Gu San
    b. Mu Li San
    c. Dang Gui Liu Huang Tang
    d. Huang Long Tang

255. Which herb treats Damp-Heat jaundice accompanied by constipation?
    a. Fan Xie Yi
    b. Mang Xiao
    c. Da Huang
    d. Yu Li Ren

256. Which of the following would you treat with Da Huang steamed with wine?
    a. Constipation caused by accumulation of Heat
    b. Burns or hot skin lesions
    c. Blood Stasis Syndrome
    d. Bleeding caused by Excess Heat

257. Da Huang does *not* performs which of the following functions?
    a. Drain Heat and move the stool
    b. Drain Heat and quell Fire
    c. Clear and detoxify Fire-Poison
    d. Soften hard lumps and dispel nodules

258. Which herb provides the *best* treatment for red eyes caused by Liver Fire and for constipation with dry stool?
    a. Da Huang
    b. Lu Hui
    c. Gan Sui
    d. Da Ji

259. Which herb drains Heat, moves stool, clears Heat, and reduces swelling?
    a. Da Huang
    b. Mang Xiao
    c. Mu Li
    d. Xuan Shen

260. Which herb treats childhood nutritional impairment?
    a. Lu Hui
    b. Fan Xie Ye
    c. Huo Ma Ren
    d. Yu Li Ren

261. Which herb treats dry intestine constipation caused by Deficient Blood and Deficient body fluids, especially in the elderly?
    a. Mang Xiao
    b. Fan Xie Ye
    c. Huo Ma Ren
    d. Qian Niu Zi

262. Yu Li Ren moistens the Intestines, moves the stool, and also performs which of the following functions?
    a. Drain Damp-Heat and treat jaundice
    b. Promote urination and reduce edema
    c. Clear the Liver and eyes
    d. Nourish the fluids and alleviate thirst

263. Da Ji expels water and also performs which of the following functions?
    a. Clear Heat and detoxify Fire-Poison
    b. Reduce swelling and dispel nodules
    c. Promote Blood circulation to remove Blood Stasis
    d. Quell Liver Fire and benefit the eyes

264. Which herb expels fluid and also expels parasites to treat scabies?
    a. Yuan Hua
    b. Da Ji
    c. Huo Ma Ren
    d. Ku Lian Gen Pi

265. Which herb has the properties of strong heat and toxicity?
    a. Shang Lu
    b. Bi Ba
    c. Ba Dou
    d. Qian Niu Zi

266. Which herb is especially effective for treating constipation caused by accumulation of Cold?
    a. Da Huang
    b. Fan Xie Ye
    c. Ba Dou
    d. Da Ji

267. What should a patient do if after taking Ba Dou diarrhea occurs and will not stop?
    a. Drink hot water
    b. Take Sheng Jiang Tang
    c. Take honey
    d. Take cold diluted gruel

268. Yuan Hua, Da Ji, and Gan Sui are each indicated for which of the following?
    a. Traumatic injuries with congested Blood
    b. Wind-Damp, or Damp-Heat painful obstruction
    c. Abdominal distension and fluid accumulation in the chest
    d. Sluggish Cold

269. Which is the best combination to treat Excess Syndrome of Interior Heat accompanied by constipation with dry stool?
    a. Da Huang and Fan Xie Ye
    b. Da Huang and Liu Hui
    c. Da Huang and Huo Ma Ren
    d. Da Huang and Mang Xiao

270. Which herb treats amenorrhea caused by Blood Stasis accompanied by immobile abdominal masses?
    a. Da Huang
    b. Mang Xiao
    c. Gan Sui
    d. Yu Li Ren

271. Which herb treats lung abscesses, pain in the chest, pharyngitis, abundant expectoration, and tachypnea?
    a. Da Huang
    b. Qian Niu Zi
    c. Gan Sui
    d. Ba Dou

272. Shang Lu performs which of the following functions?
    a. Promote Blood circulation to remove Blood Stasis
    b. Clear Heat and quell Liver Fire
    c. Expel intestinal parasites and reduce Stagnation
    d. Expel water through the urethra and stool; reduce sores and carbuncles

273. Qian Niu Zi does *not* perform which of the following functions?
    a. Expel water
    b. Expel intestinal parasites
    c. Promote Blood
    d. Act as a purgative

274. Which of the following is *not* antagonistic with Gan Cao?
    a. Da Ji
    b. Yuan Hua
    c. Gan Sui
    d. Shang Lu

275. Which of the following functions is *not* performed by purgative formulas?
    a. Move the stool
    b. Potently purge the accumulation of Heat
    c. Purge the sluggish Cold
    d. Clear Heat and detoxify Fire-Poison

276. Da Cheng Qi Tang does *not* contain which of the following?
    a. Da Huang
    b. Mang Xiao
    c. Hou Po
    d. Yu Li Ren

277. Which of the following herbs serve as the chief (monarch or *jun*) component in Da Cheng Qi Tang?
    a. Mang Xiao
    b. Da Huang
    c. Da Huang and Mang Xiao
    d. Da Huang and Hou Po

278. Which of the following is an indication for the use of Xiao Cheng Qi Tang?
    a. A light case of Heat accumulation in the Yangming with a feeling of fullness in the chest or upper abdomen with distention and hardness
    b. A heavy case of Heat accumulation in the Yangming with a feeling of fullness in the chest or upper abdomen with distention and hardness
    c. Excess-Dry-Heat Syndrome of the Interior with no feeling of fullness in the upper abdomen
    d. None of the above

279. Da Cheng Qi Tang is *not* indicated for which of the following?
    a. Constipation with occasional watery discharge caused by accumulation of Heat
    b. Excess Syndrome of Interior Heat
    c. Yangming hollow organ Excess Syndrome
    d. Syndrome of accumulation of Stagnant Blood in the Lower Energizer

280. Which formula does *not* contain Mang Xiao, Da Huang, and Gan Cao?
    a. Tiao Wei Cheng Qi Tang
    b. Tao Ren Chen Qi Tang
    c. Xin Chia Huang Lung Tang
    d. Da Xian Xiong Tang

281. What is the composition of Da Xian Xiong Tang?
    a. Da Huang, Mang Xiao, and Gan Sui
    b. Da Huang, Mang Xiao, and Yuan Hua
    c. Da Huang, Mang Xiao, and Fan Xie Ye
    d. Da Huang, Mang Xiao, and Da Ji

282. What is the composition of Wen Pi Tang?
    a. Si Ni Tang with the addition of Da Huang and Mang Xiao
    b. Si Ni Tang with the addition of Da Huang and Ren Shen
    c. Si Ni Tang with the addition of Da Huang and Shao Yao
    d. Si Ni Tang with the addition of Da Huang and Bai Zhu

283. Wen Pi Tang performs which of the following functions?
    a. Warm and recuperate the Spleen Yang, purge Cold and sluggishness
    b. Warm and recuperate the Spleen and Kidneys, purge Cold-Excess and sluggishness
    c. Warm the Spleen and Stomach, purge Cold-Excess and sluggishness
    d. Warm the Kidney and Stomach, purge Cold-Excess and sluggishness

284. Which formula warms the body, dispels Cold, and purges accumulation?
    a. Li Zhong Tang
    b. Shih Zao Tang
    c. Da Huang Fu Zi Tang
    d. Da Huang Mu Dan Tang

285. Which formula treats this pattern: constipation, Cold-pain in the abdomen, cold hands and feet, chronic red-and-white dysentery, deep-wiry pulse?
    a. Li Zhong Tang
    b. Da Huang Fu Zi Tang
    c. Wen Pi Tang
    d. Da Jian Zhong Tang

286. Which formula treats this pattern: acute sharp pain in the abdomen, fullness and distention of the abdomen, a pale face, dyspnea, lockjaw, constipation?
    a. Wen Pi Tang
    b. Da Huang Fu Zi Tang
    c. San Wu Bei Ji Wang
    d. Da Jian Zhong Tang

287. Ma Zi Ren Wan can be produced by adding Huo Ma Ren, Bai Shao and Xing Ren to which formula?
    a. Da Cheng Chi Tang
    b. Tiao Wei Cheng Chi Tang
    c. Xiao Wei Cheng Chi Tang
    d. Zhen Yi Tang

288. Which statement is *not* correct regarding Ma Zi Ren Wan?
    a. Huo Ma Ren moisturizes the Intestines and relaxes the bowels
    b. Da Huang Quells Heat and relaxes the bowels
    c. Xing Ren moisturizes the Intestines and lowers the adverse rising Qi
    d. Hou Po and Zhi Shi promote the Qi and expand the chest

289. Which formula does *not* contain Da Huang?
    a. Da Xian Xiong Tang
    b. Ma Zi Ren Wan
    c. Zhou Che Wan
    d. Ji Chuan Jian

290. When is the best time to take Shih Zao Tang?
    a. After a meal
    b. Before a meal
    c. Before going to bed
    d. On an empty stomach in the morning

291. Shih Zao Tang is *not* indicated for which of the following symptoms?
    a. Pain in the hypochondria when coughing
    b. Fullness and rigidity in the upper abdomen
    c. Retching and deficient breath
    d. Afternoon fever

292. Da Zao does *not* perform which of the following functions in Shih Zao Tang?
    a. Reduces the poison of harsh expellants
    b. Reduces the damage to the healthy energy
    c. Supplements the Qi and protects the Stomach
    d. Strengthens the Middle Energizer and benefits the Qi

293. What are the two "Pi" ingredients in Zhou Che Wan?
    a. Gui Pi and Sang Bai Pi
    b. Fu Ling Pi and Sheng Jiang Pi
    c. Chen Pi and Qing Pi
    d. Mu Dan Pi and Dang Gua Pi

294. Which type of edema is treated with Zhou Che Wan?
    a. Excess of both the body and the Qi
    b. Excess of both the Exterior and Interior of the body
    c. Failure of the Yang
    d. Superficial Stagnation of Wind-Damp evil

295. Which formula treats this pattern: constipation with dry stool, swelling, fullness and hardness of the abdomen, tiredness from Deficient Qi, dry mouth and throat, a dark red tongue with yellow fur, or a tongue with dry fissures?
    a. Tiao Wei Cheng Chi Tang
    b. Huang Lung Tang
    c. Xin Chia Huang Lung Tang
    d. Zhen Yi Tang

296. Xin Chia Huang Lung Tang does *not* contain which of the following?
    a. Zhen Yi Tang
    b. Tiao Wei Cheng Chi Tang
    c. Ren Shen and Hai Shen
    d. Sha Shen and Da Zao

297. Zhen Yi Cheng Qi Tang can be produced by adding which herbs to Zhen Yi Tang?
    a. Da Huang and Mang Xiao
    b. Da Huang and Zhi Shi
    c. Da Huang and Hou Po
    d. Da Huang and Huo Ma Ren

298. Which formula nourishes the Yin to promote fluids and expels Heat to loosen the bowels?
    a. Xin Chia Huang Lung Tang
    b. Huang Lung Tang
    c. Ma Zi Ren Wan
    d. Zhen Yi Cheng Qi Tang

299. Which formula would you select to treat a patient with Yangming Heat Syndrome marked by Heat accumulation and Deficient Yin causing constipation, where decoctions aimed at increasing fluids have been tried to no good effect?
    a. Zhen Yi Cheng Qi Tang
    b. Zhen Yi Tang
    c. Da Cheng Qi Tang
    d. Huang Lung Tang

300. Which formula treats this pattern: watery diarrhea with undigested food in the stool that is green or yellow-brown and foul smelling, abdominal pain, a feeling of hardness and lumps upon palpation, dry mouth and tongue, slippery-Excess pulse?
    a. Da Cheng Chi Tang
    b. Tiao Wei Cheng Chi Tang
    c. Bai Tou Weng Tang
    d. Ge Gen Huang Lian Huang Qin Tang

301. What are the properties of Fu Ling?
    a. Sweet, bland and cool
    b. Sweet, bitter and cool
    c. Sweet, bland and neutral
    d. Sweet, bitter and neutral

302. Fu Ling is *not* indicated for which of the following?
    a. Difficult urination and edema
    b. Dizziness, palpitation, and cough caused by congested fluid
    c. Loss of appetite, diarrhea, and lassitude caused by Deficient Spleen
    d. Summer Heat thirst and diarrhea caused by Damp-Heat evil

303. Which herb strengthens the Spleen, drains Damp, clears Heat, and expels pus?
    a. Fu Ling
    b. Bai Zhu
    c. Yi Yi Ren
    d. Zi Xie

304. Which herb promotes urination, leaches out Damp, and eliminates arthralgia?
    a. Yi Yi Ren
    b. Mu Gua
    c. Che Qian Zi
    d. Ze Xie

305. Which herb treats intestinal and lung abscesses?
    a. Yu Xing Cao
    b. Zi Hua Di Ding
    c. Jie Geng
    d. Yi Yi Ren

306. Which herb promotes urination, leaches out Damp, and promotes lactation?
    a. Yi Yi Ren
    b. Che Qian Zi
    c. Mu Tong
    d. Chuan Shan Jia

307. Which herb promotes urination, brings Heat downward, treats stranguria caused by Heat, and treats erosion of the mucous membrane in the oral cavity?
    a. Zhu Ling
    b. Mu Tong
    c. Hua Shi
    d. Fu Ling

308. Che Qian Zi does *not* perform which of the following functions?
    a. Promote urination
    b. Clear away Liver Fire to treat eye diseases
    c. Clear Heat and expel Phlegm
    d. Clear Heat and detoxify Fire-Poison

309. Che Qian Zi is *not* indicated for which of the following?
    a. Edema and stranguria
    b. Coughing caused by Lung Heat
    c. Damp-Heat diarrhea
    d. Exudative skin damage

310. Which herb treats Damp-Heat in the Bladder and stranguria with painful micturition?
    a. Fu Ling
    b. Che Qian Zi
    c. Zhu Ling
    d. Ma Huang

311. Zhu Ling performs which of the following functions?
    a. Expel Wind-Damp
    b. Clear Heat and dry Damp
    c. Drain Damp
    d. Eliminate Damp with fragrant drugs

312. Which of the following would *best* treat stranguria caused by Damp-Heat?
    a. Fu Ling
    b. Zhu Ling
    c. Ze Xie
    d. Hua Shi

313. Which of the following would *best* treat urinary dysfunction accompanied by dry stool?
    a. Qu Mai
    b. Bian Xu
    c. Dong Kui Zi
    d. Tong Cao

314. Which herb is especially effective for treating dermal diseases?
    a. Dong Gua Pi
    b. Di Fu Zi
    c. Ze Xie
    d. Chi Xiao Dou

315. Which herb is especially effective for treating stranguria complicated by hematuria?
    a. Hua Shi
    b. Zhu Ling
    c. Di Fu Zi
    d. Shi Wai

316. Which of the following is the *best* indication for the use of Jin Qian Cao?
    a. Stranguria caused by Heat or urinary stones
    b. Stranguria caused by Heat and complicated by hematuria
    c. Stranguria complicated by hematuria and induced by overstrain
    d. None of the above

317. Which herb promotes urination, eliminates Damp, and treats jaundice?
    a. Hai Jin Sha
    b. Long Dan Cao
    c. Jin Qian Cao
    d. Dan Zhu Ye

318. Which of the following herbs would *best* treat liver and gallbladder stones?
    a. Jin Qian Cao
    b. Chai Hu
    c. Bei Xie
    d. Che Qian Zi

319. Which of the following herbs would *best* treat Damp-Heat jaundice?
    a. Jin Qian Cao
    b. Yin Chen Hao
    c. Hai Jin Sha
    d. Chuan Xin Lian

320. Which herb is especially effective for treating cloudy urine?
    a. Shi Wei
    b. Hua Shi
    c. Bei Xie
    d. Che Qian Cao

321. Which herb promotes diuresis to eliminate Damp from the Lower Energizer, expels Wind-Damp, and treats cloudy urine?
    a. Yi Yi Ren
    b. Mu Tong
    c. Yu Mi Xu
    d. Bei Xie

322. Deng Xin Cao performs which of the following functions?
    a. Promote urination and lactation
    b. Clear Heat and expel Phlegm
    c. Promote urination and expel Wind-Damp
    d. Promote urination and clear Heart Heat to expel irritability

323. Bian Xu performs which of the following functions?
    a. Promote urination, eliminate swelling, expel Phlegm, and stop cough
    b. Promote urination, detoxify Fire-Poison, and expel pus
    c. Promote urination, eliminate swelling, clear Heat, and promote lactation
    d. Promote urination, clear Damp-Heat in the Bladder, expel parasites, and stop itching

324. Which two herbs each promote urination, treat stranguria, and expel stones?
    a. Fu Ling and Bei Xie
    b. Hua Shi and Chi Xiao Dou
    c. Yi Yi Ren and Ze Xie
    d. Shi Wei and Hai Jin Sha

325. What is the mechanism by which Yin Chen Hao expels jaundice?
    a. Clear Heat and dry Damp
    b. Disperse and rectify the depressed Liver Qi
    c. Clear away Heat and promote diuresis
    d. Promote diuresis to eliminate Damp

326. Bei Xia and Zhu Ling are both indicated for which of the following?
    a. Leukorrhea caused by Damp-Heat with turbid urine
    b. Palpitation, insomnia and forgetfulness
    c. Edema caused by Deficient Spleen
    d. Loss of appetite and diarrhea caused by Deficient Spleen

327. Fu ling and Yi Yi Ren each perform which of the following functions?
    a. Promote urination, leach out Damp, and expel pus
    b. Promote urination, leach out Damp, and expel jaundice
    c. Promote urination, leach out Damp, and strengthen the Spleen
    d. Promote urination, leach out Damp, and promote lactation

328. Mu Tong and Tong Cao each perform which of the following functions?
    a. Promote urination, clear Heat, and promote lactation
    b. Promote urination, clear Heat, and restrain lactation
    c. Promote urination, clear Heat, and expel Wind-Damp
    d. Promote urination, clear Heat, and release summer-Heat

329. Fu Ling performs which of the following functions?
    a. Promote urination, leeches out Damp, and expel arthralgia and expel pus
    b. Promote urination, strengthen the Spleen, and calm the Spirit
    c. Promote urination, clear Lung Heat, and eliminate Phlegm
    d. Promote urination, clear summer-Heat, and stop diarrhea

330. Shi Wei performs which of the following functions?
    a. Clear Heat, promote urination, and stop diarrhea
    b. Clear Heat, promote urination, and expel pus
    c. Clear Heat, promote urination, and expel arthralgia
    d. None of the above

331. Which herb expels Wind-Damp and treats Damp evil stagnating in the Spleen?
    a. Qiang Huo
    b. Xiang Ru
    c. Cao Dou Kou
    d. Cang Zhu

332. Which herb dries Damp, strengthens the Spleen, and releases Exterior conditions?
    a. Xiang Ru
    b. Bai Zhu
    c. Cang Zhu
    d. Cao Dou Kou

333. Which herb is especially effective for treating night blindness?
    a. Cang Zhu
    b. Ju Hua
    c. Gou Qi Zi
    d. Sang Ye

334. Which of the following is an indication for the use of Cang Zhu?
    a. Cold pain in the abdomen, vomiting, and diarrhea
    b. Damp evil stagnating in the Middle Energizer
    c. Accumulation of undigested food, abdominal distention and pain
    d. Incoordination between the Liver and Stomach, vomiting, and loss of appetite

335. What are the properties of Hou Po?
    a. Bitter, acrid, and warm
    b. Bitter, acrid, and neutral
    c. Bitter, sweet, and warm
    d. Acrid, sweet, and cool

336. Which of the following would you treat with Bai Dou Kou?
    a. Vomiting caused by Stomach-Heat
    b. Vomiting caused by Stomach-Cold
    c. Vomiting caused by Deficient Stomach
    d. Morning sickness

337. Hou Po does *not* perform which of the following functions?
    a. Move the Qi and transform Damp
    b. Resolve Stagnation and relieve asthma
    c. Calm the Liver
    d. Warm and transform Phlegm

338. Bai Dou Kou does *not* perform which of the following functions?
    a. Move the Qi and transform Damp
    b. Warm the Middle Energizer
    c. Alleviate vomiting
    d. Invigorate the Yang

339. Sha Ren does *not* perform which of the following functions?
    a. Move the Qi and transform Damp
    b. Warm the Middle Energizer
    c. Calm the fetus
    d. Wakes the patient from unconsciousness

340. Which herb enters the Spleen and Stomach meridians?
    a. Dong Gua Ren
    b. Sha Ren
    c. Xing Ren
    d. Yu Li Ren

341. Sha Ren is used to treat diarrhea associated with which of the following?
    a. Spleen-Cold
    b. Damp-Heat
    c. Intense Heat evil
    d. Summer-Heat-Damp

342. Which herb transforms Damp, releases summer-Heat, and stops vomiting?
    a. Huo Xiang
    b. Pei Lan
    c. Huang Qin
    d. Hua Shi

343. Which herb *best* treats this pattern: aversion to cold, fever, swelling of the abdomen, vomiting and diarrhea, dirty greasy tongue fur?
    a. Pei Lan
    b. Huo Xiang
    c. Xiang Ru
    d. Zi Su Ye

344. Which herb treats vomiting caused by Damp evil Stagnation?
    a. Cang Zhu
    b. Bai Zhu
    c. Cao Guo
    d. Huo Xiang

345. Which herb transforms Damp, releases Summer Heat, and is especially useful to treat halitosis accompanied by a sweet taste in the mouth, excess saliva, and greasy tongue fur?
    a. Pei Lan
    b. Sha Ren
    c. Hou Po
    d. Bai Dou Kou

346. Huo Xiang treats vomiting caused by which of the following?
    a. Damp evil stagnating in the Spleen and Stomach
    b. Damp-Heat
    c. Deficient Spleen and Stomach
    d. Stomach-Cold

347. Sha Ren and Bai Dou Kou each are indicated for which of the following?
    a. Diarrhea caused by Spleen-Cold
    b. Morning sickness
    c. Damp evil and Qi Stagnation with incoordination between the Spleen and Stomach
    d. None of the above

348. Which two herbs each transform Damp and release Summer Heat?
    a. Sha Ren and Bai Dou Kou
    b. Huo Xiang and Pei Lan
    c. Cang Zhu and Hou Po
    d. Cao Guo and Chen Pi

349. Which herb harmonizes intermittent fever and chills, warms the Middle Energizer, and dries Damp?
    a. Qing Hao
    b. Pei Lan
    c. Cao Guo
    d. Chang Shan

350. Which herb is very effective at clearing Damp-Heat Poison, clears Heat, and also treats syphilis and hot skin lesions?
    a. Fu Ling
    b. Tu Fu Ling
    c. Di Fu Zi
    d. Zhu Ling

351. Which herb does *not* treat Damp evil Stagnation injuring the Middle Energizer?
    a. Hou Po
    b. Huo Xiang
    c. Chen Pi
    d. Yu Mi Xu

352. How should Sha Ren be decocted?
    a. Separately from other herbs
    b. Before other herbs are added
    c. In a wrapping
    d. It is added after other herbs

353. Formulas that expel Damp are *not* indicated for which of the following?
    a. Damp evil Stagnation and incoordination between the Spleen and Stomach
    b. Evils of Damp and Heat blended and stagnated within the body
    c. Evils of Damp and Heat blended together and attacking the Lower Energizer
    d. Failure of the Spleen to transport and convert Phlegm caused by Damp evil Stagnation

354. What are the important components of Ping Wei San?
    a. Hou Po, Chen Pi, Cang Zhu, and Da Zao
    b. Hou Po, Chen Pi, Gan Cao, and Bai Zhu
    c. Hou Po, Chen Pi, Gan Cao, and Cang Zhu
    d. Hou Po, Chen Pi, Gan Cao, and Sheng Jiang

355. Huo Xiang Cheng Qi San is composed of Er Chen Tang and which other herbs?
    a. Huo Xiang and Zi Su Ye
    b. Bai Zhi and Bai Zhu
    c. Hou Po and Jie Geng
    d. All of the above

356. Huo Xiang Zheng Qi San is *not* indicated for which of the following?
    a. Fever, aversion to cold and headache
    b. Chest distension, abdominal fullness and pain
    c. Nausea, vomiting, borborygmus and diarrhea
    d. Dizziness and arcus senilis

357. Which formula treats this pattern: abdominal fullness, loss of appetite, nausea and vomiting, belching, acid regurgitation, white greasy tongue fur, moderate pulse?
    a. Huo Xiang Zheng Qi San
    b. Ping Wei San
    c. Shi Pi Yin
    d. Bu Huan Jin Zheng Qi San

358. Which two herbs are added to Ping Wei San to produce Bu Huan Jin Zheng Qi San?
    a. Ban Xia and Fu Ling
    b. Xiang Ru and Sheng Jiang
    c. Huo Xiang and Ban Xia
    d. Huo Xiang and Sheng Jiang

359. Yin Chen Hao Tang does *not* contain which of the following?
    a. Yin Chen Hao
    b. Zhi Zi
    c. Da Huang
    d. Huang Qin

360. Yin Chen Hao Tang does *not* perform which of the following functions?
    a. Move the Qi
    b. Clear Heat
    c. Resolve Damp
    d. Reduce jaundice

361. What is the main indication for the use of Yin Chen Hao Tang?
    a. Urinary difficulty
    b. Abdominal distention
    c. Yellow greasy tongue fur and a deep-rapid pulse
    d. Whole body jaundice with color that resembles a fresh tangerine

362. Yin Chen Hao Tang treats jaundice caused by which of the following?
    a. Overabundance of both Heat and Damp
    b. Mild Heat and Damp
    c. Damp-Heat where the Damp is stronger than the Heat
    d. None of the above

363. Which of the following is *not* one of the "three Ren" ingredients in San Ren Tang?
    a. Xing Ren
    b. Bai Dou Kou
    c. Yi Yi Ren
    d. Dong Gua Ren

364. Da Huang performs which of the following functions in Yin Chen Hao Tang?
    a. Resolve Damp and reduce jaundice
    b. Clear Heat and dry Damp
    c. Quell Fire and detoxify Poison
    d. Clear Heat, expel Blood Stasis, and move the stool

365. San Ren Tang performs which of the following functions?
    a. Resolve Damp, promote diuresis, clear Heat, and detoxify Poison
    b. Eliminate Heat and Damp and open the inhibited activities of Qi
    c. Clear Heat, resolve Damp, and regulate the Qi and the Middle Energizer
    d. Clear Heat, resolve Damp, and reduce jaundice

366. San Ren Tang is *not* indicated for which of the following?
    a. Headache and intolerance of cold
    b. Recessive fever
    c. Feeling of oppression in the chest
    d. Epigastric distending pain

367. Xing Ren performs which of the following functions in San Ren Tang?
    a. Moisturizes the intestine
    b. Open the inhibited energy
    c. Eliminate Damp evil
    d. Expel Phlegm

368. Gan Lu Xiao Du Dan does *not* contain which of the following?
    a. Hua Shi, Yin Chen Hao, and Mu Tong
    b. Huang Qin, Lian Qiao, and Chuan Bei Mu
    c. She Gan, Shi Chang Pu, and Huo Xiang
    d. Fu Ling, Tong Cao, and Bo He

369. San Ren Tang, Gan Lu Xiao Du Dan, Huang Qin Hua Shi Tang, and Hou Po Xia Ling Tang each perform which of the following functions?
    a. Eliminate Heat and Damp
    b. Eliminate Cold and Damp
    c. Diaphoretics
    d. Eliminate Dry

370. Which formula resolves Damp, transforms turbidity, clears Heat, and detoxifies Poison?
    a. Lian Po Yin
    b. San Ren Tang
    c. Gan Lu Xiao Du Dan
    d. None of the above

371. Which formula clears Heat, transforms Damp, regulates the Qi, and harmonizes the Middle Energizer?
    a. Gan Lu Xiao Du Dan
    b. Lian Po Yin
    c. Ping Wei San
    d. Huo Xiang Zheng Qi San

372. Lian Po Yin does *not* contain which of the following?
    a. Chen Pi and Sheng Jiang
    b. Huang Lian and Hou Po
    c. Zhi Zi and Dan Dou Chi
    d. Chi Chang Pu, Ban Xia, and Lu Gen

373. Lian Po Yin is *not* indicated for which of the following?
    a. Simultaneous vomiting and diarrhea
    b. Distention and a stifling sensation in the chest and epigastrium
    c. Dark and scanty urine
    d. A feeling of heaviness and pain in the entire body

374. Which of the following herbs do *not* serve to promote urination and unblock painful urinary dysfunction in the formula Ba Zheng San?
    a. Mu Tong and Bian Xu
    b. Qu Mai and Che Qian Zi
    c. Hua Shi
    d. Ze Xie

375. Which herb does not serve to clear Heat and quell Fire in Ba Zheng San?
    a. Da Huang
    b. Huang Bai
    c. Zhi Zi
    d. Deng Xin Cao

376. Which formula would best treat this pattern: weakness or atrophy of the lower extremities, red hot swollen painful feet or knees, scanty yellow urine, yellow greasy tongue fur?
    a. Ba Zheng San
    b. Er Miao San
    c. Ji Ming San
    d. Fang Ji Huang Qi Tang

377. Which formula would best treat this pattern: dark, turbid, scanty, difficult and painful urination, dry mouth and throat, yellow greasy tongue fur, slippery-rapid pulse?
    a. Dao Chi San
    b. Ba Zheng San
    c. Gan Lu Xiao Du Dan
    d. Xiao Ji Yin Zi

378. Which formula would best treat this pattern: throbbing pulsation just below the umbilicus, vomiting, frothy saliva, vertigo, shortness of breath, coughing?
    a. Er Chen Tang
    b. Ling Gui Zhu Gan Tang
    c. Wu Ling San
    d. Zhen Wu Tang

379. What is added to Er Miao San to produce San Miao Wan?
    a. Che Qian Zi
    b. Yi Yi Ren
    c. Fu Ling
    d. Niu Xi

380. What is added to San Miao Wan to produce Si Miao Wan?
    a. Fu Ling
    b. Yi Yi Ren
    c. Zhu Ling
    d. Hua Shi

381. Wu Ling San Which does *not* contain which of the following?
    a. Gui Zhi
    b. Mu Tong
    c. Ze Xie and Fu Ling
    d. Zhu Ling and Bai Zhu

382. Wu Ling San is *not* indicated for which of the following?
    a. Superficial syndrome and retention of fluid in the body
    b. Diarrhea caused by sudden turmoil disorder
    c. Phlegm retention disease and throbbing pulsation just below the umbilicus
    d. Dysuria caused by evils of Damp and Heat blended together and attacking the Lower Energizer

383. Si Ling San can be created by subtracting which herb from Wu Ling San?
    a. Ze Xie
    b. Fu Ling
    c. Bai Zhu
    d. Gui Zhi

384. Zhu Ling San does *not* contain which of the following?
    a. Ze Xie
    b. E Jiao
    c. Bai Shao
    d. Hua Shi

385. Wei Ling Tang performs which of the following functions?
    a. Clear Heat and promote urination
    b. Strengthen the Spleen and promote urination
    c. Dispel Damp and regulate the flow of Qi in the Stomach
    d. Promote urination and drain Damp

386. Zhu Ling Tang performs which of the following functions?
    a. Promote urination, clear Heat, and nourish the Yin
    b. Promote urination, drain Damp, and nourish the Yin
    c. Promote urination, strengthen the Spleen, and nourish the Yin
    d. None of the above

387. Zhu Ling Tang is *not* indicated for which of the following?
    a. Urinary difficulty, fever, and thirst with a desire to drink
    b. Irritability or insomnia
    c. Diarrhea accompanied by cough or nausea
    d. Throbbing pulsations just below the umbilicus

388. Which formula is *not* used to clear Heat and promote urination?
    a. Gan Lu Xiao Du Dan
    b. San Ren Tang
    c. Wu Pi San
    d. Yin Chen Hao Tang

389. Fang Ji Huang Qi Tang does *not* contain which of the following?
    a. Bai Zhu
    b. Gan Cao
    c. Sheng Jiang
    d. Fu Ling

390. E Jiao performs which of the following functions in Zhu Ling Tang?
    a. Nourish the Blood and Yin
    b. Moisturize dryness and enrich the Yin
    c. Clear Heat and enrich the Yin
    d. Tonify the Blood and stop bleeding

391. Which formula would best treat the following pattern: sweating, aversion to wind and cold, heavy sensation in the body, superficial edema, urinary difficulty, pale tongue with white fur, floating pulse?
    a. Gui Zhi Tang
    b. Fang Ji Huang Qi Tang
    c. Yu Ping Feng San
    d. Wu Pi San

392. Wu Pi San does *not* contain which of the following?
    a. Fu Ling Pi
    b. Di Gu Pi
    c. Sang Bai Pi and Da Fu Pi
    d. Sheng Jiang Pi and Chen Pi

393. Which formula would best treat the following pattern: generalized edema with a sensation of heaviness, distention and fullness in the epigastrium and abdomen, rapid respiration, urinary difficulty, white greasy tongue fur, deep-moderate pulse?
    a. Wu Ling San
    b. Zhu Ling Tang
    c. Wu Pi San
    d. Zhen Wu Tang

394. Which formula would best treat the following pattern: full feeling in the chest and hypochondria, Deficient Qi, vertigo, cough, palpitations, white slippery tongue fur, wiry-slippery pulse?
    a. Er Chen Tang
    b. Ling Gan Wu Wei Jiang Xin Tang
    c. Ling Gui Zhu Gan Tang
    d. Zhi Shou San

395. Zhen Wu Tang does *not* contain which of the following?
    a. Fu Ling and baked Fu Zi
    b. Bai Zhu and Bai Shao Yao
    c. Sheng Fu Zi
    d. Sheng Jiang

396. Bai Shao Yao performs which of the following functions in Zhen Wu Tang?
    a. Preserve the Yin and alleviate pain
    b. Nourish the Blood
    c. Prevent excessive urination
    d. Calm the rising Liver Yang

397. Which of the formulas below would you select to treat Deficient Yang of the Spleen and Kidneys with generalized edema caused by water retention?
    a. Ling Gui Zhu Gan Tang
    b. Feng Ji Huang Qi Tang
    c. Feng Ji Fu Ling Tang
    d. Zhen Wu Tang

398. How can the formula for Zhen Wu Tang be altered to produce the formula for Fu Zi Tang?
    a. Add Fu Zi
    b. Subtract Sheng Jiang and add Fu Zi
    c. Subtract Sheng Jiang and add Ren Shen
    d. Subtract Bai Zhu and add Ren Shen

399. Which formula would best treat a 40-year-old female patient with these symptoms: edema (more severe below the waist), fullness and distention of the chest and abdomen, a heavy sensation in the body, loss of appetite, cold extremities, scanty urine, loose stool, thick greasy tongue fur, deep-slow pulse?
    a. Zhen Wu Tang
    b. Shi Pi Yin
    c. Ling Gui Zhu Gan Tang
    d. Shen Qu Wan

400. Which formula warms the Yang, strengthens the Spleen, moves the Qi, and promotes urination?
    a. Wu Ling San
    b. Ling Gui Zhu Gan Tang
    c. Zhen Wu Tang
    d. Shi Pi Wan

401. Bai Xie Fen Qing Yin does *not* contain which of the following?
    a. Yi Zhi Ren and Fu Ling
    b. Shi Chang Pu and Wu Yao
    c. Sheng Jiang
    d. Gan Cao

402. Which formula treats Damp seeping into the Bladder causing cloudy urine or gonorrhea accompanied by frequent urination that is white and mucoid?
    a. Sang Piao Xiao San
    b. Jin Suo Gu Jing Wan
    c. Bei Xie Fen Qin Yin
    d. Mu Li San

403. Which herb expels Wind-Damp, relaxes and activates the tendons, and removes Deficiency-Heat?
    a. Mu Gua
    b. Qin Jiao
    c. Du Huo
    d. Huang Bai

404. Which herb expels Wind-Damp and releases Exterior conditions?
    a. Sang Zhi
    b. Du Huo
    c. Fang Ji
    d. Wei Ling Xian

405. Which herb would you select to treat Wind-Cold-Damp pain obstruction, especially in the lower back and leg?
    a. Wei Ling Xian
    b. Du Huo
    c. Qiang Huo
    d. Fang Feng

406. Which herb would *best* treat arthralgia of the Heat type?
    a. Fang Feng
    b. Du Huo
    c. Qin Jiao
    d. Hai Feng Tang

407. Which herb expels Wind-Damp and removes jaundice?
    a. Yin Chen Hao
    b. Jin Qian Cao
    c. Haung Qin
    d. Qin Jiao

408. Which of the following is strongest at relaxing and activating the tendons and stopping pain?
    a. Wei Ling Xian
    b. Qin Jiao
    c. Xi Xian Cao
    d. Luo Shi Teng

409. Which herb expels Wind-Damp, activates the meridians, and relieves convulsions?
    a. Bai Hua She
    b. Mu Gua
    c. Bai Fu Zi
    d. Sang Zhi

410. Which of the following is an indication for Sang Zhi?
    a. Arthralgia in the upper extremities
    b. Arthralgia in the lower extremities
    c. Arthralgia of the Cold type
    d. Arthralgia of the Damp type

411. Which herb does *not* treat insufficiency of the Liver and Kidneys accompanied by weakness and atrophy of the sinews and bones?
    a. Hu Gu
    b. Sang Ji Sheng
    c. Sang Zhi
    d. Xu Duan

412. Which herb is best for treating diarrhea, vomiting, and spasm and cramping of the calves?
    a. Ban Xia
    b. Mu Gua
    c. Huang Lian
    d. Yi Yi Ren

413. Which herb does *not* treat both endogenous and exogenous Wind evil?
    a. Fang Feng
    b. Can Sha
    c. Xi Xian Cao
    d. Wu Shao She

414. Which herb comforts the sinews, activates the meridians, harmonizes the Stomach, and transforms Damp?
    a. Luo Shi Teng
    b. Mu Gua
    c. Kuan Jin Teng
    d. Bai Hua She

415. Which is herb is best for treating Damp-Heat type arthralgia and edema?
    a. Fang Ji
    b. Du Huo
    c. Wei Ling Xian
    d. Qin Jiao

416. Which herb promotes urination, reduces swelling, expels Wind-Damp, and strengthens the sinews?
    a. Sang Zhi
    b. Wu Jia Pi
    c. Bai Hua She
    d. Wei Ling Xian

417. Which herb expels Wind-Damp and tonifies the Liver and Kidneys?
    a. Qin Jiao
    b. Hu Gu
    c. Sang Ji Sheng
    d. Xu Duan

418. Which herb treats spontaneous abortion caused by Deficient Kidneys?
    a. Huang Qin
    b. Bai Zhu
    c. Sang Ji Sheng
    d. Qin Jiao

419. Which herb does *not* activate the meridians?
    a. Hai Feng Teng
    b. Qian Nian Jian
    c. Hai Tong Pi
    d. Wei Ling Xian

420. Which of the following functions do Wu Shao She and Bai Hua She *not* have in common?
    a. Expel Wind
    b. Activates the meridians
    c. Strengthen the sinews and bones
    d. Relieve convulsions

421. Which two herbs each expel Wind-Damp and dredge the meridian passage?
    a. Can Sha and Sang Ji Sheng
    b. Qin Jiao and Fang Ji
    c. Sang Zhi and Bai Hua She
    d. Xi Xian Cao and Wu Jia Pi

422. Which two herbs each expel Wind-Damp and strengthen the sinews and bones?
    a. Du Huo and Qin Jiao
    b. Sang Zhi and Mu Gua
    c. Qian Nian Jian and Wei Ling Xian
    d. Wu Jia Pi and Sang Ji Sheng

423. Which herb treats vaginal bleeding during pregnancy and spontaneous abortion?
    a. Sang Shen
    b. Wu Jia Pi
    c. Sang Ji Sheng
    d. Sang Bai Pi

424. Which herb cools the Blood, reduces abscesses, expels Wind-Damp, and activates the meridians?
    a. Luo Shi Teng
    b. Xi Xian Can
    c. Hong Teng
    d. Kuan Jin Teng

425. Which herb expels Wind-Damp, pacifies the Liver, clears Heat, and can be used to lower blood pressure?
    a. Xi Xian Cao
    b. Sang Zhi
    c. Can Sha
    d. Fang Ji

426. Which herb does *not* treat Wind-Damp-Heat painful obstruction?
    a. Hai Tong Pi
    b. Wei Ling Xian
    c. Luo Shi Teng
    d. Fang Ji

427. Qing Huo Sheng Shi Tang does *not* contain which of the following?
    a. Qiang Huo and Chuan Xiong
    b. Du Huo and Man Jing Zi
    c. Fang Feng, Gao Ben, and Gan Cao
    d. Bai Zhi, Xi Xin, and Wei Ling Xian

428. Du Huo Ji Sheng Tang does *not* perform which of the following functions?
    a. Treat rheumatic pain
    b. Clear Damp-Heat
    c. Tonify the Liver and Kidneys
    d. Replenish the Qi and Blood

429. Which herbs in Du Huo Ji Sheng tonify the Liver and Kidneys?
    a. Gou Ji and Xu Duan
    b. Tu Si Zi and Huang Jing
    c. Sang Shen, He Shou Wu, and Gou Qi Zi
    d. Sang Ji Sheng, Du Zhong, and Huai Niu Xi

430. Which formula treats this pattern: heavy and painful head, general sensation of heaviness, back or generalized pain, difficulty in rotating or bending the trunk, white tongue fur, floating pulse?
    a. Du Huo Ji Sheng Tang
    b. Qiang Huo Sheng Shi Tang
    c. Ma Huang Jia Zhu Tang
    d. Juan Bi Tang

431. Which of the following serves as the chief (monarch or *jun*) component in Qiang Huo Sheng Shi Tang?
    a. Qiang Huo and Fang Feng
    b. Qiang Huo and Du Huo
    c. Chuan Xiong and Man Jing Zi
    d. Qiang Huo

432. Juan Bi Tang does *not* contain which of the following?
    a. Qiang Huo, Du Huo, Sang Ji Sheng
    b. Qiang Huo, Jiang Huang, Huang Qi
    c. Dang Gui, Chi Shao Yao, Fang Feng
    d. Dang Gui, Sheng Jiang, Gan Cao

433. Which formula would best treat the following pattern: a heavy painful sensation at fixed locations in the lower back and lower extremities accompanied by weakness and stiffness, intolerance of cold, attraction to warmth, pale tongue with white fur, thin-weak pulse?
    a. Du Huo Ji Sheng Tang
    b. Qiang Huo Sheng Shi Tang
    c. Bu Yang Huan Wu Tang
    d. Dang Gui Si Ni Tang

434. Which herbs in the formula for Du Huo Ji Sheng Tang serve to nourish the Blood and promote Blood circulation?
    a. Shu Di Huang, Dang Gui, and Chi Shao Yao
    b. Shu Di Huang, Dang Gui, Bai Shao Yao, and Chuan Xiong
    c. Sheng Di Huang, Dang Gui, Bai Shao Yao, and Chuan Xiong
    d. Sheng Di Huang, Dang Gui, Bai Shao Yao, and E Jiao

435. Ji Ming San does *not* contain which of the following?
    a. Bing Lang, Mu Gua, and Chen Pi
    b. Zi Su Ye, Jie Geng, and Wu Zhu Yu
    c. Sheng Jiang
    d. Gan Jiang

436. Which formula is used to treat wet beriberi?
    a. Du Huo Ji Sheng Tang
    b. Chuan Pi Tang
    c. Ji Ming San
    d. Zhen Wu Tang

437. Which herb would you select to treat a case where Qi has collected in the patient's chest leading to a sensation of distension, constriction, pain, or diaphragmatic pressure?
    a. Zhe Bei Mu
    b. Gua Lou
    c. Chen Pi
    d. Tian Nan Xing

438. Which herb treats hemiplegia caused by accumulation of Wind-Phlegm?
    a. Ban Xia
    b. Bai Fu Zi
    c. Shi Jue Ming
    d. Gou Teng

439. Ban Xia does *not* perform which of the following functions?
    a. Dry Damp and transform Phlegm
    b. Harmonize the Stomach and stop vomiting
    c. Warm the Middle Energizer and stop diarrhea
    d. Dissipate nodules and reduce distension

440. Which two herbs are often used with Ban Xia to treat Damp-Phlegm?
    a. Bai Zhu and Fo Shou
    b. Bai Dou Kou and Cao Dou Kou
    c. Fu Ling and Chen Pi
    d. Cang Zhu and Yi Yi Ren

441. Which herb treats migraine caused by accumulation of Wind-Phlegm?
    a. Gao Ben
    b. Qiang Huo
    c. Tian Nan Xing
    d. Bai Fu Zi

442. Which herb treats tremors, seizures, or stroke induced by Hot-Phlegm?
    a. Tian Nan Xing
    b. Bai Fu Zi
    c. Dan Nan Xing
    d. Gou Teng

443. Which herb treats vomiting from Stomach-Heat caused by the accumulation of Phlegm and Heat?
    a. Tian Zhu Huang
    b. Zhu Li
    c. Zhu Ru
    d. Zhu Ye

444. Which herb treats cough with copious sputum, or abnormal rising of Qi caused by the failure of the Spleen to resolve Damp?
    a. Fu Ling
    b. Qian Hu
    c. Ban Xia
    d. Jie Geng

445. Which herb treats morning sickness and globus hystericus, nodules, and goiters?
    a. Ban Xia
    b. Kun Bu
    c. Hai Zao
    d. Huang Qin

446. Which herb treats cough with copious sputum accompanied by a feeling of oppression in the chest and a sore throat or loss of voice?
    a. Ban Xia
    b. Niu Bang Xi
    c. Bai Fu Zi
    d. Jie Geng

447. Which herb treats lung abscesses, pain in the chest, and Hot-Phlegm with blood and pus?
    a. Lu Gen
    b. Pu Gong Ying
    c. Chuan Bai Mu
    d. Jie Geng

448. Which is the best herb to redirect the Stomach Qi downward in Cold-Deficient Stomach or Spleen patterns, or in Damp Spleen conditions with vomiting and hiccups?
    a. Jie Geng
    b. Qian Hu
    c. Bai Qian
    d. Xuan Fu Hua

449. Which is the best herb to clear Lung and Stomach Heat, transform Phlegm, unbind the Qi in the chest, and dissipate nodules?
    a. Xing Ren
    b. Sang Bai Pi
    c. Gua Lou
    d. Chuan Bei Mu

450. Which herb can be substituted for Bei Mu to treat coughing caused by Hot-Phlegm?
    a. Jie Geng
    b. Zhu Ru
    c. Sang Ye
    d. Gua Lou

451. Which herb is used primarily to treat Exterior conditions caused by Wind-Heat and nodules caused by Phlegm-Heat?
    a. Chuan Bei Mu
    b. Ban Xia
    c. Xing Ren
    d. Zhe Bei Mu

452. Which herb warms the Lungs, expels Phlegm, dissipates nodules, reduces swelling, and alleviates pain?
    a. Bai Jie Zi
    b. Su Zi
    c. Bai Fu Zi
    d. Fu Hai Shi

453. Which herb quells Lung Heat and alleviates coughing and wheezing?
    a. Jie Geng
    b. Sang Bai Pi
    c. Zi Wan
    d. Su Zi

454. Hai Zao and Kun Bu each perform which of the following functions?
    a. Warm the Lungs and expel Phlegm
    b. Dry Damp and transform Phlegm
    c. Clear Heat and reduce Phlegm nodules
    d. None of the above

455. Sang Bai Pi and Ting Li Zi each perform which of the following functions?
    a. Clear Lung Heat and alleviate wheezing; promote urination and reduce edema
    b. Moisten the Lungs and stop cough; promote urination
    c. Warm the Lungs and stop cough; promote urination
    d. None of the above

456. Which herb is used when Cold-Phlegm collects in the meridians causing such symptoms as joint pain, numbness, and body aches?
    a. Bai Jie Zi
    b. Ban Xia
    c. Bei Mu
    d. Xuan Fu Hua

457. What are the properties of Jie Geng?
    a. Bitter, acrid, and cool
    b. Bitter, acrid, and neutral
    c. Bitter and cold
    d. Bitter, acrid, and warm

458. Jie Geng does *not* perform which of the following functions?
    a. Circulate the Lung Qi and expel Phlegm
    b. Benefit the throat
    c. Dissipate nodules
    d. Promote the discharge of pus

459. Which herb treats both wheezing with swelling and wheezing with shortness of breath caused by Excess-Lung-Heat Syndrome?
    a. Qian Hu
    b. Bai Qian
    c. Sang Bai Pi
    d. Ban Xia

460. Zhe Bei Mu performs which of the following functions?
    a. Clear Heat, transform Phlegm, and dissipate nodules
    b. Clear Heat, transform Phlegm, and stop convulsions
    c. Clear Heat, transform Phlegm, and stop vomiting
    d. Clear Heat, transform Phlegm, and release Exterior Wind-Heat

461. Which herb cools the Heart, stops convulsions, clears Heat and transforms Phlegm?
    a. Zhu Ru
    b. Tian Zhu Huang
    c. Zhu Ye
    d. Zhi Zi

462. Which herb inhibits adverse rising of Qi, expels Phlegm, and calms the Liver to stop convulsions?
    a. Xuan Fu Hua
    b. Meng Shi
    c. Jiang Can
    d. Zhe Bei Mu

463. Which of the following indicates the use of Xing Ren?
    a. Many kinds of cough and wheezing syndromes
    b. Chronic cough caused by Deficient Lung
    c. Lung Heat coughing
    d. Dryness coughing caused by Deficient Yin

464. Su Zi is especially effective at accomplishing which of the following?
    a. Clear the Lungs and transform Phlegm
    b. Moisten the Lungs and transform Phlegm
    c. Redirect the Qi downward and dissolve Phlegm
    d. Dry Damp and transform Phlegm

465. Sang Bai Pi does *not* perform which of the following functions?
    a. Promote urination and reduce edema
    b. Expel Phlegm and redirect the Qi downward
    c. Tonify the Yin and moisten the Lung
    d. Lower blood pressure

466. Which of the following is an important indication for the use of Bai Bu?
    a. Coughing caused by Wind-Heat
    b. Coughing caused by Cold-Phlegm
    c. Coughing caused by Wind-Cold
    d. Coughing caused by tuberculosis

467. Which herb treats Excess-type edema and fluid accumulation in the chest and abdomen?
    a. Xuan Fu Hua
    b. Sang Bai Pi
    c. Ting LI Zi
    d. Bai Qian

468. Pi Pa Ye performs which of the following functions?
    a. Promote urination and reduce swelling
    b. Harmonize the Stomach and redirect the Stomach Qi downward
    c. Disperse Wind and clear Heat
    d. Promote urination and leach out Damp

469. Taking too large a dosage of Ma Dou Ling causes which of the following?
    a. Pain in the abdomen
    b. Edema
    c. Vomiting
    d. Spasms

470. Bai Guo performs which of the following functions?
    a. Dry Damp and stop itching
    b. Eliminate Damp and stop vaginal discharge
    c. Promote fluids and stop thirst
    d. Strengthen the Spleen and stop diarrhea

471. Which herb is astringent, neutral, expels Phlegm, and stops wheezing?
    a. Xing Ren
    b. Sang Bai Pi
    c. Qian Hu
    d. Bai Guo

472. Which herb treats wheezing with styptic pectoralis, eliminates Damp, astringes, and treats vaginal discharge and turbid urine?
    a. Ma Dou Ling
    b. Xing Ren
    c. Bai Guo
    d. Qian Shi

473. Which herb clears Lung Heat, moistens the Lungs, and nourishes Lung Yin?
    a. Sha Shen
    b. Chuan Bei Mu
    c. Gua Lou Pi
    d. Yin Guo

474. Which herb treats constrained Lung Qi, Phlegm-Heat cough, sore throat, and hoarseness?
    a. Xing Ren
    b. Fu Hai Shi
    c. Ju Hua
    d. Pang Da Hai

475. Which two herbs each expel Phlegm, redirect the Lung Qi downward, and treat a cough that produces copious sputum?
    a. Chuan Bei Mu and Jie Geng
    b. Qian Hu and Bai Qian
    c. Ban Xia and Zhu Ru
    d. Xing Ren and Gua Lou

476. Bai Jie Zi, Su Zi, and Bai Fu Zi each perform which of the following functions?
    a. Moisten the Intestines
    b. Disperse Wind
    c. Stop wheezing
    d. Transform Phlegm

477. Which two herbs each moisten the Lungs, transform Phlegm, and stop coughing and wheezing?
    a. Chuan Bei Mu and Jie Geng
    b. Bai Bu and Gua Lou
    c. Qian Hu and Zhu Ru
    d. Hai Zao and Xing Ren

478. Ban Xia and Tian Nan Xing have similar functions, but Ban Xia is especially effective for treating which of the following?
    a. Phlegm-Damp in the Stomach and Spleen
    b. Wind-Phlegm in the meridians
    c. Stop wheezing
    d. None of the above

479. Tian Nan Xing is especially effective for treating which of the following?
    a. Phlegm-Damp in the Stomach and Spleen
    b. Wind-Phlegm in the meridians
    c. Wheezing
    d. None of the above

480. Zhu Ru and Pi Pa Ye each perform which of the following functions?
    a. Stop coughing with styptic pectorals
    b. Harmonize the Stomach, redirect Stomach Qi downward, and stop vomiting
    c. Clear Heat and dissipate nodules
    d. None of the above

481. Zi Wan and Kuan Dong Hua prepared with honey each perform which of the following functions?
    a. Clear Lung-Heat and expel Phlegm; stop coughing
    b. Moisten the Lungs and expel Phlegm; stop coughing
    c. Styptic pectorals and expel Phlegm; stop coughing
    d. None of the above

482. Which of the following functions do Fu Hai Shi and Hai Ge Ke *not* have in common?
    a. Warm the Lungs and expel Phlegm
    b. Clear the Lungs and expel Phlegm
    c. Soften hardness and dissipate nodules
    d. Promote urination

483. Which two herbs each transform Phlegm and dissipate goiters?
    a. Hai Ge Ke and Hai Zao
    b. Zhu Ru and Tian Hua Fen
    c. Bai Qian and Bai Jie Zi
    d. Yin Guo and Tian Zhu Huang

484. Which two herbs each transform Phlegm, are slightly warm, and moisten the Lungs?
    a. Xing Ren and Yin Gue
    b. Sang Bai Pi and Ting Li Zi
    c. Ma Dou Ling and Mu Hu Die
    d. Bai Bu and Zi Wan

485. Which herb expels Phlegm, redirects the Qi downward, and stops coughing?
    a. Bai Qian
    b. Jie Geng
    c. Bai Fu Zi
    d. Guo Lou

486. Which herb clears Heat and transforms Phlegm obstructing the Heart orifices?
    a. Chuan Bei Mu
    b. Zhu Ru
    c. Zhu Li
    d. Zhu Ye

487. Which herb reduces toxicity, expels goiters, cools the Blood and stops bleeding?
    a. Bai Fu Zi
    b. Huang Yao Zi
    c. Fu Hai Shi
    d. Hai Zao

488. Which herb moistens the Lungs, stops coughing, expels parasites and kills lice?
    a. Zi Wan
    b. Kuan Dong Hua
    c. Chuan Bei Mu
    d. Bai Bu

489. Meng Shi does *not* perform which of the following functions?
    a. Moisten the Lung
    b. Direct the Qi downward and reduce Phlegm
    c. Calm the Liver
    d. Control palpitations and seizures

490. Which herb treats voice loss?
    a. Ban Xia
    b. Jie Geng
    c. Chuan Bai Mu
    d. Zhu Ru

491. Ban Xia and Zhu Ru each perform which of the following functions?
    a. Transform Phlegm and promote urination
    b. Transform Phlegm and regulate the Qi
    c. Transform Phlegm and stop vomiting
    d. Transform Phlegm and stop bleeding

492. Formulas that treat Phlegm do *not* perform which of the following functions?
    a. Dry Damp and expel Phlegm
    b. Clear Heat and transform Phlegm
    c. Moisten Dry and transform Phlegm
    d. Warm and transform Damp-Phlegm

493. Er Chen Tang does *not* perform which of the following functions?
    a. Strengthen the Spleen and nourish the Blood
    b. Dry Damp and transform Phlegm
    c. Regulate the Qi
    d. Harmonize the Middle Energizer

494. Which of the following serves as the chief (monarch or *jun*) component in Er Chen Tang?
    a. Ban Xia
    b. Ju Hong
    c. Fu Ling
    d. Ban Xia and Zhi Gan Cao

495. Which modification of Er Chen Tang is *not* correct?
    a. For Hot-Phlegm, add Zhu Ru and Tian Zhu Huang
    b. For Cold-Phlegm, add Gan Jiang and Xi Xin
    c. For Wind-Phlegm, add Tian Nan Xing and Bai Fu Zi
    d. For stubborn Phlegm, add Da Huang and Mang Xiao

496. Dao Tan Tang can be created by subtracting Wu Mei from Er Chen Tang and adding:
    a. Tian Nan Xing and Zhi Shi
    b. Tian Nan Xing and Zhi Ke
    c. Tian Nan Xing and Gua Lou
    d. Chuan Bei Mu and Fu Hai Shi

497. How would you adapt Er Chen Tang to create Di Tan Tang?
    a. Add Zhi Shi, Zhu Ru, and Tian Nan Xing
    b. Subtract Wu Mei; add Dan Nan Xing, Zhi Shi, Zhu Ru, Ren Shen, Shi Chang Pu, and Da Zao
    c. Add Zhi Shi, Tian Nan Xing, and Ren Shen
    d. Add Zhi Ke, Zhu Ru, Shi Chang Pu, and Da Zao

498. Which formula would you select to treat this pattern: cough that produces copious white sputum, tongue with moist white fur, slippery pulse?
    a. Wen Dan Tang
    b. Xiao Qing Long Tang
    c. Er Chen Tang
    d. Zhi Sou San

499. Which formula treats internal obstruction caused by severe Phlegm, stiffness of the tongue, and speech impairment?
    a. Di Tan Tang
    b. Dao Tan Tang
    c. Wen Dan Tang
    d. Er Chen Tang

500. Wen Dan Tang does *not* contain which of the following?
    a. Ban Xia and Chen Pi
    b. Zhi Ke and Tian Nan Xing
    c. Zhi Shi and Zhu Ru
    d. Fu Ling and Gan Cao

501. Wen Dan Tang does *not* perform which of the following functions?
    a. Dry Damp and transform Phlegm
    b. Regulate the Qi and transform Phlegm
    c. Clear the Gallbladder
    d. Harmonize the Stomach

502. Wen Dan Tang is *not* indicated for which of the following?
    a. Coughing with yellow sputum
    b. Insomnia and anxiety
    c. Nausea and vomiting
    d. Seizures with copious sputum

503. Zhu Ru performs which of the following functions in Wen Dan Tang?
    a. Clear Heat and Phlegm, and stop vomiting
    b. Break up Stagnant Qi and reduce accumulation
    c. Direct the Qi downwards and unblock the bowels
    d. Transform Phlegm and expel focal distention

504. Which two herbs do Dao Tan Tang and Di Tan Tang *not* have in common?
    a. Ban Xia and Ju Hong
    b. Fu Ling and Zhi Shi
    c. Dan Nang Xing and Da Zao
    d. Gan Cao and Sheng Jiang

505. Qing Qi Hua Tan Wan is *not* indicated for which of the following?
    a. Insomnia caused by vexation
    b. Coughing of yellow viscous sputum
    c. A feeling of fullness in the chest and diaphragm
    d. Difficulty breathing

506. Which formula does *not* contain Er Chen Tang?
    a. Wen Dan Tang
    b. Di Tan Tang
    c. Ban Xia Bai Zhu Tian Ma Tang
    d. Qing Qi Hua Tan Wan

507. Which herb is part of the formula for Xiao Xian Xiong Tang?
    a. Gua Lou Pi
    b. Quan Gua Lou
    c. Gua Lou Ren
    d. None of the above

508. Xiao Xian Xiong Tang does *not* perform which of the following functions?
    a. Moisten the Lungs and transform Phlegm
    b. Clear Heat and transform Phlegm
    c. Expand the chest
    d. Dissipate clumps

509. Xiao Xian Xiong Tang is *not* indicated for which of the following?
    a. Focal distention in the chest and epigastrium
    b. Pain when pressed
    c. Coughing up of yellow and viscous sputum
    d. Loose stool

510. Xiao Xian Xiong Tang and Qing Qi Hua Tan Wan both treat Phlegm-Heat accumulating in the Interior. Which of the following indications is specific for Xiao Xian Xiong Tang?
    a. Stagnation of Phlegm-Heat in the Lung
    b. Phlegm accumulating in the hypochondriac region
    c. Phlegm-Heat accumulating in the epigastrium
    d. None of the above

511. Gun Tan Wan does *not* contain which of the following?
    a. Mu Xiang
    b. Chen Xiang
    c. Meng Shi
    d. Da Huang and Huang Qin

512. Gun Tan Wan performs which of the following functions?
    a. Regulate the Qi and drive out Phlegm
    b. Clear Heat and drive out Phlegm
    c. Dry Damp and drive out Phlegm
    d. Drain Fire and drive out Phlegm

513. Gun Tan Wan is *not* indicated for which of the following?
    a. Mania-withdrawal and palpitations with anxiety caused by Excess-Heat and lingering Phlegm
    b. Severe, continuous palpitations which can lead to coma; or coughing and wheezing with thick viscous sputum
    c. Focal distention and a stifling sensation in the chest and epigastrium; or dizziness, vertigo, tinnitus and/or constipation
    d. Yellowish urine with pain during micturition

514. Which two herbs are *not* part of the formula for Bei Mu Gua Lou San?
    a. Bei Mu and Gua Lou
    b. Ban Xia and Chen Pi
    c. Tian Hua Fen and Fu Ling
    d. Ju Hong and Jie Geng

515. Which formula does *not* contain Jie Geng or Gan Cao?
    a. Zhi Sou San
    b. Yin Qiao San
    c. Huang Long Tang
    d. Bei Mu Gua Lou San

516. Which formula does *not* release Exterior conditions?
    a. Zhi Sou San
    b. Ding Chuan Tang
    c. Wu Ling San
    d. Ling Gan Wu Wei Jiang Xin Tang

517. Ling Gan Wu Wei Jiang Xin Tang is *not* indicated for which of the following?
    a. Coughing with profuse sputum
    b. Phlegm that is thin, watery, and white
    c. Yellow and greasy tongue fur
    d. A wiry-slippery pulse

518. Ling Gan Wu Wei Jiang Xin Tang performs which of the following functions?
    a. Warm the Yang and transform congested fluids
    b. Warm the Spleen and transform Phlegm
    c. Warm the Lungs and transform congested fluids
    d. Warm the Spleen and transform congested fluids

519. Which formula would best treat a cough with deep-seated sputum where it is difficult to expectorate and the throat is dry and sore?
    a. Ling Gan Wu Wei Jiang Xin Tang
    b. Xiao Xian Xiong Tang
    c. San Zi Yang Qin Tang
    d. Bei Mu Gua Lou San

520. Which formula would you select to treat this pattern: Deficient Spleen Yang with ascendent Yin, Stagnation of fluids, Damp-Phlegm collecting and forming congested fluids, inability of the Lung Qi to descend leading to dyspnea and coughing?
    a. Ding Chuan Tang
    b. Xiao Qing Long Tang
    c. Su Zi Jiang Qi Tang
    d. Ling Gan Wu Wei Jiang Xin Tang

521. San Zi Yang Qin Tang does *not* contain which of the following?
    a. Wu Wei Zi
    b. Bai Jie Zi
    c. Su Zi
    d. Lai Fu Zi

522. San Zi Yang Qin Tang is *not* indicated for which of the following?
    a. Coughing and wheezing
    b. Copious sputum with focal distention in the chest
    c. Dizziness and vertigo
    d. Loss of appetite with digestive difficulties

523. Ban Xia Bai Zhu Tian Ma Tang can be formed by adapting Er Chen Tang in what way?
    a. Remove Fu Ling; add Bai Zhu and Tian Ma
    b. Remove Fu Ling; add Sheng Jiang and Bai Zhu
    c. Remove Fu Ling; add Cang Zhu and Tian Ma
    d. Add Bai Zhu and Tian Ma

524. Which of the following indicates the use of Ban Xia Bai Zhu Tian Ma Tang?
    a. Headache caused by Wind-Phlegm
    b. Headache caused by Wind-Cold
    c. Headache caused by Deficient Blood
    d. Headache caused by Excess Liver Yang

525. Which formula dries Damp, transforms Phlegm, and calms the Liver to stop Wind?
    a. Er Chen Tang
    b. Wen Dan Tang
    c. Di Tan Tang
    d. Ban Xia Bai Zhu Tian Ma Tang

526. Which formula directs the Qi downward, relaxes the diaphragm, and reduces Stagnation of Phlegm and food?
    a. Gun Tan Wan
    b. Ling Gan Wu Wei Jiang Xin Tang
    c. Ban Xia Bai Zhu Tian Ma Tang
    d. San Zi Yang Qin Tang

527. Which formula would you select to treat this pattern: Wind-Phlegm with dizziness or vertigo, headache, stifling sensation in the chest, nausea or vomiting, greasy white tongue fur, wiry-slippery pulse?
    a. Dao Tan Tang
    b. Ban Xia Bai Zhu Tian Ma Tang
    c. Ling Gan Wu Wei Jiang Xin Tang
    d. Er Chen Tang

528. Which herbs in Ding Xian Wan serve to extinguish Wind and stop spasms?
    a. Quan Xie, Tian Ma, and Shi Jue Ming
    b. Quan Xie, Tian Ma, and Jiang Can
    c. Quan Xie, Tian Ma, and Wu Gong
    d. Quan Xie, Tian Ma, and Bai Ji Li

529. Which formula does *not* contain Ban Xia and Chen Pi?
    a. Qing Qi Hua Tan Wan
    b. Zhi Sou San
    c. Xing Su San
    d. Bao He Wan

530. Which of the following is *not* contained in Zhi Sou San?
    a. Jie Geng and Jing Jie
    b. Ban Xia and Fu Ling
    c. Zi Wan Bai Bu
    d. Bai Qian, Gan Cao, and Chen Pi

531. Zhi Sou San does *not* perform which of the following functions?
    a. Stop coughing and transform Phlegm
    b. Expel the evil factors from the Exterior
    c. Disseminate Lung Qi
    d. Relieve food Stagnation and direct rebellious Qi downward

532. Which formula treats epilepsy in children caused by accumulation of Phlegm-Heat?
    a. Wen Dan Tang
    b. Gun Tan Tang
    c. Ding Xian Wan
    d. Di Tan Tang

533. Which formula does *not* contain Dan Nan Xing, Ban Xia, and Chen Pi?
    a. Di Tan Tang
    b. Dao Tan Tang
    c. Qing Qi Hua Tan Tang
    d. Ding Xian Wang

534. Which formula would you select to treat this pattern: cough, itchy throat, slight aversion to cold, fever, thin white tongue fur?
    a. Ling Gan Wu Wei Jiang Xin Tang
    b. Gui Zhi Tang
    c. Zhi Sou San
    d. Dao Tan Tang

535. Which of the following is a basic formula for drying Damp and expelling Phlegm?
    a. Wen Dan Tang
    b. Er Chen Tang
    c. Dao Tan Tang
    d. Ling Gan Wu Wei Jiang Xin Tang

536. Which formula is *not* used to moisten Dry and transform Phlegm?
    a. Xiao Xian Xiong Tang
    b. Qing Qi Hua Tan Wan
    c. Gun Tan Wan
    d. Bei Mu Gua Lou San

537. Which herb treats accumulation caused by meat or greasy food with accompanying symptoms of abdominal distention and pain or diarrhea?
    a. Mai Ya
    b. Gu Ya
    c. Ji Nei Jin
    d. Shan Zha

538. Which herb relieves food Stagnation, transforms Blood Stasis, and dissipates clumps?
    a. Shen Qu
    b. Mai Ya
    c. Shan Zha
    d. Ji Nei Jin

539. What method is used to process Shen Qu?
    a. Water processing
    b. Fire processing
    c. Frostation processing
    d. Fermentation processing

540. Mai Ya does *not* perform which of the following functions?
    a. Reduce food stagnation
    b. Inhibit lactation
    c. Facilitate the smooth flow of Liver Qi
    d. Move water and reduce edema

541. Lai Fu Zi does *not* perform which of the following functions?
    a. Reduce food Stagnation and transform accumulation
    b. Spread and regulate Liver Qi
    c. Cause Qi to Descend
    d. Reduce Phlegm

542. Ji Nei Jin does *not* perform which of the following functions?
    a. Nourish and tonify Liver and Kidney Yin
    b. Reduce food Stagnation
    c. Dissolve stones
    d. Stop enuresis

543. Which meridians are entered by Gu Ya?
    a. Spleen, Stomach, and Liver
    b. Spleen, Stomach, and Bladder
    c. Spleen, Stomach, and Lung
    d. Spleen and Stomach

544. Shan Zha does *not* perform which of the following functions?
    a. Reduce food Stagnation
    b. Strengthen the Spleen and Stomach
    c. Transform Blood Stasis
    d. Stop diarrhea

545. Which herb relieves food Stagnation, causes the Qi to descend, and reduces Phlegm?
    a. Shen Qu
    b. Gu Ya
    c. Shan Zha
    d. Lai Fu Zi

546. Which herb relieves food Stagnation, transforms hardness, and dissolves stones?
    a. Lai Fu Zi
    b. Shen Qu
    c. Ji Nei Jin
    d. Mai Ya

547. Which herb transforms food Stagnation, secures the Essence, and stops enuresis?
    a. Ji Nei Jin
    b. Shen Qu
    c. Shan Zha
    d. Liu Ji Nu

548. Shan Zha does *not* perform which of the following functions?
    a. Transform Blood Stasis
    b. Cause the Qi to descend
    c. Stop diarrhea
    d. Lower elevated serum cholesterol

549. Bao He Wan does *not* contain which of the following?
    a. Mai Ya and Zhi Shi
    b. Shan Zha and Shen Qu
    c. Lai Fu Zi and Chen Pi
    d. Ban Xia, Fu Ling, and Lian Qiao

550. Bao He Wan performs which of the following functions?
    a. Reduce food Stagnation and strengthen the Spleen
    b. Reduce food Stagnation and harmonize the Stomach
    c. Reduce food Stagnation and drain Heat
    d. Reduce food Stagnation and eliminate Phlegm

551. Bao He Wan is *not* indicated for which of the following?
    a. Fullness and pain in the abdomen
    b. Rotten smelling belching and acid regurgitation
    c. Weight loss and weakness of the extremities
    d. Nausea and vomiting or diarrhea

552. Which statement is false?
    a. Shen Qu serves as the chief (monarch or *jun*) component in Bao He Wan
    b. Da Huang serves as the chief (monarch or *jun*) component in Zhi Shi Dao Zhi Wan
    c. Zhi Shi serves as the chief (monarch or *jun*) component in Zhi Shi Xiao Pi Wan
    d. Bai Zhu serves as the chief (monarch or *jun*) component in Zhi Zhu Wan

553. Which of the following is *not* true of how herbs function in the formula Bao He Wan?
    a. Shan Zha reduces all types of food Stagnation, especially that caused by meat and fatty foods
    b. Shen Qu reduces food Stagnation; Lai Fu Zi reduces food accumulation and causes the Qi to descend
    c. Ban Xia and Chen Pi promote movement of Qi, transform Stagnation, and harmonize the Stomach
    d. Lian Qiao clears Heat from the Upper Energizer

554. Zhi Shi Dao Zhi Wan does *not* contain which of the following?
    a. Shan Zha and Mai Ya
    b. Zhi Shi and Da Huang
    c. Shen Qu, Fu Ling, and Ze Xie
    d. Huang Qin, Huang Lian, and Bai Zhu

555. Zhi Shi Dao Zhi Wan does *not* perform which of the following functions?
    a. Reduce food Stagnation
    b. Cause the Qi to descend
    c. Clear Heat
    d. Dispel Damp

556. Zhi Shi Dao Zhi Wan is *not* indicated for which of the following?
    a. Fullness and pain in the abdomen
    b. Nausea and vomiting
    c. Dysentery or constipation
    d. Oliguria with reddish urine

557. Zhi Shi Dao Zhi Wan is indicated for symptoms caused by which if the following?
    a. Accumulation of food caused by Deficient Spleen
    b. Accumulation of food caused by Qi Stagnation of the Spleen and Stomach
    c. Accumulation of food transformed into Damp-Heat that obstructs the Stomach and Intestines
    d. None of the above

558. Which herbs do Mu Xiang Bing Lang Wan and Zhou Che Wan *not* have in common?
    a. Huang Lian and Zhi Shi
    b. Mu Xiang and Bing Lang
    c. Chen Pi and Qing Pi
    d. Da Huang and Qian Niu Zi

559. Mu Xiang Bing Lang Wan is *not* indicated for which of the following?
    a. Fullness and pain in the abdomen
    b. Red-white dysenteric diarrhea
    c. Tenesmus or constipation
    d. White, greasy tongue fur

560. Which formula contains all of the herbs in the formula Si Jun Zi Tang?
    a. Zhi Shi Xiao Pi Wan
    b. Zhi Shi Dao Zhi Wan
    c. Mu Xiang Bing Lang Wan
    d. Bao He Wan

561. Da An Wan consists of the herbs in Bao He Wan plus which of the following?
    a. Mai Ya
    b. Bai Zhu
    c. Gan Cao
    d. Huang Lian

562. Which formula best treats Deficient Spleen and Stomach, obstruction of Qi, and food Stagnation?
    a. Bao He Wan
    b. Zhi Shi Dao Zhi Wan
    c. Zhi Zhu Wan
    d. Jian Pi Wan

563. Which formula is used to strengthen the Spleen, harmonize the Stomach, reduce food Stagnation, and stop diarrhea?
    a. Zhi Zhu Wan
    b. Bao He Wan
    c. Da An Wan
    d. Jian Pi Wan

564. Which formula promotes the movement of Qi, purges accumulation, guides out Stagnation and drains Heat?
    a. Bao He Wan
    b. Zhi Zhu Wan
    c. Zhi Shi Dao Zhi Wan
    d. Mu Xiang Bing Lang Wan

565. Which formula reduces distention, eliminates fullness, strengthens the Spleen, and harmonizes the Stomach?
    a. Jian Pi Wan
    b. Xiang Sha Liu Jun Zi Tang
    c. Zhi Shi Xiao Pi Wan
    d. Bao He Wan

566. Which formula would you select to treat this pattern: reduced appetite with difficulty in digestion, bloating and focal distention of the epigastrium and abdomen, loose and watery diarrhea, greasy and slightly yellow tongue fur, Deficient-frail pulse?
    a. Bao He Wan
    b. Zhi Zhu Wan
    c. Jian Pi Wan
    d. Shen Ling Bai Zhu San

567. Which formula would you select to treat this pattern: focal distention and fullness in the upper epigastrium, lack of appetite, fatigue and weakness, wan complexion, irregular bowel movements?
    a. Zhi Zhu Wan
    b. Ping Wei San
    c. Zhi Shi Xiao Pi Wan
    d. Zhi Shi Dao Zhi Wan

568. Chen Pi does *not* perform which of the following functions?
    a. Reduce food Stagnation
    b. Dry Damp and transform Phlegm
    c. Regulate the Qi and improve the transporting function of the Spleen
    d. Adjust the Middle Energizer and relieve the diaphragm

569. Chen Pi is *not* indicated for which of the following?
    a. Middle Energizer Stagnation of Qi
    b. Abdominal distention and fullness
    c. Lack of appetite and loose and watery diarrhea
    d. Nausea and vomiting

570. Which herb spreads Liver Qi and powerfully promotes the movement of Qi?
    a. Chen Pi
    b. Mu Xiang
    c. Qing Pi
    d. Zhi Shi

571. Which herb enters the Lung and Spleen meridians?
    a. Qing Pi
    b. Chen Pi
    c. Zhi Shi
    d. Xiang Fu

572. Which herb breaks up Stagnant Qi, reduces accumulation, transforms Phlegm, and expels focal distention?
    a. Chen Pi
    b. Hou Po
    c. Zhi Shi
    d. Fo Shou

573. Which portion of Qing Pi is used medicinally?
    a. The peel
    b. The immature fruit
    c. The mature fruit
    d. None of the above

574. Which portion of Zhi Shi is used medicinally?
    a. Peel
    b. Seed
    c. Immature fruit
    d. Mature fruit

575. Which herb treats epigastric or abdominal distention, fullness, bloating, belching, nausea and vomiting caused by Stagnant Qi of the Spleen or Stomach?
    a. Chen Pi
    b. Ban Xia
    c. Hou Po
    d. Fu Ling

576. Which of the following herbs would you select to treat the following pattern: a stifling sensation in the chest, abdominal distention, loss of appetite, fatigue, loose stool caused by Damp turbidity obstructing the Middle Energizer, cough with copious sputum?
    a. Qing Pi
    b. Chen Pi
    c. Su Zi
    d. Pei Lan

577. Chuan Lian Zi does *not* perform which of the following functions?
    a. Promote the movement of Qi
    b. Stop pain
    c. Kill parasites
    d. Disperse Cold

578. Fo Shou does *not* perform which of the following functions?
    a. Spread and regulate Liver Qi
    b. Promote the movement of Blood
    c. Harmonize the Stomach
    d. Transform Phlegm

579. Which herb spreads Liver Qi, breaks up Stagnant Qi, dissipates clumps, and reduces Stagnation?
    a. Chen Pi
    b. Zhi Shi
    c. Fo Shou
    d. Qing Pi

580. Which herb has bitter, acrid, and slightly cold properties?
    a. Chen Pi
    b. Qing Pi
    c. Fo Shou
    d. Zhi Shi

581. Which herb dries Damp and transforms Phlegm, calms the adverse rising energy by keeping it downward, stops vomiting, regulates the Qi, and strengthens the Spleen?
    a. Hou Po
    b. Bai Zhu
    c. Mu Xiang
    d. Chen Pi

582. Which herb promotes the movement of Qi, alleviates pain, and is known especially for adjusting and regulating Stagnation of the Spleen or Stomach?
    a. Qing Pi
    b. Mu Xiang
    c. Xiang Fu
    d. Chuan Lian Zi

583. Wu Yao does *not* perform which of the following functions?
    a. Promote the movement of Qi
    b. Harmonize the Middle Energizer
    c. Alleviate pain
    d. Warm the Kidney

584. Which herb helps the Kidneys to grasp Qi, promotes the movement of Qi, and alleviates pain?
    a. Mu Xiang
    b. Wu Yao
    c. Chen Xiang
    d. Bu Gu Zhi

585. Which herb treats frequent urination or urinary incontinence caused by insufficiency of Kidney Yang and Cold from Deficient Bladder?
    a. Mu Xiang
    b. Gan Jiang
    c. Wu Yao
    d. Wu Zhu Yu

586. Which herb treats asthma and wheezing caused by the Kidney's inability to grasp Qi?
    a. Wu Yao
    b. Mu Xiang
    c. Chen Xiang
    d. Xiang Fu

587. Which herb treats lack of appetite, epigastric or abdominal pain or distention, nausea and vomiting, and bloating and belching caused by Spleen or Stomach Qi Stagnation?
    a. Qing Pi
    b. Zhi Ke
    c. Chen Xiang
    d. Mu Xiang

588. Which herb treats Liver and Stomach Qi Stagnation, rib or flank distention and pain, and belching or vomiting?
    a. Qing Pi
    b. Fo Shou
    c. Zhi Ki
    d. Chen Xiang

589. Which herb promotes the movement of Qi, relieves toxicity, and stops pain?
    a. Guang Mu Xiang
    b. Chen Pi
    c. Fo Shou
    d. Qing Mu Xiang

590. Xiang Fu performs which of the following functions?
    a. Nourish the Liver
    b. Clear Liver Heat
    c. Calm the Liver
    d. Disperse depressed Liver Qi

591. Which two herbs each are used to treat obstruction in the chest (*xiong bi*)?
    a. Fo Shou and Chuan Lian Zi
    b. Li Zhi He and Chen Xiang
    c. Mu Xiang and Xiang Fu
    d. Tan Xiang and Xie Bai

592. Which herb spreads and regulates Liver Qi, regulates menstruation, and alleviates pain?
    a. Chen Xiang
    b. Bai Shao
    c. Xiang Fu
    d. Jin Ling Zi

593. Which herb treats dysmenorrhea, irregular menstruation, and swelling and pain of the breast?
    a. Mu Xiang
    b. Wu Yao
    c. Xiang Fu
    d. Zhi Shi

594. Which herb treats flank, rib, and abdominal hernial pain, and for painful and swollen testes, especially when there are signs of Heat?
    a. Li Zhi He
    b. Wu Yao
    c. Chuan Lian Zi
    d. Xiang Fu

595. Which herb treats abdominal pain caused by accumulation of parasites?
    a. Wu Yao
    b. Mu Xiang
    c. Chuan Lian Zi
    d. Li Zhi He

596. Which herb is *not* from a plant in the citrus family?
   a. Xiang Fu
   b. Fo Shou
   c. Qing Pi
   d. Zhi Ke

597. Which herb comes from the same plant as Chen Pi?
   a. Zhi Shi
   b. Zhi Ke
   c. Qing Pi
   d. Li Zhi He

598. Which herb unblocks the Yang, disperses lumps, promotes the movement of Qi, reduces Qi Stagnation, and is one of the best treatments for pain in the chest, flank, or upper back?
   a. Ban Xia
   b. Zhi Shi
   c. Xie Bai
   d. Gui Zhi

599. Xie Bai performs which of the following functions?
   a. Strengthen the Yang
   b. Recuperate the depleted Yang
   c. Lift the Yang
   d. Unblock the Yang

600. Which herb regulates the Qi and stops pain, disperses Cold and Stagnation, and is especially effective for treating swollen and painful testes?
   a. Chuan Lian Zi
   b. Li Zhi He
   c. Shan Zha
   d. Mu Xiang

601. Xiang Fu, Mu Xiang, and Wu Yao each perform which of the following functions?
   a. Spread and regulate Liver Qi
   b. Promote the movement of Qi and disperse Stagnation
   c. Regulate the Qi and stop pain
   d. Direct the Qi downward and stop vomiting

602. Which two herbs treat the following pattern: chest pain radiating to the back, shortness of breath, asthma, white greasy tongue fur, slippery-wiry pulse?
   a. Xie Bai and Cong Bai
   b. Xie Bai and Gua Lou
   c. Xiang Fu and Chuan Lian Zi
   d. Zhi Ke and Ban Xia

603. Which herb enters the meridians of the Upper, Middle, and Lower Energizer, promotes the movement of Qi, stops pain, warms the Kidneys, and expels Cold?
   a. Qing Pi
   b. Zhi Ke
   c. Wu Yao
   d. Xiang Fu

604. Which herb that regulates the Qi is often used to treat prolapse of the organs?
   a. Chen Pi
   b. Xiang Fu
   c. Zhi Shi
   d. Mu Xiang

605. Which herb is used to unblock the Yang, expel Cold, release the Exterior, and induce sweating?
    a. Gui Zhi
    b. Xie Bai
    c. Chen Xiang
    d. Cong Bai

606. Which herb that regulates the Qi does *not* have cold properties?
    a. Zhi Shi
    b. Zhi Ke
    c. Chuan Lian Zi
    d. Li Zhi He

607. Chen Pi does *not* perform which of the following functions?
    a. Regulate the Qi
    b. Warm the Middle Energizer
    c. Adjust the Middle Energizer
    d. Dry Damp

608. Formulas that regulate the Qi are *not* indicated for which of the following?
    a. Raising the Stomach Qi
    b. Raising the Lung Qi
    c. Coordinating the Liver and the Stomach
    d. Clearing the depressed Liver Qi

609. Yue Ju Wan does *not* contain which of the following?
    a. Cong Zhu
    b. Bai Zhu
    c. Chuan Xiong and Xiang Fu
    d. Zhi Zi and Shen Qu

610. Which herb serves as the chief (monarch or *jun*) component of Yue Ju Wan?
    a. Chuan Xiong
    b. Cong Zhu
    c. Xiang Fu
    d. Shen Qu

611. Yue Ju Wan performs which of the following functions?
    a. Promote the movement of Qi and alleviate pain
    b. Promote the movement of Qi and dissipate clumps
    c. Promote the movement of Qi and release constraint
    d. None of the above

612. Which formula does *not* contain Wu Zhu Yu?
    a. Wen Jing Tang
    b. Jin Ling Zi San
    c. Si Shen Wan
    d. Ji Ming San

613. Jin Ling Zi San does *not* perform which of the following functions?
    a. Spread Liver Qi
    b. Invigorate the Blood
    c. Stop pain
    d. Dispel Blood Stasis

614. Which are the six depressive syndromes treated by Yue Ju Wan?
    a. Phlegm, Damp, water, Fire, Qi, and Blood constraint
    b. Phlegm, Damp, food, Fire, Qi, and Blood constraint
    c. Phlegm, Damp, food, Fire, Qi, and water constraint
    d. Phlegm, Damp, food, Cold, Qi, and water constraint

615. Which of the six depressive syndromes does Yue Ju Wan treat *most effectively*?
    a. Fire constraint
    b. Food constraint
    c. Qi constraint
    d. Phlegm or Damp constraint

616. Which formula would you select to treat this pattern: intermittent epigastric and hypochondriac pain, bitter taste in mouth, pain which worsens upon ingesting hot food, red tongue with yellow fur, wiry-rapid pulse?
    a. Yue Ju Wan
    b. Long Dan Xie Gan Tang
    c. Jin Ling Zi San
    d. Zuo Jin Wan

617. What is the pathogenesis of the syndrome for which Jin Ling Zi San is indicated?
    a. Deficient Yin of the Liver and Kidneys; disorder of the Liver Qi
    b. Depression of Liver Qi Transforming to Fire Syndrome; Qi and Blood unable to flow smoothly
    c. Excessive Fire in the Liver meridian
    d. None of the above

618. Ban Xia Hou Po Tang does *not* contain which of the following?
    a. Gan Jiang
    b. Sheng Jiang
    c. Ban Xia and Hou Po
    d. Fu Ling and Zi Su Ye

619. Ban Xia Hou Po Tang does *not* perform which of the following functions?
    a. Soften hard masses and stop pain
    b. Promote the movement of Qi and dissipate clumps
    c. Direct rebellious Qi downward
    d. Transform Phlegm

620. Ban Xia Hou Po Tang is *not* indicated for which of the following?
    a. A feeling of something caught in the throat that can neither be swallowed nor ejected
    b. A stifling sensation in the chest and hypochondria
    c. Menstrual pain
    d. Coughing or vomiting

621. Which of the following serves as the chief (monarch or *jun*) component in Ban Xia Hou Po Tang?
    a. Hou Po
    b. Ban Xia
    c. Zi Su Ye
    d. Fu Ling and Ban Xia

622. Which herb is part of the formula for Zhi Shi Gua Lou Gui Zhi Tang?
    a. Qing Pi
    b. Mu Xiang
    c. Chen Pi
    d. None of the above

623. Which formula treats painful obstruction of the chest that is so severe the patient is unable to lie down comfortably and there are severe symptoms of Phlegm accumulation?
    a. Gua Lou Xie Bai Bai Jiu Tang
    b. Gua Lou Xie Bai Ban Xia Tang
    c. Zhi Shi Gua Lou Gui Zhi Tang
    d. Ban Xia Hou Po Tang

624. Which formula unblocks the Yang, dissipates clumps, expels Phlegm, and directs Qi downward?
    a. Ban Xia Hou Po Tang
    b. Gua Lou Xie Bai Ban Xia Tang
    c. Zhi Shi Gua Lou Gui Zhi Tang
    d. Gua Lou Xie Bai Bai Jiu Tang

625. Ju He Wan does *not* perform which of the following functions?
    a. Expel Cold and alleviate pain
    b. Promote the movement of Qi and alleviate pain
    c. Soften hardness
    d. Dissipate clumps

626. Tian Tai Wu Yao San does *not* contain which of the following?
    a. Chen Pi and Rou Gui
    b. Wu Yao and Mu Xiang
    c. Xiao Hai Xiang, Qing Pi, and Gao Liang Jiang
    d. Bing Lang, Jin Ling Zi, and Ba Dou

627. Tian Tai Wu Yao San does *not* perform which of the following functions?
    a. Promote the movement of Qi and spread Liver Qi
    b. Scatter Cold
    c. Warm the Liver and Kidney
    d. Alleviate pain

628. Nuan Gan Jian does *not* contain which of the following?
    a. Dang Gui and Gou Ji Zi
    b. Xiao Hui Xiang, Rou Gui, and Wu Yao
    c. Qing Pi, Mu Xiang, and Fo Shou
    d. Fu Ling, Sheng Jiang, and Chen Xiang

629. Hou Po Wen Zhong Tang does *not* contain which of the following?
    a. Hou Po and Cao Dou Kou
    b. Bai Zhu and Ren Shen
    c. Chen Pi and Mu Xiang
    d. Gan Jiang, Fu Ling, and Zhi Gan Cao

630. Hou Po Wen Zhong Tang does *not* perform which of the following functions?
    a. Warm the Middle Energizer and promote the movement of Qi
    b. Direct the Qi downward
    c. Dry Damp
    d. Eliminate fullness

631. Which formula treats hernia resulting from Liver and Kidney Yin Cold causing the Qi to stagnate?
    a. Tian Tai Wu Yao San
    b. Ju He Wan
    c. Dao Qi Tang
    d. Nuan Gan Jian

632. Which formula treats inguinal hernia caused by the Stagnation of Cold evil and Qi?
    a. Tian Tai Wu Yao San
    b. Ju He Wan
    c. Nuan Gan Jian
    d. Dao Qi Tang

633. Which formula would be indicated for Damp-Cold injuring the Spleen and Stomach?
    a. Liang Fu Wan
    b. Hou Po Wen Zhong Tang
    c. Li Zhong Wan
    d. Liu Jun Zi Tang

634. Su Zi Jiang Qi Tang does *not* contain which of the following?
    a. Shu Di Huang and Chai Hu
    b. Su Zi and Ban Xia
    c. Dang Gui and Gan Cao
    d. Hou Po, Qian Hu, and Rou Gui

635. Su Zi Jiang Qi Tang does *not* perform which of the following functions?
    a. Direct rebellious Qi downward
    b. Clear Heat and strengthen the Lung
    c. Arrest wheezing and stop coughing
    d. Warm and transform Phlegm

636. Which formula does *not* direct the Stomach Qi downward to treat the adverse rising of Stomach Qi?
    a. Su Zi Jiang Qi Tang
    b. Xuan Fu Dai Zhe Tang
    c. Ding Xiang Shi Di Tang
    d. Ju Pi Zhu Ru Tang

637. Ding Chuan Tang does *not* contain which of the following?
    a. Yin Xing and Ma Huang
    b. Sheng Jiang and Fu Ling
    c. Su Zi, Gan Cao, and Kuan Dong Hua
    d. Xing Ren, Sang Bai Pi, Huang Qi, and Ban Xia

638. Ding Chuan Tang is *not* indicated for which of the following?
    a. Direct rebellious Qi downward and strengthen the Lung
    b. Disseminate and redirect the Lung Qi
    c. Arrest wheezing
    d. Clear Heat and transform Phlegm

639. Si Mo Tang does *not* contain which of the following?
    a. Su Zi
    b. Ren Shen
    c. Bing Lang
    d. Chen Xiang and Wu Yao

640. Which formula promotes the movement of Qi, directs rebellious Qi downward, expands the chest, and dissipates clumps?
    a. Su Zi Jiang Qi Tang
    b. Si Mo Tang
    c. Xuan Fu Dai Zhe Tang
    d. Nuan Gan Jian

641. Which formula would you select to treat this pattern: coughing and wheezing with copious, thick, or yellow sputum, labored breathing, greasy yellow tongue fur, slippery-rapid pulse?
    a. Qing Qi Hua Tan Wan
    b. Bei Mu Gua Lou San
    c. Ding Chuan Tang
    d. Xie Bai San

642. Which formula treats rising up of Stomach Qi caused by constraint and clumping of Liver Qi attacking the Stomach?
    a. Xuan Fu Dai Zhe Tang
    b. Si Mo Tang
    c. Ju Pi Zhu Ru Tang
    d. Ding Xiang Shi Di Tang

643. Which formula treats wheezing caused by Wind-Cold constraining the Exterior and Phlegm-Heat smoldering in the Interior?
    a. Zhi Sou San
    b. Qing Qi Hua Tan Wan
    c. Ding Chuan Tang
    d. None of the above

644. Which herbs do Ju Pi Zhu Ru Tang, Ding Xiang Shi Di Tang, and Xuan Fu Dai Zhe Tang have in common?
    a. Ren Shen and Sheng Jiang
    b. Ban Xia and Chen Pi
    c. Sheng Jiang and Da Zao
    d. Gan Cao and Xing Ren

645. Vomiting caused by which of the following is an indication for Xuan Fu Dai Zhe Tang?
    a. Stomach-Heat
    b. Stomach Deficiency-Cold
    c. Damp obstruction and Qi Stagnation
    d. Phlegm turbidity obstructing the Interior combined with weak and Deficient Stomach Qi

646. Xuan Fu Hua performs which of the following functions in the formula Xuan Fu Dai Zhe Tang?
    a. Dissolve Phlegm and promote urination
    b. Open the inhibited Lung energy and dissolve Phlegm
    c. Open the inhibited Lung energy and promote urination
    d. Drive the rebellious Qi downward and dissolve Phlegm

647. Ju Pi Zhu Ru Tang does *not* contain which of the following?
    a. Gan Jiang and Fu Ling
    b. Chen Pi and Zhu Ru
    c. Sheng Jiang and Gan Cao
    d. Ren Shen and Dao Zao

648. Ding Xiang Shi Di Tang does *not* perform which of the following functions?
    a. Warm the Middle Energizer and augment the Qi
    b. Direct rebellious Qi downward
    c. Regulate the Stomach energy and clear Heat
    d. Stop hiccough

649. Which formula treats hiccups and retching caused by Deficient Stomach and Heat?
    a. Si Mo Tang
    b. Ding Xiang Shi Di Tang
    c. Ju Pi Zhu Ru Tang
    d. Su Zi Jiang Qi Tang

650. Which formula treats fullness in the chest and persistent belching where the Stomach is Cold but *not* suffering from Deficiency?
    a. Ding Xiang Shi Di Tang
    b. Ju Pi Zhu Ru Tang
    c. Shi Di Tang
    d. Xuan Fu Dai Zhe Tang

651. Which herb cools the blood, stops bleeding, and is used to treat carbuncles, sores, swellings, and hypertension?
    a. Xiao Ji
    b. Di Yu
    c. Da Ji
    d. Bai Mao Gen

652. Which herb is used primarily to treat blood in the urine?
    a. Da Ji
    b. Xiao Ji
    c. Di Yu
    d. Bai Mao Gen

653. Which herb cools the Blood, stops bleeding, relieves toxicity, and is used to treat sores, ulcers, and injuries from burns?
    a. Da Ji
    b. Ce Bai Ye
    c. Di Yu
    d. Zong Lu Tan

654. Which two herbs treat blood in the stool and bleeding hemorrhoids caused by Damp-Heat in the Large Intestine?
    a. Qian Cao Gen and Bai Mao Gen
    b. Xue Yu Tan and Ai Ye
    c. Di Yu and Huai Jiao
    d. Ou Jie and Fu Long Gan

655. Xue Yu Tan performs which of the following functions?
    a. Restrain the leakage of blood and stop bleeding
    b. Cool the Blood and stop bleeding
    c. Dispel Blood Stasis and stop bleeding
    d. None of the above

656. Bai Mao Gen does *not* perform which of the following functions?
    a. Cool the Blood and stop bleeding
    b. Expel Phlegm and stop bleeding
    c. Quell Heat
    d. Promote urination

657. Which herb cools the Blood, stops bleeding, and reduces blood pressure?
    a. Bai Mao Gen
    b. Di Yu
    c. Huai Hua Mi
    d. Zi Zhu Cao

658. Huai Hua Mi is especially effective for treating which type of bleeding?
    a. Bleeding in the upper portion of the body
    b. Bleeding in the lower portion of the body
    c. Bleeding in the urine
    d. Nose bleeds

659. Ce Bai Ye does *not* perform which of the following functions ?
    a. Cool the Blood
    b. Promote urination
    c. Expel Phlegm
    d. Stop coughing

660. What is the special function of Ai Ye?
    a. Cool the Blood and stop bleeding
    b. Warm the menstruation and stop bleeding
    c. Restrain the leakage of blood and stop bleeding
    d. Transform Blood Stasis and stop bleeding

661. Which herb is used especially to warm the Middle Energizer and stop vomiting, bleeding, and diarrhea?
    a. Xue Yu Tan
    b. Ou Jie
    c. Lian Fang
    d. Fu Long Gan

662. Which herb transforms Blood Stasis, stops bleeding, and is taken directly as a powder?
    a. Yan Hu Suo
    b. Xiao Ji
    c. San Qi
    d. Xian He Cao

663. Which herb retains the Essence and stops bleeding, diarrhea, and pain?
    a. Qian Cao Gen
    b. Jiang Xiang
    c. Lian Fang
    d. Wu Zei Gu

664. What is the particular use of Pao Jiang?
    a. Stop pain
    b. Stop itching
    c. Stop bleeding
    d. Stop vomiting

665. Which of the following is *not* used to stop bleeding?
    a. Lu Jiao
    b. E Jiao
    c. Dong Chong Xia Cao
    d. Huang Jing

666. Which herb must be charred before it can be used to stop bleeding?
    a. Da Ji
    b. Qian Cao Gen
    c. Ce Bai Ye
    d. Guan Zhong

667. Bai Ji performs which of the following functions?
    a. Transform Blood Stasis and stop bleeding
    b. Stop coughing and expel Phlegm
    c. Reduce swelling and generate flesh
    d. Promote urination and alleviate pain

668. Which of the following is *not* used to stop bleeding?
    a. Sang Ye
    b. Jing Jie
    c. Wu Ling Zhi
    d. Hong Hua

669. Which of the following would *best* treat hematemesis caused by Hot-Blood and adverseness (adverse movement???) of Qi?
    a. San Qi
    b. Da Ji
    c. Xian He Cao
    d. Dai Zhe Shi

670. Xian He Cao performs which of the following functions?
    a. Alleviate diarrhea and kill parasites
    b. Clear Heat and promote urination
    c. Relieve toxicity and promote urination
    d. Cool the Blood and promote urination

671. Which herb is incompatible with Wu Tou?
    a. Xue Yu Tan
    b. Zong Lu Tan
    c. Di Yu Tan
    d. Bai Ji

672. Which herb treats Blood Stasis, swelling, and pain caused by traumatic injuries?
    a. Su Mu
    b. Hong Hua
    c. San Qi
    d. Wang Bu Liu Xing

673. Which herb would you select to stop bleeding, transform Blood Stasis, and alleviate pain?
    a. Bai Ji
    b. Di Yi
    c. Ai Ye
    d. San Qi

674. Which herb treats any bleeding caused by Hot Blood, and also treats lochioschesis, pain from trauma, and joint pain?
    a. San Qi
    b. Hong Hui
    c. Pu Huang
    d. Qian Cao Gen

675. Which herb cools the Blood, stops bleeding, and promotes Blood circulation to remove Blood Stasis?
    a. Hua Rui Shi
    b. Bai Mao Gen
    c. Qian Cao Gen
    d. Zong Lu Tan

676. Which portion of Pu Huang has medicinal use?
    a. Root
    b. Flower
    c. Leaf
    d. Pollen

677. Which herb treats internal bleeding accompanied by vomiting or coughing up of blood and internal Blood Stasis?
    a. Ai Ye
    b. Ce Bai Ye
    c. Bai Ji
    d. Hua Rui Shi

678. Which herb treats menorrhagia, metrorrhagia, and metrostaxis caused by Deficiency-Cold in the Lower Energizer, and also treats eczema and pruritis?
    a. Ai Ye
    b. Hua Rui Shi
    c. Bai Ji
    d. Ou Jie

679. Which herb best treats prolonged menstrual bleeding and uterine bleeding caused by Deficiency-Cold?
    a. Pu Huang
    b. Di Yu
    c. Xue Yu Tan
    d. Ai Ye

680. Fu Long Gan does *not* perform which of the following functions?
    a. Warm the Middle Energizer and stop bleeding
    b. Stop vomiting
    c. Stop diarrhea
    d. Stop coughing

681. Which herb would you select to treat a woman in her forties with the following symptoms: pale blood in the stool, pale complexion, cold extremities, pale tongue, thin pulse?
    a. Xue Yu Tan
    b. Fu Long Gan
    c. Di Yu
    d. Zong Lu Tan

682. Which herb treats vomiting or coughing up of blood?
    a. Pu Huang
    b. Ou Jie
    c. Ce Bai Ye
    d. Qian Cao Gen

683. Which herb restrains leakage of Blood, stops bleeding, invigorates the Blood, and dispels Blood Stasis?
    a. Xian He Cao
    b. Bai Ji
    c. Pu Huang
    d. Ce Bai Ye

684. Which herb treats metrorrhagia involving pale blood, pale tongue, and thin pulse?
    a. Qian Cao Gen
    b. Ou Jie Tan
    c. Pu Huang
    d. Pao Jiang

685. How must large doses of Fu Long Gan be prepared for use in decoctions?
    a. Cooked before decocting
    b. Cooked after decocting
    c. Infused in warm boiled water
    d. Cooked separately from the rest of the herbs

686. Which herb is derived from the center of the ashes after Zi Cao has been burned?
    a. Gan Jiang
    b. Gao Liang Jiang
    c. Rou Dou Kou
    d. Fu Long Gan

687. Da Ji and Xiao Ji each perform which of the following functions?
    a. Warm menstruation and stop bleeding
    b. Disperse Blood Stasis and stop bleeding
    c. Cool the Blood and stop bleeding
    d. Restrain the leakage of Blood and stop bleeding

688. Which two herbs each dispel Blood Stasis and stop bleeding?
    a. Bai Ji and Qian Cao Gen
    b. Huai Hua Mi and San Qi
    c. Pu Huang and Qian Cao Gen
    d. Ce Bai Ye and Hua Rui Shi

689. Which two herbs each do *not* cool the Blood or stop bleeding?
    a. Di Yu and Qian Cao Gen
    b. Ce Bai Ye and Bai Mao Gen
    c. Da Ji and Huai Hua Mi
    d. Ou Ji and Fu Long Gan

690. Bai Mao Gen and Lu Gen each perform which of the following functions?
    a. Cool the Blood and stop bleeding
    b. Quell Fire and relieve toxicity
    c. Clear the Liver and brighten the eyes
    d. Quell Heat and promote urination, especially in Heat patterns with thirst

691. Which two herbs would best treat blood in the urine caused by Blood-Heat?
    a. Di Yu and Huai Hua Mi
    b. Xiao Ji and Bai Mao Gen
    c. Zi Zhu and Hua Rui Shi
    d. Xian He Cao and San Qi

692. Which herb disperses Blood, stops bleeding, and promotes urination, especially in cases where there is blood in the urine?
    a. San Qi
    b. Hua Rui Shi
    c. Pu Huang
    d. Xue Yu Tan

693. Hua Rui Shi performs which of the following functions?
    a. Disperse Blood Stasis and stop bleeding
    b. Cool the Blood and stop bleeding
    c. Promote healing and generate flesh
    d. Sedate the Heart and calm the Spirit

694. Which herb does *not* cool the Blood, stop bleeding, clear Heat, and promote urination?
    a. Bai Moa Gen
    b. Xiao Ji
    c. Di Yu
    d. Da Ji

695. Which herb does *not* restrain the leakage of Blood and stop bleeding?
    a. Bai Ji
    b. Hua Rui Shi
    c. Zong Lu Tan
    d. Wu Zie Gu

696. Which herb restrains the leakage of Blood, stops bleeding, reduces swelling, and generates flesh, especially in cases where there is bleeding from the Lungs and Stomach?
    a. Xian He Cao
    b. Di Yu
    c. Bai Ji
    d. Huai Jiao

697. Which herb restrains the leakage of Blood, stops bleeding, and is most effective aged and carbonized?
    a. Chen Pi
    b. Zong Lu Tan
    c. Xian He Cao
    d. Er Cha

698. Which herb treats Stagnant Qi, Blood Stasis, and pain (chest, abdominal, extremity, and all other types)?
    a. Qing Pi
    b. Xiang Fu
    c. Yan Hu Suo
    d. Ru Xiang

699. Which herb treats arthralgia pain and headaches?
    a. Ru Xiang
    b. Mu Xiang
    c. Tan Xiang
    d. Chuan Xiong

700. Which herb expels Wind, alleviates pain, invigorates the Blood, and promotes the movement of Qi?
    a. Dan Shen
    b. Yu Jin
    c. Mo Yao
    d. Chuan Xiong

701. Which herb invigorates the Blood, promotes movement of Qi, benefits the Gallbladder, and reduces jaundice?
    a. San Leng
    b. Chuan Xiong
    c. Yu Jin
    d. Ru Xiang

702. Chuan Xiong has which of the following properties?
    a. Bitter and cold
    b. Acrid and warm
    c. Acrid and cool
    d. Sour and warm

703. Which herb breaks up Blood Stasis, promotes the movement of Qi, unblocks menstruation, alleviates pain, and is used especially in cases of Wind-Damp-Cold arthralgia pain in the shoulder and brachia?
    a. Chuan Xiong
    b. Hong Hua
    c. Jiang Huang
    d. E Zhu

704. Of the herbs that invigorate the Blood, which ones also reduce swelling and generate flesh?
    a. San Leng and E Zhu
    b. Dan Shen and Bai Zhi
    c. Chuang Xiong and Hong Hua
    d. Ru Xiang and Mo Yao

705. Which herb best treats Blood-Heat Stagnation, dysmenorrhea, or postpartum abdominal pain?
    a. Chuan Xiong
    b. Dan Shen
    c. Jiang Huang
    d. Ru Xiang

706. Which herb invigorates, nourishes, and cools the Blood, breaks up Blood Stasis, reduces abscesses, and tranquilizes?
    a. Chuang Xiong
    b. Chi Shan
    c. Dan Shen
    d. Yuan Zhi

707. Which herb does *not* move the Qi and invigorate the Blood?
    a. Chuan Xiong
    b. Jiang Huang
    c. Yu Jin
    d. Dan Shen

708. Which herb invigorates the Blood, breaks up Blood Stasis, promotes urination, and reduces swelling?
    a. E Zhu
    b. Tao Ren
    c. Tong Cao
    d. Yu Mu Cao

709. Which herb treats pain in the abdomen, amenorrhea, and abdominal masses caused by Qi Stagnation and Blood Stasis?
    a. Yu Jin
    b. Jiang Huang
    c. E Zhu
    d. Chuan Xiong

710. Which herb treats postpartum abdominal pain and lochiostasis?
    a. Jue Ming Zi
    b. Su Mu
    c. Chuan Xiong
    d. Chong Wei

711. Which herb promotes movement of Qi, tonifies the Blood, invigorates the meridians, and relaxes sinews?
    a. Chuan Xiong
    b. Su Mu
    c. Ji Xue Teng
    d. Dang Gui

712. Which herb treats traumatic injuries, pain caused by Blood Stasis, and constipation caused by dry Intestines?
    a. Yu Jin
    b. Hong Hua
    c. Ru Xiong
    d. Tao Ren

713. Which herb supplements and restores the Liver and Kidneys, invigorates the Blood, and expels Blood Stasis?
    a. Mo Yao
    b. Tao Ren
    c. Niu Xi
    d. Dan Shen

714. Which herb treats amenorrhea, dysmenorrhea, postpartum abdominal pain caused by Blood Stasis, and epigastric pain?
    a. Yi Mu Cao
    b. Xue Jie
    c. Wu Ling Zhi
    d. Niu Xi

715. Which herb disperses and transforms Blood Stasis, alleviates pain, and stops bleeding?
    a. Yan Hu Suo
    b. Chuan Shan Jia
    c. Wu Ling Zhi
    d. Bai Ji

716. Niu Xi does *not* perform which of the following functions?
    a. Invigorate the Blood and expel Blood Stasis
    b. Expel Wind and Damp
    c. Strengthen the sinews and bones
    d. Promote diuresis to eliminate Damp from the Lower Energizer

717. Which of the following herbs disperse Blood Stasis, unblock menstruation, promote lactation, reduce swelling, and promote the discharge of pus?
    a. Wang Bu and Liu Xing
    b. Chuan Shan Jia
    c. Niu Xi
    d. Jie Geng

718. Niu Xi is *not* indicated for which of the following?
    a. Dysmenorrhea, amenorrhea, and lochioschesis
    b. Pain and soreness affecting the lower back and knees
    c. Nosebleed, vomiting of blood, toothaches, and bleeding gums
    d. Scrofula or Phlegm nodules

719. Which herb is used to renew sinews, join bones, and break up and drive out Blood Stasis?
    a. Niu Xi
    b. Chuan Shan Jia
    c. Tu Bie Chong
    d. Xu Duan

720. Which herb dissolves unformed pus and promotes the healing of suppurative lesions?
    a. Tu Bie Chong
    b. Huang Qi
    c. Chuan Shan Jia
    d. Lu Rong

721. Which herb invigorates the Blood, drives out Blood Stasis, alleviates pain, and stops bleeding?
    a. Lian Fang
    b. Jiang Xiang
    c. Ze Lan
    d. Tu Bie Chong

722. Which herb is used primarily to treat traumatic injuries?
    a. Wang Bu Liu Xing
    b. Su Mu
    c. Liu Ji Nu
    d. Zi Ran Tong

723. San Leng and E Zhu each perform which of the following functions?
    a. Nourish and circulate the Blood
    b. Expel Blood Stasis and stop bleeding
    c. Break up Blood Stasis, expel Damp, and alleviate pain
    d. Break up Blood Stasis, promote the movement of Qi, and alleviate pain

724. Ru Xiang and Mo Yao each perform which of the following functions?
    a. Invigorate the Blood, dispel Blood Stasis, cool the Blood, and stop bleeding
    b. Invigorate the Blood, alleviate pain, reduce swelling, and generate flesh
    c. Invigorate the Blood, alleviate pain, promote urination, and reduce swelling
    d. None of the above

725. Which three herbs each invigorate the Blood and promote the movement of Qi?
    a. Chuan Xiong, Yu Jin, and Mu Xiang
    b. Wu Yao, Mo Yao, and Ru Xiang
    c. Yu Jin, Ru Xiang, and E Zhu
    d. Yan Hu Suo, Niu Xi, and Chuan Xiong

726. Which of the herbs that invigorate the Blood and dispel Blood Stasis are used especially for galactostasis?
    a. Niu Xi and Ze Lan
    b. Chuan Xiong and Wu Ling Zhi
    c. Wang Bu Liu Xing and Chuan Shan Jia
    d. Wang Bu Liu Xing and Hong Hua

727. Which herb induces the downward movement of Blood?
    a. Niu Xi
    b. Hong Hua
    c. Dan Shen
    d. Chuan Xiong

728. Which herb is often combined with Wu Ling Zhi to invigorate the Blood and alleviate pain?
    a. Hong Hua
    b. Pu Huang
    c. Tao Ren
    d. Chuan Shan Jia

729. Which herb has a function similar to that of Hu Zhang?
    a. Dan Shen
    b. Da Huang
    c. Yi Mu Cao
    d. Yu Jin

730. Tao Ren does *not* perform which of the following functions?
    a. Invigorate the Blood
    b. Dispel Blood Stasis
    c. Moisten the Intestines
    d. Reduce swelling

731. Yu Jin does *not* perform which of the following functions?
    a. Invigorate the Blood and promote the movement of Qi
    b. Clear the Heart and cool the Blood
    c. Expel Damp evil and alleviate pain
    d. Benefit the Gallbladder and reduce jaundice

732. Tao Ren Cheng Qi Tang does *not* contain which of the following?
    a. Da Huang
    b. Mang Xiao
    c. Gui Zhi and Gan Cao
    d. Gan jiang and Hong Hua

733. Da Huang performs which of the following functions in Tao Ren Cheng Qi Tang?
    a. Invigorate the Blood and break up Blood Stasis
    b. Drain Heat and move the stool
    c. Attack and purge Blood Stasis and cleanse pathogenic Heat
    d. Clear Heat and detoxify Fire-Poison

734. Which of the following yields Xue Fu Zhu Yu Tang?
    a. Combine Tao Hong Si Wu Tang with Si Ni San and add Niu Xi and Jie Geng
    b. Combine Tao Hong Si Wu Tang with Si Ni San and add Niu Xi
    c. Combine Si Wu Tang with Si Ni San and add Hong Hua and Niu Xi
    d. Combine Si Wu Tang with Si Ni San and add Tao Ren

735. Xue Fu Zhu Yu Tang does *not* perform which of the following functions?
    a. Invigorate Blood circulation and remove stasis
    b. Promote the movement of Qi
    c. Nourish the Blood
    d. Alleviate pain

736. Tao Ren Cheng Qi Tang performs which of the following functions?
    a. Invigorate Blood circulation and remove stasis
    b. Eliminate Heat and move the stool
    c. Break up Blood Stasis and drain Heat
    d. None of the above

737. Tao Ren Cheng Qi Tang is *not* indicated for which of the following?
    a. Acute abdominal pain
    b. Urinary incontinence
    c. Increased body temperature at night
    d. Squamous and dry skin

738. Which formula would you select to treat this pattern: pain in the chest and hypochondria, palpitations, restless sleep, irritability, dark spots on the sides of the tongue, wiry-tight pulse?
    a. Tao Hong Si Wu Tang
    b. Shao Fu Zhu Yu Tang
    c. Xue Fu Zhu Yu Tang
    d. Dan Shen Yin

739. Xue Fu Zhu Yu Tang is *not* indicated for which of the following?
    a. Chronic pain in the chest
    b. Chronic headache
    c. Acute abdominal pain
    d. Dark spots on the sides of the tongue

740. Jie Geng performs which of the following functions in Xue Fu Zhu Yu Tang?
    a. Circulates the Lung Qi and expel Phlegm
    b. Promote the discharge of pus
    c. Benefit the throat
    d. Direct the effect of other herbs upwards in order to treat the upper region of the body

741. Niu Xi performs which of the following functions in Xue Fu Zhu Yu Tang?
    a. Invigorate the Blood and expel Blood Stasis
    b. Invigorate the Blood and promote urination
    c. Clear Damp-Heat in the Lower Energizer
    d. Improve the circulation by eliminating Blood Stasis and inducing the downward movement of Blood

742. Which formula invigorates the Blood, dispels Blood Stasis, warms the menses, and alleviates pain?
    a. Shao Fu Zhu Yu Tang
    b. Ge Xia Zhu Yu Tang
    c. Shen Tong Zhu Yu Tang
    d. Shi Xiao San

743. Which formula consists of the following herbs: Wu Ling Zhi, Dang Gui, Chuan Xiong, Tao Ren, Mu Dan Pi, Chi Shao, Wu Yao, Yan Hu Suo, Gan Cao, Xiang Fu, Hong Hua, and Zhi Ke?
    a. Shao Fu Zhu Yu Tang
    b. Ge Xia Zhu Yu Tang
    c. Shen Tong Zhu Yu Tang
    d. Shi Xiao San

744. Which formula treats various types of painful obstruction caused by the obstruction of Qi and Blood in the meridians and collaterals?
    a. Ge Xia Zhu Yu Tang
    b. Shao Fu Zhu Yu Tang
    c. Shen Tong Zhu Yu Tang
    d. Xue Fu Zhu Yu Tang

745. Fu Yuan Huo Xue Tang does *not* contain which of the following?
    a. Tao Ren and Hong Hua
    b. Chuan Xiong and Zhi Shi
    c. Dang Gui, Chuan Shan Jia, and Da Huang
    d. Chai Hu, Gan Cao, and Gua Lou Gen

746. Which formula would you select to treat a patient who fell from a high place two days ago and has now begun experiencing intense pain in the hypochondria?
    a. Qi Li San
    b. Shi Xiao San
    c. Fu Yuan Huo Xue Tang
    d. Huo Luo Xiao Ling Dan

747. Which formula invigorates Blood, dispels Blood Stasis, spreads Liver Qi, and unblocks the meridians?
    a. Shi Xiao San
    b. Xue Fu Zhu Yu Tang
    c. Fu Yuan Huo Xue Tang
    d. Da Huang Zhe Chong Wan

748. Qi Li San does *not* contain which of the following?
    a. Ru Xiang and Mo Yao
    b. Dang Gui and Chi Shao
    c. Xue Jie, Hong Hua, and She Xiang
    d. Bing Pian, Zhu Sha, and Er Cha

749. Which herb serves as the chief (monarch or *jun*) component of Bu Yang Huan Wu Tang?
    a. Huang Qi
    b. Dang Gui
    c. Chuan Xiong
    d. Hong Hua

750. Which formula invigorates the Blood, dispels Blood Stasis, alleviates pain and stops bleeding?
    a. Qi Li San
    b. Shi Xiao San
    c. Bu Yang Huan Wu Tang
    d. Sheng Hua Tang

751. Bu Yang Huan Wu Tang does *not* perform which of the following functions?
    a. Tonify the Qi
    b. Invigorate the Blood
    c. Alleviate pain
    d. Unblock the meridians

752. Bu Yang Huan Wu Tang is *not* indicated for which of the following?
    a. Hemiplegia and paralysis
    b. Slurred speech
    c. Facial paralysis
    d. Delirium and excessive thirst

753. Shi Xiao San does *not* perform which of the following functions?
    a. Invigorate the Blood and dispel Blood Stasis
    b. Disperse accumulation
    c. Warm the menses
    d. Alleviate pain

754. Shi Xiao San is particular effective for treating which of the following?
    a. Blood Stasis in the Liver meridian
    b. Blood Stasis with a Cold pattern
    c. Blood Stasis with Deficient Blood
    d. Blood Stasis and severe Stagnation of Qi

755. Shi Xiao San is *not* indicated for which of the following?
    a. Postpartum abdominal pain
    b. Severe pain in epigastric region and the middle of the abdomen
    c. Acute, colicky pain in the lower abdomen
    d. A feeling of cold pain in the lower abdomen

756. Dan Shen Yin does *not* contain which of the following?
    a. Dan Shen
    b. Tan Xiang
    c. Chen Pi
    d. Sha Ren

757. Which formula treats Blood Stasis and Qi Stagnation accompanied by abdominal or epigastric pain?
    a. Shi Xiao San
    b. Qi Li San
    c. Fu Yuan Huo Xue Tang
    d. Dan Shen Yin

758. Which formula does *not* contain both Tao Ren and Dang Gui?
    a. Bu Yang Huan Wu Tang
    b. Fu Yuan Huo Xue Tang
    c. Xue Fu Zhu Yu Tang
    d. Wen Jing Tang

759. Wen Jing Tang does *not* perform which of the following functions?
    a. Warm the menses and dispel Cold
    b. Tonify the Spleen
    c. Nourish the Blood
    d. Dispel Blood Stasis

760. Which formula contains Wu Zhu Yu, Gui Zhi, Dang Gui, Bai Shao Yao, Ren Shen, E Jiao, and Chuan Xiong?
    a. Wen Jing Tang
    b. Fu Yuan Huo Xue Tang
    c. Bu Yang Huan Wu Tang
    d. Da Huang Zhe Chong Wan

761. Sheng Hua Tang does *not* contain which of the following?
    a. Dang Gui
    b. Hong Hua
    c. Chuan Xiong and Tao Ren
    d. Pao Jiang and Gan Cao

762. Sheng Hua Tang does *not* perform which of the following functions?
    a. Invigorate the Blood, transform and dispel Blood Stasis
    b. Warm the menses
    c. Nourish the Blood
    d. Alleviate pain

763. A heavy dosage of which herb serves as the chief (monarch or *jun*) component in Sheng Hua Tang?
    a. Dang Gui
    b. Chuan Xiong
    c. Tao Ren
    d. Pao Jiang

764. Huo Luo Xiao Ling Dan does *not* contain which of the following?
    a. Chuan Xiong
    b. Dang Gui
    c. Dan Shen
    d. Ru Xiang and Mo Yao

765. Huo Luo Xioa Ling Dan does *not* perform which of the following functions?
    a. Invigorate the Blood and dispel Blood Stasis
    b. Promote the movement of Qi
    c. Unblock the collaterals
    d. Alleviate pain

766. Which of the following herbs does *not* dispel Blood Stasis in the formula Gui Zhi Fu Ling Wan?
    a. Hong Hua
    b. Chi Shao
    c. Mu Dan Pi
    d. Tao Ren

767. Which formula would you select to treat a pregnant woman who complains of mild, persistent uterine bleeding that is purple or dark and accompanied by abdominal pain that increases with pressure?
    a. Wen Jing Tang
    b. Jiao Ai Tang
    c. Gui Zhi Fu Ling Wan
    d. Da Huang Zhe Chong Wan

768. Which formula invigorates the Blood, transforms Blood Stasis, and reduces fixed abdominal masses?
    a. Da Huang Zhe Chong Wan
    b. Gui Zhi Fu Ling Wan
    c. Dan Shen Yin
    d. Shi Xiao San

769. Which formula breaks up and dispels Blood Stasis and generates new Blood?
    a. Gui Zhi Fu Ling Wan
    b. Da Huang Zhe Chong Wan
    c. Dan Shen Yin
    d. Wan Jing Tang

770. Which formula would you select to treat this pattern: emaciation, abdominal fullness, loss of appetite, skin that is dry, rough and scaly, eyes that have a dull and dark appearance?
    a. Da Huang Zhe Chong Wan
    b. Wen Jing Tang
    c. Huo Luo Xiao Ling Dan
    d. Sheng Hua Tang

771. Shi Hui San does *not* contain which of the following?
    a. Da Ji and Xiao Ji
    b. Dang Gui and Bai Shao
    c. He Ye, Ce Bai Ye, Bai Mao Gen, and Qian Cao Gen
    d. Zhi Zi, Da Huang, Mu Dan Pi, and Zong Lu Pi

772. Shi Hui San is often used to treat bleeding caused by reckless movement of Hot-Blood which spills out of the meridians. Which of the following symptoms would *not* be present in such a case?
    a. Vomiting
    b. Spitting
    c. Coughing
    d. Blood in the stool

773. Shi Hui San performs which of the following functions?
    a. Clear Heat and stop bleeding
    b. Cool the Blood and stop bleeding
    c. Warm the menses and stop bleeding
    d. Dispel Blood Stasis and stop bleeding

774. Which of the following is *not* a function performed by Da Huang and Zhi Zi in the formula Shi Hui San?
    a. Clear Liver Heat
    b. Lead Heat downward
    c. Prevent Heat from rising
    d. Cool the Blood

775. Si Sheng Wan does *not* contain which of the following?
    a. Sheng He Ye
    b. Sheng Pi Pa Ye
    c. Sheng Ce Bai Ye
    d. Sheng Ai Ye and Sheng Di Huang

776. Which of the following is *not* a function performed by Sheng He Ye in the formula Si Sheng Wan?
    a. Cool the Blood
    b. Clear Heat
    c. Stop bleeding
    d. Dispel Blood Stasis

777. Which formula would you select to treat coughing up of blood-streaked sputum that is difficult to expectorate and is caused by Liver Fire attacking and scorching the Lungs?
    a. Si Sheng Wan
    b. Ke Xue Fang
    c. Qing Qi Hua Tan Wan
    d. Bei Mu Gua Lou San

778. Which formula would you select to treat this pattern: a nosebleed that has continued for two days and produces bright red blood, dry mouth and throat, red tongue, wiry-rapid pulse?
    a. Si Sheng Wan
    b. Ke Xue Fang
    c. Shi Hui San
    d. Jiao Ai Tang

779. Ke Xue Fang does *not* contain which of the following?
    a. Huang Qin
    b. Qing Dai
    c. Zhi Zi and Gua Lou Ren
    d. Fu Hai Shi and He Zi

780. Qing Dai and Zhi Zi perform which of the following functions in the formula Ke Xue Fang?
    a. Clear the Liver, drain Fire, and cool the Blood
    b. Clear the Liver and detoxify the Blood
    c. Detoxify Poison and cool the Blood
    d. Cool the Blood and stop bleeding

781. Huai Hua San does *not* contain which of the following?
    a. Fang Feng
    b. Huai Hua
    c. Ce Bai Ye
    d. Jing Jie Sui and Zhi Ke

782. Huai Hua San does *not* perform which of the following functions?
    a. Cool the Intestines and stop bleeding
    b. Disperse Wind
    c. Nourish the Blood and tonify the Qi
    d. Promote the movement of Qi downward

783. Which formula would you select to treat bleeding that is caused by a toxin formed because Wind-Heat became lodged—or Damp-Heat accumulated—in the Intestines and Stomach?
    a. Shi Hui San
    b. Si Sheng Wan
    c. Huai Hua San
    d. Huang Tu Tang

784. Huai Hua San is *not* indicated for which of the following?
    a. Bleeding before passage of stool
    b. Bleeding following the passage of stool
    c. Bleeding caused by hemorrhoids
    d. Menorrhagia caused by Deficient Spleen Qi

785. What formula is the basis of Xiao Ji Yin Zi?
    a. Si Sheng San
    b. Dao Chi San
    c. Shi Hui San
    d. Bi Yu San

786. Which formula cools Blood, stops bleeding, promotes urination, and unblocks painful urinary dysfunction?
    a. Wu Ling San
    b. Ba Zheng San
    c. Zhu Ling Tang
    d. None of the above

787. Which formula would you be very unlikely to select to treat vomiting of blood or nosebleeds?
    a. Si Sheng San
    b. Huai Hua San
    c. Shi Hui San
    d. Huang Lian Jie Du Tang

788. Which formula would select to treat this pattern: blood in the urine, frequent urgent urination that is accompanied by burning and pain, red tongue, rapid pulse?
    a. Xiao Ji Yin Zi
    b. Wu Ling San
    c. Dao Chi San
    d. None of the above

789. Which herbs in the formula Xiao Ji Yin Zi cool the Blood and stop bleeding?
    a. Xiao Ji, Ou Jie, Pu Huang, and Wu Ling Zhi
    b. Xiao Ji, Ou Jie, Pu Huang, and Di Yu
    c. Xiao Ji, Ou Jie, Pu Huang, and Sheng Di Huang
    d. Xiao Ji, Ou Jie, Pu Huang, and Mu Dan Pi

790. Huang Tu Tang does *not* contain which of the following?
    a. Gan Di Huang
    b. Fu Ling
    c. Gan Cao, Zao Xin Tu, and E Jiao
    d. Bai Zhu, Fu Zi, and Huang Qin

791. Huang Tu Tang does *not* perform which of the following functions?
    a. Warm the Yang and strengthen the Spleen
    b. Nourish the Blood
    c. Stop bleeding
    d. Nourish the Qi

792. Which formula would you select to treat this pattern: blood in the stool, vomiting/spitting up of blood or abnormal uterine bleeding of pale red blood, cold extremities, wan complexion, pale tongue with white fur, deep-thin-forceless pulse?
    a. Jioa Ai Tang
    b. Huai Hua San
    c. Xiao Ji Yin Zi
    d. None of the above

793. Jiao Ai Tang and Wen Jing Tang each contain which of the following ingredients?
    a. E Jiao, Ai Ye, Sheng Di Huang, Chuan Xiong, and Dang Gui
    b. E Jiao, Bai Shao, Gan Cao, Chuan Xiong, and Dang Gui
    c. E Jiao, Bai Shao, Ren Shen, Chuan Xiong, and Dang Gui
    d. E Jiao, Bai Shao, Gan Cao, Chuan Xiong, and Huang Qin

794. Jiao Ai Tang does *not* perform which of the following functions?
    a. Invigorate the Qi to accelerate hemostasis
    b. Enrich the Blood and stop bleeding
    c. Regulate menstruation
    d. Calm the fetus

795. Which statement is true about the functions herbs perform in Jiao Ai Tang?
    a. Gan Di Huang, Bai Shao, Dang Gui, and Chuan Xiong enrich the Blood and regulate menstruation
    b. E Jiao and Ai Ye stop bleeding and nourish the Blood
    c. E Jiao and Bai Shao stop bleeding
    d. Chuan Xiong and Gan Cao alleviate pain

796. Which formula would you *not* select to invigorate the Blood and dispel Blood Stasis?
    a. Tao He Cheng Qi Tang
    b. Xue Fu Zhu Yu Tang
    c. Jiao Ai Tang
    d. Dan Shen Yin

797. Jiao Ai Tang is *not* indicated for which of the following?
    a. Bleeding during pregnancy
    b. Excessive menstruation
    c. Irregular menstruation
    d. Abdominal pain with uterine bleeding

798. Herbs that warm the Interior do *not* perform which of the following functions?
    a. Warm the Middle Energizer
    b. Expel Cold and alleviate pain
    c. Nourish Yin and assist the Yang
    d. Warm the Fire and assist the Yang

799. What are the properties of Fu Zi?
    a. Sour, warm, and toxic
    b. Sweet and neutral
    c. Acrid, hot, and toxic
    d. Acrid, sweet, hot, and toxic

800. What are the properties of Chuan Wu?
    a. Acrid, Hot, and toxic
    b. Acrid, bitter, warm, and very toxic
    c. Acrid, sweet, hot, and toxic
    d. Acrid and hot

801. Which herb is often used with Fu Zi to recuperate the depleted Yang and rescue the patient from danger?
    a. Gui Zhi
    b. Gan Jiang
    c. Gao Liang Jiang
    d. Sheng Jiang

802. Fu Zi is *not* indicated for which of the following?
    a. Damp-Cold painful obstruction
    b. Profuse perspiration caused by Yang Exhaustion
    c. Spontaneous perspiration caused by Deficient Yang
    d. Damp evil stagnating in the Middle Energizer

803. Which of the following *best* treats Cold pain in the sinews caused by Cold evil?
    a. Sang Zhi
    b. Gui Zhi
    c. Fang Feng
    d. Fu Zi

804. The most commonly used dosages of prepared Cao Wu fall within which of the following ranges?
    a. 3.0–15.0 grams
    b. 1.5–4.5 grams
    c. 0.5–2.0 grams
    d. 3.0–10.0 grams

805. Which meridians does Gan Jiang enter?
    a. Heart, Spleen, Stomach, and Lung
    b. Spleen and Lung
    c. Spleen and Stomach
    d. Stomach and Lung

806. Which of the following herbs has acrid and hot properties?
    a. Sheng Jiang
    b. Gan Jiang
    c. Pao Jiang
    d. Jiang Pi

807. What is the special function of Pao Jiang?
    a. Warm the Middle Energizer and expel Cold
    b. Warm the Stomach and stop vomiting
    c. Warm the Lungs and transform Phlegm
    d. Warm the meridians and stop bleeding

808. Which herb treats pain caused by a Cold Syndrome that manifests itself as a hernia?
    a. Gan Jiang
    b. Wu Zhu Yu
    c. Mu Xiang
    d. Chuan Lian Zi

809. Which herb treats Cold Syndromes of the Spleen and Stomach with symptoms of Cold pain in the abdomen, vomiting, and diarrhea?
    a. Wu Yao
    b. Xi Xin
    c. Gan Jiang
    d. Sheng Jiang

810. Which herb is usually taken as a powder?
    a. Xi Xin
    b. Bo He
    c. Bai Zhi
    d. Rou Gui

811. Which herb warms the Middle Energizer, rescues the devastated Yang, warms the Lungs, and transforms Phlegm?
    a. Rou Gui
    b. Fu Zi
    c. Gan Jiang
    d. Bai Jie Zi

812. Rou Gui does *not* perform which of the following functions?
    a. Warm the Fire and assist the Yang
    b. Expel Cold evil and alleviate pain
    c. Warm the Lungs and transform Phlegm
    d. Warm and unblock the meridians and vessels

813. Which herb is especially effective for treating Taiyang headaches?
    a. Wu Zhu Yu
    b. Bai Zhi
    c. Xi Xin
    d. Chuan Xiong

814. The most commonly used dosages of Rou Gui fall within which of the following ranges?
    a. 10-15 grams
    b. 5-10 grams
    c. .5-1 grams
    d. 1.5-4.5 grams

815. Which herb warms the Liver and disperses the depressed Liver Qi?
    a. Rou Gui
    b. Chuan Jiao
    c. Ding Xiang
    d. Wu Zhu Yu

816. Which herb is especially effective for treating Jueyin headaches?
    a. Gan Jiang
    b. Bai Zhi
    c. Wu Zhu Yu
    d. Cong Zhu

817. Which two herbs are usually used with Wu Zhu Yu to treat Cold syndromes with pain in the abdomen?
    a. Sheng Jiang and Ren Shen
    b. Mu Xiang and Xiang Fu
    c. Bai Zhu and Wu Wei Zi
    d. Xiao Hui Xiang and Wu Yao

818. Which herb warms the Lungs, transforms Phlegm, and disperses and unblocks the Qi of the nasal orifice?
    a. Gan Jiang
    b. Xin Yi Hua
    c. Bai Zhi
    d. Xi Xin

819. Xi Xin is *not* indicated for which of the following?
    a. Headache caused by an Exterior Cold pattern
    b. Headache caused by Deficient Yin
    c. Headache caused by nasal congestion
    d. Headache caused by Wind-Damp evil

820. Which herb treats abdominal pain caused by roundworms?
    a. Wu Zhu Yu
    b. Bi Ba
    c. Hua Jiao
    d. Xiao Hui Xiang

821. Which herb warms the Middle Energizer, directs rebellious Qi downward, warms the Kidneys, and aids the Yang?
    a. Cheng Pi
    b. Ding Xiang
    c. Fu Zi
    d. Hou Po

822. Which herb kills parasites, warms the Middle Energizer, and alleviates pain?
    a. Ding Xiang
    b. Mu Xiang
    c. Hua Jiao
    d. Chuan Lian Zi

823. Which herb treats Cold hernial pain and pain caused by orchidoptosis?
    a. Ding Xiang
    b. Hua Jiao
    c. Xiao Hui Xiang
    d. Gao Liang Jiang

824. Which herb treats Cold pain in the abdomen and vomiting or diarrhea?
    a. Xiao Hui Xiang
    b. Ding Xiang
    c. Gao Liang Jiang
    d. Xi Xin

825. What is a common use of Gan Jiang with Fu Zi?
    a. Recuperate the depleted Yang and rescue the patient from danger
    b. Aid Spleen Yang and warm the Kidney Yang
    c. Strongly recuperate the depleted Yang, rescue the patient from danger, and reduce the poisonous nature of Fu Zi
    d. None of the above

826. Gan Jiang and Gao Liang Jiang each perform which of the following functions?
    a. Warm the Middle Energizer and alleviate pain
    b. Warm the meridians and stop bleeding
    c. Warm the Lungs and transform Phlegm
    d. None of the above

827. Which two herbs each warm the Interior, disperse Cold, and spread Liver Qi?
    a. Gao Liang Jiang and Ding Xiang
    b. Hua Jiao and Rou Gui
    c. Xiao Hui Xiang and Wu Zhu Yu
    d. Fu Zi and Bi Ba

828. Bi Ba and Bi Cheng Qie each perform which of the following functions?
    a. Warm the Lungs and transform Phlegm
    b. Warm the meridians and stop bleeding
    c. Warm the Kidneys and fortify the Yang
    d. Warm the Middle Energizer and alleviate pain

829. Which statement is true of Fu Zi and Rou Gui?
    a. They are very acrid, very hot, and sweet
    b. They are generally used as a powder
    c. They recuperate the depleted Yang and rescue the patient from danger
    d. They warm the Fire and assist the Yang

830. Which herb is acrid, hot, and slightly toxic?
    a. Hua Jiao
    b. Ding Xiang
    c. Xiao Hui Xiang
    d. Gao Liang Jiang

831. Which herb is especially effective for treating Shao Yang headache?
    a. Bai Zhi
    b. Xi Xin
    c. Chai Hu
    d. Man Jing Zi

832. Li Zhong Wan does *not* contain which of the following?
    a. Ren Shen
    b. Bai Zhu
    c. Sheng Jiang and Fu Ling
    d. Gan Jiang and Zhi Gan Cao

833. Wu Zhu Yu Tang does *not* contain which of the following?
    a. Wu Zhu Yu Tang
    b. Gan Jiang
    c. Ren Shen
    d. Sheng Jiang and Da Zao

834. Wu Zhu Yu Tang does *not* perform which of the following functions?
    a. Warm and tonify the Liver and Stomach
    b. Rescue the devastated Yang
    c. Direct the rebellious Qi downward
    d. Stop vomiting

835. Which formula warms and tonifies the Middle Energizer, directs Qi downward, and stops vomiting?
    a. Wu Zhu Yu Tang
    b. Li Zhong Wan
    c. Xiao Jian Zhong Tang
    d. Do Jian Zhong Tang

836. Li Zhong Wan is *not* indicated for which of the following?
    a. Diarrhea with watery stool caused by Deficiency-Cold of the Spleen and Stomach
    b. Bleeding caused by Deficient Yang
    c. Chest pain caused by Middle Energizer Cold from Deficiency
    d. Abdominal pain and distension caused by Damp-Cold of the Spleen and Stomach and Qi Stagnation

837. Which of the following is *not* a function performed by Wu Zhu Yu in the formula Wu Zhu Yu Tang?
    a. Expel Cold and dry Damp
    b. Direct rebellious Qi downward
    c. Warm the Stomach
    d. Warm the Liver

838. What is added to Gui Zhi Tang in order to make Xiao Jian Zhong Tang?
    a. 30 grams of Yi Tang
    b. 30 grams of Yi Tang and 9 grams of Gui Zhi
    c. 30 grams of Yi Tang and 9 grams of Sheng Jiang
    d. 30 grams of Yi Tang and 9 grams of Bai Shao

839. Xiao Jian Zhong Tang performs which of the following functions?
    a. Warm and tonify the Middle Energizer; moderate spasmodic abdominal pain
    b. Warm and tonify the Middle Energizer; direct rebellious Qi Downward
    c. Warm and tonify the Middle Energizer
    d. Warm and tonify the Middle Energizer; strengthen the Spleen and Stomach

840. Xiao Jian Zhong Tang is *not* indicated for which of the following?
    a. Intermittent, spasmodic abdominal pain that eases with local application of warmth and pressure
    b. Low-grade fever, palpitations, and irritability
    c. Cold and sore extremities with nonspecific discomfort
    d. Night sweats and a burning sensation of the five centers

841. Da Jian Zhong Tang does *not* contain which of the following?
    a. Bai Zhu
    b. Ren Shen
    c. Chuan Jian
    d. Gan Jiang and Yi Tang

842. Da Jian Zhong Tang does *not* perform which of the following functions?
    a. Warm and tonify the Middle Energizer
    b. Tonify the Spleen and Stomach
    c. Direct rebellious Qi downward
    d. Alleviate pain

843. Which formula would you select to treat this pattern: abdominal pain that has continued for more than a month and is eased by warmth and pressure, pale tongue with white fur, thin-wiry-moderate pulse?
    a. Li Zhong Wan
    b. Xiao Jian Zhong Tang
    c. Da Jian Zhong Tang
    d. Wu Zhu Yu Tang

844. Which statement is false?
    a. Gan Jiang serves as the chief (monarch or *jun*) component of Li Zhong Wan
    b. Bai Shao serves as the chief (monarch or *jun*) component of Xiao Jian Zhong Tang
    c. Wu Zhu Yu serves as the chief (monarch or *jun*) component of Wu Zhu Yu Tang
    d. Chuan Jiao serves as the chief (monarch or *jun*) component of Da Jian Zhong Tang

845. Which of the following is *not* classified as a formula that warms the Middle Energizer?
    a. Li Zhong Wan
    b. Xiao Jian Zhong Tang
    c. Wu Zhu Yu Tang
    d. Hui Yang Jiu Ji Tang

846. What is the pathogenesis for an abdominal pain syndrome that indicates Da Jian Zhong Tang?
    a. Weakness and Deficient Middle Energizer Yang, with Yin or Cold which is ascendant in the Interior
    b. Incoordination between the Liver and Spleen
    c. Disorder of the Liver Qi
    d. Stagnation of the Qi and Blood

847. What differentiates Si Ni Tang from Tong Mai Si Ni Tang?
    a. The dosage of Zhi Gan Cao
    b. The dosage of Gan Jiang
    c. The dosage of Fu Zi
    d. The dosages of Gan Jiang and Fu Zi

848. Which formula would you select to treat this pattern: very cold extremities, aversion to cold, preference for sleeping with the knees drawn up, vomiting, diarrhea, lethargy with a constant desire to sleep, lack of thirst, submerged-thin or submerged-faint pulse?
    a. Si Ni Tang
    b. Si Ni San
    c. Tong Mai Si Ni Tang
    d. Shan Fu Tang

849. Which herb is *not* part of the formula for Si Ni Tang?
    a. Xi Xian
    b. Sheng Fu Zi
    c. Gan Jiang
    d. Zhi Gan Cao

850. Tong Mai Si Ni Tang is *not* indicated for which of the following symptoms?
    a. Sweating, shortness of breath and dizziness
    b. A faint or hidden pulse
    c. No aversion to cold, with a flushed face
    d. Cold extremities

851. What is a function of the formula Shen Fu Tang?
    a. Supplement the Qi and nourish the Yin
    b. Restore the Yang, strongly tonify the source Qi, and rescue the Qi from collapse caused by devastated Yang
    c. Invigorate the Qi and strengthen the resistance of the body's surface
    d. Strengthen the Middle Energizer and benefit the Qi

852. Which of the following yields the formula for Hui Yang Jiu Ji Tang?
    a. Combining Si Ni Tang with Du Shen Tang
    b. Combining Er Chen Tang with Si Jun Zi Tang
    c. Combining Si Ni Tang with Liu Ju Zi Tang and adding Rou Gui, Wu Wei Zi, and She Xiang
    d. None of the above

853. Which formula would you select to treat this pattern: cold extremities, sweating, weak breathing, dizziness, and a faint pulse that is almost imperceptible?
    a. Si Ni Tang
    b. Si Ni San
    c. Shen Fu Tang
    d. Zhu Fu Tang

854. Hui Yang Jiu Ji Tang is *not* indicated for which of the following?
    a. Cold extremities and a lethargic state with a constant desire to sleep
    b. Vomiting, diarrhea and abdominal pain
    c. Cyanosis of the fingernails and lips
    d. Anxiety with palpitation

855. Hai Xi Dan does *not* perform which of the following functions?
    a. Warm the Kidney Yang
    b. Expel Yin-Cold
    c. Warm the Spleen Yang
    d. Relieve wheezing from Deficiency

856. Hei Xi Dan is *not* indicated for which of the following?
    a. Deficiency-Cold in the lower source and sterility caused by Blood deficiency-Cold
    b. Deficiency-Cold in the lower source with impotence caused by Deficient Kidney Yang
    c. Deficiency-Cold in the lower source with Deficiency wheezing caused by Kidney energy failing to aid the Lungs in regulating inspiration
    d. Deficiency-Cold in the lower source with pain in the abdomen during pregnancy caused by an overabundance of Yin-Cold

857. Dang Gui Si Ni Tang can be created by adapting Gui Zhi Tang in which of the following ways?
    a. Remove Sheng Jiang; add Dang Gui, Xi Xin, and Mu Tong
    b. Add Dang Gui, Xi Xin, and Mu Tong
    c. Add Dang Gui, Xi Xin, and Shui Di
    d. Add Dang Gui, Xi Xin, and Bai Shao

858. Dang Gui Si Ni Tang does *not* perform which of the following functions?
    a. Break up Blood Stasis and unblock Stagnation
    b. Warm the meridians and disperse Cold
    c. Nourish the Blood
    d. Unblock the blood vessels

859. Dang Gui Si Ni Tang is *not* indicated for which of the following?
    a. Cold hands and feet
    b. Arthralgia-pain of the extremities
    c. Pale tongue with a white coating
    d. Pain in the abdomen with diarrhea

860. Mu Tong performs which of the following functions in the formula Dang Gui Si Ni Tang?
    a. Leads the herbs which nourish the Blood to the Heart
    b. Prevents injury of the Yin caused by the warm and dry nature of Xi Xin and Gui Zhi
    c. Protects against the lifting and releasing qualities of Xi Xin
    d. Facilitates the flow in the meridians and vessels

861. Which herb treats extreme collapse of Qi where the pulse is so faint as to be almost imperceptible?
    a. Huang Qi
    b. Dan Shen
    c. Fu Zi
    d. Ren Shen

862. What dosage of Ren Shen is commonly used in decoctions for treatment of collapse?
    a. 1-3 grams
    b. 3-6 grams
    c. 6-10 grams
    d. 15-30 grams

863. Which herb tonifies the Qi, nurtures the Yin, clears Fire, and generates fluids?
    a. Tai Zi Shen
    b. Dang Shen
    c. Xi Yang Shen
    d. Xuan Shen

864. Which herb strengthens the Qi and generates fluids?
    a. Dang Shen
    b. Huang Qi
    c. Tai Zi Shen
    d. Shan Yao

865. Which herb treats Deficient Qi accompanied by Deficient body fluids, fatigue, lack of appetite, and thirst?
    a. Huang Qi
    b. Bai Zhu
    c. Sheng Di Huang
    d. Tai Zi Shen

866. Which herb tonifies the Qi, raises the Yang, augments the protective Qi, stabilizes the Exterior, promotes the discharge of pus, generates flesh, promotes urination, and reduces edema?
    a. Ren Shen
    b. Tai Zi Shen
    c. Huang Qi
    d. Shan Yao

867. Which herb treats collapse of the Middle Energizer Qi and prolapse disorders of the rectum caused by chronic diarrhea?
    a. Sheng Ma
    b. Dang Shen
    c. Bai Zhu
    d. Huang Qi

868. What meridians does Huang Qi enter?
    a. Lung and Kidney
    b. Liver and Stomach
    c. Lung and Spleen
    d. Heart and Kidney

869. Which herb tonifies the Spleen, augments the Qi, dries Damp, promotes urination, stops sweating, and calms the fetus?
    a. Bai Zhu
    b. Huang Qi
    c. Shan Yao
    d. Ren Shen

870. Which herb tonifies the Kidneys and treats spermatorrhea and frequent urination?
    a. Dang Shen
    b. Shan Yao
    c. Huang Qi
    d. Gan Cao

871. Shan Yao does *not* perform which of the following functions?
    a. Nourish the Blood and calm the Spirit
    b. Tonify the Qi of the Lungs, Kidneys and Spleen
    c. Nourish the Yin
    d. Stabilize and bind

872. Which herb eliminates Damp evil, regulates the Middle Energizer, and strengthens the Spleen?
    a. Hou Po
    b. Xiang Ru
    c. Bian Dou
    d. Gan Cao

873. Which herb relieves poisoning from food or herbs?
    a. Sheng Jiang
    b. Gan Cao
    c. Shan Yao
    d. Ming Fan

874. Yi Tang does *not* perform which of the following functions?
    a. Tonify the Spleen and augment the Qi
    b. Tonify the Middle Energizer Qi and alleviate pain
    c. Moisten the Lungs and stop coughs
    d. Promote fluids and stop thirst

875. Shan Yao and Bian Dou each perform which of the following functions?
    a. Tonify the Qi and nourish the Yin
    b. Tonify the Spleen and stop diarrhea
    c. Tonify the Kidneys and stabilize and bind
    d. Promote fluids and stop thirst

876. Which herb treats Deficiency-Cold of the Chong and Ren meridians, stabilizes the Dai meridian, and treats leukorrhea?
    a. Lu Rong
    b. Qian Shi
    c. Long Gu
    d. Mu Li

877. What function does Ba Ji Tian have in addition to tonifying the Kidneys and fortifying the Yang?
    a. Expel Cold evil and stop pain
    b. Disperse Wind and expel Damp-Cold
    c. Tonify the Spleen and moisten the Lungs
    d. Stabilize the Essence and reserve the urine

878. Which herb tonifies Kidney Yang, tonifies the Governing Vessel, augments the Essence and Blood, and strengthens the sinews and bone?
    a. Gou Ji
    b. Rou Cong Rong
    c. Dong Chong Xia Cao
    d. Lu Rong

879. Which herb tonifies the Yang, moistens the Intestines, and unblocks the bowels?
    a. Lu Rong
    b. Ba Ji Tian
    c. Bu Gu Zhi
    d. Rou Cong Rong

880. What is the contraindication for Xian Mao?
    a. Diarrhea
    b. Deficient Spleen and Stomach
    c. Deficient Yin patterns with Heat signs
    d. Deficient Lung Qi

881. What are the properties of Du Zhong?
    a. Salty and warm
    b. Bitter and warm
    c. Sweet and warm
    d. Sour and warm

882. Which herb tonifies the Kidneys, fortifies the Yang, and expels Wind-Damp?
    a. Yin Yang Huo
    b. Du Zhong
    c. Bu Gu Zhi
    d. Rou Cong Rong

883. Which herb treats Deficient Kidney Yang, abdominal or flank distention and pain, and hernial disorders caused by Damp-Cold?
    a. Rou Cong Rong
    b. Bu Gu Zhi
    c. Xu Duan
    d. Hu Lu Ba

884. Which herb tonifies the Liver and Kidneys, strengthens the sinews and bones, and calms the fetus?
    a. Lu Rong
    b. Du Zhong
    c. Tu Si Zi
    d. Yi Zhi Ren

885. Which herb tonifies the Liver and Kidneys, strengthens the sinews and bones, and promotes the movement of Blood?
    a. Sang Ji Sheng
    b. Xu Duan
    c. Ba Ji Tian
    d. Hu Lu Ba

886. Which herb tonifies the Kidneys, promotes the mending of the sinews and bones, and stimulates the growth of hair?
    a. Bu Gu Zhi
    b. Gu Sui Bu
    c. Sang Ji Sheng
    d. Du Zhong

887. Which herb treats chronic diarrhea caused by Deficient Kidneys?
    a. Ge Gen
    b. Bu Gu Zhi
    c. Lian Zi
    d. Cao Dou Kou

888. Which of the following does *not* calm the fetus?
    a. Bu Gu Zhi
    b. Huang Qin
    c. Sang Ji Sheng
    d. Sha Ren

889. Which herb treats daily occurrence of diarrhea before dawn resulting from Deficient Kidneys and Spleen?
    a. Dang Shen
    b. Bai Zhu
    c. Sha Yuan Zi
    d. Bu Gu Zhi

890. Which herb warms the Kidneys, retains the Essence, warms the Spleen, and stops excessive salivation?
    a. Bu Gu Zhi
    b. Wu Wei Zi
    c. Sha Yuan Zi
    d. Yi Zhi Ren

891. Dong Chong Xia Cao performs which of the following functions?
    a. Tonify the Liver and the Kidneys
    b. Tonify the Spleen and the Lungs
    c. Tonify the Spleen and the Liver
    d. Tonify the Lungs and the Kidneys

892. Which herb augments the Kidneys and Lungs, transforms Phlegm, and stops bleeding?
    a. E Jiao
    b. Ge Jie
    c. Hu Tao Ren
    d. Dong Chong Xia Cao

893. Which herb warms and augments the Lungs and Kidneys, moistens the Intestines, and unblocks the bowels?
    a. Rou Cong Rong
    b. Ge Jie
    c. Huo Ma Ren
    d. Hu Tao Ren

894. Which herb augments the Qi and Essence, and nourishes the Blood?
    a. Hai Er Shen
    b. Shan Yao
    c. Huang Jing
    d. Zi He Che

895. Which herb tonifies the Yang, augments the Yin, secures the Essence, reserves urine, improves eyesight, and stops diarrhea?
    a. Zi He Qi
    b. Ba Ji Tian
    c. Tu Si Zi
    d. Sha Yuan Ji Li

896. Which herb treats Deficient Liver and Kidneys and weakness, soreness, or numbness of the lower back, spine, or leg which is caused by Wind-Cold-Damp evil?
    a. Du Zhong
    b. Gou Ji
    c. Wei Ling Xian
    d. Hu Gu

897. Which herb has a function similar to that of Rou Cong Rong?
    a. Suo Yang
    b. Ba Ji Tian
    c. Hu Tao Ren
    d. Tu Si Zi

898. Hu Lu Ba does *not* perform which of the following functions?
    a. Warms the Kidney Yang
    b. Disperse Damp and Cold
    c. Alleviate pain
    d. Tonify the Liver and Kidneys

899. Which herb tonifies the Kidneys, secures the Essence, nourishes the Liver, and improves eyesight?
    a. Gou Qi Zi
    b. Sha Yuan Zi
    c. Bai Ji Li
    d. Qian Shi

900. Which herb treats Deficient Blood, Cold Blood, and Blood Stasis?
    a. Shu Di Huang
    b. He Shou Wu
    c. E Jiao
    d. Dang Gui

901. What function does Dang Gui have when it is prepared with wine?
    a. Strengthens the ability to tonify the Blood
    b. Strengthens the ability to promote the movement of Blood and dispel Blood Stasis
    c. Strengthens the ability to moisten the Intestines and unblock the bowels
    d. None of the above

902. Which herb would you select to treat a patient with a pallid complexion caused by Deficient Blood, which is accompanied by palpitations, insomnia, night sweats, recurring fever, tinnitus, and deafness resulting from Deficient Kidney Yin?
    a. Shan Yu Rou
    b. Dang Gui
    c. Shu Di Huang
    d. Suan Zao Ren

903. Which herb when used raw treats Fire toxin, malarial disorders, and moistens the Intestines; and when used roasted tonifies and augments the Essence and Blood?
    a. Di Huang
    b. Niu Xi
    c. He Shou Wu
    d. Sha Yuan Zi

904. Which herb calms and curbs Liver Yang, nourishes the Blood, and preserves the Yin?
    a. Gou Qi Zi
    b. Bai Shao Yao
    c. Ju Hua
    d. He Shou Wu

905. Which herb nourishes the Yin, moistens the Lungs, nourishes the Blood, and stops bleeding?
    a. Tian Men Dong
    b. Yu Zhu
    c. E Jiao
    d. Huang Jing

906. Which of the following is *not* a function of Long Yan Rou?
    a. Tonify and augment the Lungs and Kidneys
    b. Tonify and augment the Heart and Spleen
    c. Nourish the Blood
    d. Calm the Spirit

907. Which treats pain and spasms in the abdomen?
    a. E Jiao
    b. Dang Gui
    c. Bai Shao
    d. Long Yan Rou

908. Which herb treats Deficient Heart Yin, irritability, palpitations, and insomnia?
    a. Huang Lian
    b. Zhi Zi
    c. Dan Zhu Ye
    d. Mai Men Dong

909. Which herb nourishes the Yin of the Lungs and Stomach and clears Heat of the Lungs and Stomach?
    a. Shui Ye
    b. Huang Qin
    c. Gou Qi Zi
    d. Sha Shen

910. Which herb would best treat Deficient Yin of the Stomach?
    a. Sha Shen
    b. Tian Men Dong
    c. Mai Men Dong
    d. Shi Hu

911. Which herb nourishes Stomach Yin, generates fluids, nourishes Kidney Yin, and clears Deficiency-Fire?
    a. Tian Men Dong
    b. Mai Men Dong
    c. Shi Hu
    d. Sha Shen

912. Which herb tonifies the Spleen, augments the Qi, moistens the Lungs, and nourishes the Yin?
    a. Huang Jing
    b. Gan Cao
    c. Yu Zhu
    d. Huang Qi

913. Which herb clears Heat, calms the Spirit, moistens the Lungs, and stops cough?
    a. Yu Zhu
    b. Bai He
    c. Sha Shen
    d. Huang Lian

914. Which herb treats diminished visual acuity in patients with Deficient Liver and Kidneys?
    a. Gou Qi Zi
    b. Sang Ji Sheng
    c. Du Zhong
    d. Xu Duan

915. Which herb tonifies the Blood, enriches the Yin, and moistens the Intestines?
    a. Sheng Di Huang
    b. Sang Shen Zi
    c. Gou Qi Zi
    d. Bai Shao

916. Which herb treats diminished visual acuity in patients with Deficient Liver and Kidneys?
    a. Du Zhong
    b. Nu Zhen Zi
    c. Wu Wei Zi
    d. Xu Duan

917. Han Lian Cao does *not* perform which of the following functions?
    a. Moisten the Intestines
    b. Nourish and tonify the Yin of the Liver and Kidneys
    c. Cool the Blood
    d. Stop bleeding

918. Which herb dissipates nodules, nourishes the Yin, and anchors the Yang?
    a. Gui Ban
    b. Long Gu
    c. Bie Jia
    d. Shi Jue Ming

919. Which herb nourishes Kidney Yin and is classified as an herb that clears the Lungs and promotes fluids?
    a. Sha Shen
    b. Tian Men Dong
    c. Mai Men Dong
    d. Lu Gen

920. Which herb moistens the Lungs, nourishes the Yin, augments the Stomach, generates fluids, clears the Heart, and eliminates irritability?
    a. Tian Men Dong
    b. Lu Gen
    c. Tian Hua Fen
    d. Mai Men Dong

921. Which herb nourishes the Yin, anchors the Yang, benefits the Kidneys, strengthens the bones, nourishes the Blood, and tonifies the Heart?
    a. Shu Di
    b. Huang Jing
    c. Bie Jia
    d. Gui Ban

922. Huang Qi and Bai Zhu each perform which of the following functions?
    a. Alleviate sweating and promote urination
    b. Augment the Qi and raise the Yang
    c. Promote the discharge of pus and generate flesh
    d. None of the above

923. Gan Cao and Da Zao each perform which of the following functions?
    a. Tonify the Middle Energizer and augment the Qi; moderate and harmonize the harsh properties of other herbs
    b. Nourish the Blood and calm the Spirit
    c. Moisten the Lungs and stop coughing
    d. None of the above

924. Sha Shen and Mai Men Dong each perform which of the following functions?
    a. Nourish the Stomach and generate fluids
    b. Nourish the Liver and Kidney
    c. Clear the Heart and eliminate irritability
    d. Moisten the Intestines

925. Yu Zhu and Sha Shen each perform which of the following functions?
    a. Clear Heart Heat and Lung Heat
    b. Nourish the Yin of the Lungs and Stomach
    c. Clear Fire from the Liver and Gallbladder
    d. Tonify the Yin of the Liver and Kidneys

926. Xu Duan and Du Zhong each perform which of the following functions?
    a. Tonify the Liver and Kidneys and strengthen the sinews and bones
    b. Tonify the Liver and Kidneys and expel Wind-Damp
    c. Promote the movement of Blood
    d. None of the above

927. Which pair lists two herbs that tonify the Kidneys, strengthen the Yang, and moisten the Intestines?
    a. Sha Yuan Zi and Yin Yang Huo
    b. Bu Gu Zhi and Sang Ji Sheng
    c. Rou Cong Rong and Hu Tao Ren
    d. Xian Mao and Ba Ji Tian

928. Which two herbs each tonify the Yang and promote the movement of Blood?
    a. Bu Gu Zhi and Suo Yang
    b. Du Zhong and Rou Cong Rong
    c. Gou Ji and Tu Si Zi
    d. Gu Sui Bu and Xu Duan

929. Yin Yang Huo and Xian Mao each perform which of the following functions?
    a. Tonify the Spleen and augment the Qi
    b. Nourish the Kidney Yin
    c. Strengthen the sinews and bones
    d. Tonify the Kidneys and fortify the Yang

930. Ge Jie and Hu Tao Ren each perform which of the following functions?
    a. Tonify the Spleen and Lungs and promote the fluids
    b. Tonify the Spleen and Heart and moisten the Intestines
    c. Tonify the Spleen, nourish the Blood, and stop bleeding
    d. Tonify the Lungs, assist the Kidneys, and relieve asthma

931. Sha Yuan Zi and Tu Si Zi each perform which of the following functions?
    a. Benefit the Spleen and stop diarrhea
    b. Moisten the Intestines
    c. Nourish the Liver and secures the Essence
    d. Moisten the Lungs and stop coughing

932. Which herb cools the Blood, stops bleeding, and nourishes the Yin?
    a. E Jiao
    b. Nu Zhen Zi
    c. Han Lian Cao
    d. Gou Qi Zi

933. Which herb tonifies the Yang and stops diarrhea?
    a. Rou Cong Rong
    b. Suo Yang
    c. Gou Ji
    d. Bu Gu Zhi

934. Which of the following does *not* treat Deficiency-Wind stirring in the Interior?
    a. Long Gu
    b. Mu Li
    c. Gui Ban
    d. Bia Jia

935. Which of the following is *not* derived from Si Jun Zi Tang?
    a. Shen Ling Bai Zhu San
    b. Xiang Sha Liu Jun Zi Tang
    c. Bu Zhong Yi Qi Tang
    d. Yi Gong San

936. Which formula augments the Qi, strengthens the Spleen, leaches out Damp, and stops diarrhea?
    a. Si Jun Zi Tang
    b. Ping Wei San
    c. Shen Su Yin
    d. Shen Ling Bai Zhu San

937. Shen Ling Bai Zhu San is *not* indicated for which of the following?
    a. Distention with a stifling sensation in the chest and epigastrium
    b. Reduced appetite and loose stools
    c. Weakness of the extremities
    d. Irritability and insomnia

938. Bu Zhong Yi Qi Tang does *not* contain which of the following?
    a. Ren Shen, Huang Qi, and Sheng Ma
    b. Bai Zhu, Zhi Gan Cao, and Chai Hu
    c. Fu Ling and Sha Ren
    d. Dang Gui and Chen Pi

939. Which formula treats stagnation of Damp and Deficient Spleen?
    a. Bu Zhong Yi Qi Tang
    b. Si Jun Zi Tang
    c. Shen Ling Bai Zhu Sang
    d. Liu Jun Zi Tang

940. Which formula would you select to treat this pattern: spontaneous sweating, intermittent fever, thirst for warm beverages, laconic speech, shortness of breath, pale complexion, loose and watery stool, pale tongue with thin white fur, flooding-deficient pulse?
    a. Sheng Xian Tang
    b. Shen Ling Bai Zhu San
    c. Bu Zhong Yi Qi Tang
    d. Ju Yuan Jian

941. Shen Mai San does *not* contain which of the following?
    a. Sheng Di Huang
    b. Wu Wei Zi
    c. Mai Men Dong
    d. Ren Shen

942. Which herb is added to Bu Zhong Yi Qi Tang to strengthen its ability to treat collapse of Middle Energizer Qi and visceral prolapse?
    a. Chuan Xiong
    b. Fang Feng
    c. Ge Gen
    d. Zhi Ke

943. Sheng Mai San does *not* perform which of the following functions?
    a. Augment the Qi and generate the fluids
    b. Preserve the Yin
    c. Stop excessive sweating
    d. Nourish the Liver Blood

944. Which formula treats chronic cough injuring the Lungs with concurrent Deficient Qi and Deficient Yin?
    a. Mai Men Dong Tang
    b. Sheng Mai San
    c. Shen Ling Bai Zhu San
    d. Bai He Gu Jin Tang

945. Ren Shen Ge Jie San is *not* indicated for which of the following?
    a. Coughing and wheezing with thick yellow sputum
    b. Coughing of pus and blood with a sensation of Heat and irritability in the chest
    c. Dry throat with thirst
    d. Facial edema and gradual emaciation

946. Si Wu Tang is *not* derived from which of the following formulas?
    a. Ba Zhen Tang
    b. Tao Hong Si Wu Tang
    c. Jiao E Ai Tang
    d. Shi Quan Da Bu Tang

947. Si Wu Tang is *not* indicated for which of the following?
    a. Impairment of the Chong and Ren meridians with irregular menstruation
    b. Impairment of the Chong and Ren meridians with amenorrhea
    c. Impairment of the Chong and Ren meridians with restless fetus disorder
    d. Impairment of the Chong and Ren meridians with excessive leucorrhea

948. What is the ratio of Huang Qi to Dang Gui in the formula Dang Gui Bu Xue Tang?
    a. 5:1
    b. 5:2
    c. 5:3
    d. 5:4

949. Dang Gui Bu Xue Tang is *not* indicated for which of the following?
    a. A sensation of Heat in the muscles and a red face
    b. Thirst with a preference for warm beverages
    c. A full-large pulse or a slippery-strong pulse
    d. Fever and headache caused by loss of Blood

950. Which formula does *not* contain both Dang Gui and Chuan Xiong?
    a. Si Wu Tang
    b. Gui Pi Tang
    c. Wen Jing Tang
    d. Du Huo Ji Sheng Tang

951. Si Jun Zi Tang with Gui Pi Tang added does *not* contain which of the following?
    a. Dang Gui and Huang Qi
    b. Mu Xiong and Yuan Zhi
    c. Suan Zao Ren and Long Yan Rou
    d. Gui Zhi and Da Zao

952. Gui Pi Tang does *not* perform which of the following functions?
    a. Augment the Qi and tonify the Blood
    b. Stop diarrhea
    c. Strengthen the Spleen
    d. Nourish the Heart

953. Zhi Gan Cao Tang does *not* contain which of the following?
    a. Huang Qi and Bai Shao
    b. Ren Shen and Gui Zi
    c. Sheng Di, Mai Men Dong, and Da Zao
    d. E Jiao, Huo Ma Ren, and Sheng Jiang

954. Gui Pi Tang is *not* indicated for which of the following?
    a. Forgetfulness and palpitations
    b. Insomnia and dream-disturbed sleep
    c. Anxiety, phobia, feverishness, and withdrawal
    d. An uncoated tongue accompanied by dryness in the mouth and throat

955. Which herb has the largest dosage in Zhi Gan Cao Tang?
    a. Ren Shen
    b. Zhi Gan Cao
    c. Sheng Di Huang
    d. E Jiao

956. What is the main indication for the use of Zhi Gan Cao Tang?
    a. Severe palpitation
    b. Irritability and insomnia
    c. A pale, shiny tongue
    d. Emaciation and shortness of breath

957. Jia Jian Fu Mai Tang can be produced by adapting Zhi Gan Cao Tang in which way?
    a. Add Bai Shao; subtract Ren Shen, Gui Zhi, Sheng Jiang, Da Zao, and wine
    b. Add Bai Shao; subtract Ren Shen, Gui Zhi, E Jiao, Da Zao, and wine
    c. Add Bai Shao; subtract Ren Shen, Gui Zhi, Huo Ma Ren, Da Zao, and wine
    d. Add Bai Shao; subtract Ren Shen, Gui Zhi, Mai Men Dong, Da Zao, and wine

958. Ba Zhen Tang is *not* indicated for which of the following?
    a. Dizziness or vertigo
    b. Easily fatigued extremities and shortness of breath
    c. Palpitations
    d. Thin and rapid pulse

959. Which of the following functions do Shi Quan Da Bu Tang and Ren Shen Yang Ying Tang *not* have in common?
    a. Regulate the Qi and strengthen the Spleen
    b. Tonify the Blood
    c. Nourish the Heart and tranquilize
    d. Tonify the Spleen and drain Damp

960. Tai Shan Pan Shi San can be created by adapting Shi Quan Da Bu Tang in which of the following ways?
    a. Subtract Rou Gui and Fu Ling; add Xu Duan, Huang Qin, Sha Ren, and Nuo Mi
    b. Subtract Rou Gui and Fu Ling; add Xu Duan, Du Zhong, Sha Ren, and Nuo Mi
    c. Subtract Rou Gui and Fu Ling; add Xu Duan, E Jiao, Sha Ren, and Nuo Mi
    d. Subtract Rou Gui and Fu Ling; add Xu Duan, Sang Ji Sheng, Sha Ren, and Nuo Mi

961. Which formula augments the Qi, nourishes the Blood, calms the fetus, and is indicated for pregnant women with Deficient Qi and Blood, restless fetus, pale face, fatigue, and loss of appetite?
    a. Jiao E Tang
    b. Ba Zhen Tang
    c. Tai Shen Pan Shi San
    d. Wen Jing Tang

962. Which formula is derived from Liu Wei Di Huang Wan?
    a. Zuo Gui Wan
    b. You Gui Wan
    c. Da Bu Yin Wan
    d. Jin Gui Shen Qi Wan

963. Liu Wei Di Huang Wan is *not* indicated for which of the following?
    a. Soreness and weakness of the lower back, night sweats, and nocturnal emissions
    b. Light headedness, vertigo, tinnitus,, and diminished hearing
    c. Dryness of the eyes and blurry or diminished vision
    d. Hot palms and soles with hectic fever

964. Which of the following formulas is *not* derived from Liu Wei Di Huang Wan?
    a. Du Qi Wan
    b. Zuo Gui Wan
    c. Zhi Bai Di Huang Wan
    d. Qi Ju Di Huang Wan

965. Which formula treats chronic wheezing and hiccups caused by Deficient Kidney Yin?
    a. Zhi Bai Di Huang Wan
    b. Du Qi Wan
    c. Qi Ju Di Huang Wan
    d. Er Long Zuo Ci Wan

966. Zuo Gui Yin can be produced by adapting Liu Wei Di Huang Wan in which of the following ways?
    a. Remove Ze Xie and Mu Dan Pi; add Tu Si Zi and Gan Cao
    b. Remove Ze Xie and Mu Dan Pi; add Gou Qi Zi and Zhi Gan Cao
    c. Remove Ze Xie and Mu Dan Pi; add Nu Zhen Zi and Zhi Gan Cao
    d. Remove Ze Xie and Mu Dan Pi; add Gui Jiao and Zhi Gan Cao

967. Which formula would you select to treat this pattern: light-headedness, vertigo, tinnitus, soreness and weakness of the lower back and legs, nocturnal emissions, spontaneous night sweats, dry mouth and throat, shiny tongue, thin-rapid pulse?
    a. Shi Bai Di Huang Wan
    b. Qi Ju Di Huang Wan
    c. Zuo Gui Wan
    d. Er Zhi Wan

968. Da Bu Yin Wan does *not* contain which of the following?
    a. Shu Di Huang
    b. Shan Yu Rou
    c. Gui Ban
    d. Huang Bai and Zhi Mu

969. Da Bu Yin Wan performs which of the following functions?
    a. Tonify the Kidney Yin
    b. Strengthen the Liver and Kidneys
    c. Enrich the Yin cause the Fire to descend
    d. None of the above

970. Da Bu Yin Wan is *not* indicated for which of the following?
    a. Steaming bone disorder with afternoon tidal fever, night sweats, and spontaneous emissions
    b. Irritability and coughing of blood
    c. A sensation of Heat and pain or weakness in the knees and legs
    d. A thin and weak pulse

971. Which formula would you select to treat this pattern: weakness of the lower back and knees, deterioration of the sinews and bones with general reduction in function, wasting of the muscles of the legs and feet, difficulty in walking, red tongue with little fur, thin-weak pulse?
    a. Jin Gui Shen Qi Wan
    b. Zuo Gui Wan
    c. Er Zhi Wan
    d. Hu Qian Wan

972. Which statement regarding the herbs in Hu Qian Wan is false?
    a. Huang Bai and Zhi Mu drain Fire and clear Heat
    b. Shu Di, Gui Ban, and Bai Shao enrich the Yin and nourish the Blood
    c. Suo Yang warms the Yang and benefits the Essence
    d. Chen Pi and Gan Jiang warm the Middle Energizer, expel Cold, dry Damp, and dissipate Phlegm

973. Liu Wei Di Huang Wan is *not* indicated for which of the following?
    a. Weakness and soreness of the lower back and knees
    b. Spontaneous emission
    c. Premature graying or loss of hair
    d. Dryness of the throat

974. Yi Guan Jian does *not* contain which of the following?
    a. Gou Qi Zi and Sheng Di Huang
    b. Gou Ji and Bai Shao
    c. Sha Shen and Mai Men Dong
    d. Dang Gui and Chuan Lian Zi

975. Yi Guan Jian is *not* indicated for which of the following?
    a. Hypochondriac and chest pain with acid regurgitation
    b. A dry, parched mouth and throat with a red and dry tongue
    c. A thin and frail or wiry pulse
    d. Soreness and weakness in the lower back, spontaneous nocturnal emissions, and night sweats

976. Which formula does *not* strengthen the Yin and the Yang?
    a. Jin Gui Shen Qi Wan
    b. You Gui Wan
    c. Gui Lu Er Xian Jiao
    d. Yi Guan Jian

977. Shi Hu Ye Guan Wan does *not* perform which of the following functions?
    a. Extinguish Liver Wind
    b. Enrich the Yin
    c. Clear Liver Fire
    d. Improve the vision

978. Shi Hu Ye Guan Wan is *not* indicated for which of the following?
    a. Enlarged pupils and blurred vision
    b. Photophobia and excessive tearing
    c. Conjunctivitis and itching of the eye
    d. Light headedness and vertigo

979. Bu Fei E Jiao Tang does *not* contain which of the following?
    a. E Jiao
    b. Bai Shao
    c. Ma Dou Ling and Xing Ren
    d. Niu Bang Zi, Geng Mi, and Zhi Gan Cao

980. Which of the following indications do Bu Fei E Jiao Tang and Bai He Gu Jin Tang *not* have in common?
    a. A floating, thin, and rapid pulse.
    b. Coughing with blood-streaked sputum and wheezing
    c. A dry and sore throat
    d. A red tongue with little fur

981. Gui Lu Er Xian Jiao does *not* perform which of the following functions?
    a. Nourish and replenish the Yin
    b. Tonify the Essence
    c. Augment the Qi and strengthen the Yang
    d. Tonify the Spleen and warm the Kidney Yang

982. Which formula treats Deficient Yin and Deficient Yang of the Kidneys as well as Deficient Essence and Deficient Blood of the Ren and Du meridians?
    a. Gui Lu Er Xian Jiao
    b. Hu Qian Wan
    c. Qi Bao Mei Ran Dan
    d. None of the above

983. Qi Bao Mei Ran Dan does *not* contain which of the following?
    a. Shu Di Huang
    b. He Shou Wu and Fu Ling
    c. Niu Xi and Dang Gui
    d. Gou Qi Zi, Tu Si Zi, and Bu Bu Zhi

984. Qi Bao Mei Ran Dan and Liu Wei Di Huang Wan both treat soreness and weakness of the lower back and spontaneous and nocturnal emissions. What is an additional indication for Qi Bao Mei Ran Dan?
    a. Coughing with blood-streaked sputum
    b. Blurred vision
    c. Wasting of the muscles of the legs and feet with difficulty walking
    d. Premature graying of the hair and loose teeth

985. Jin Gui Shen Qi Wan performs which of the following functions?
    a. Tonify the Liver and Kidney
    b. Strengthen the Kidney Essence
    c. Warm and tonify the Kidney Yang
    d. Enrich the Kidney Yin

986. Gui Zhi and Fu Zi perform which of the following functions in Jin Gui Shen Qi Wan?
    a. Dispel Cold and eliminate Damp
    b. Warm the meridians and unblock the vessels
    c. Assist the Kidney Yang and enhance the metabolism of water
    d. None of the above

987. What is added to Jin Gui Shen Qi Wan to produce Ji Sheng Shen Qi Wan?
    a. Chuan Niu Xi and Che Qian Zi
    b. Chuan Niu Xi and Mu Tong
    c. Chuan Niu Xi and Zhu Ling
    d. Chuan Niu Xi and Tong Cao

988. Ji Sheng Shen Qi Wan and Jin Gui Shen Qi Wan both are used to warm and tonify the Kidney Yang. What is an additional function of Ji Sheng Shen Qi Wan?
    a. Warm the Spleen and stop diarrhea
    b. Warm the meridians and unblock the vessels
    c. Nourish the Blood and Essence
    d. Promote urination and reduce edema

989. Which formula warms and tonifies Kidney Yang, replenishes the Essence, and tonifies the Blood?
    a. Jin Gui Shen Qi Wan
    b. You Gui Wan
    c. Tu Su Zi Wan
    d. Zan You Dan

990. You Gui Wan is *not* indicated for which of the following?
    a. Exhaustion from long-term illness, aversion to Cold, and coolness of the extremities
    b. Impotence and spermatorrhea
    c. Incontinence and edema of the lower extremities
    d. Pain in the heels

991. Which herb stops diarrhea and generates fluids?
    a. Wu Bei Zi
    b. Rou Dou Kou
    c. He Zi
    d. Wu Mei

992. Which herb inhibits the leakage of the Lungs, binds up the Intestines, generates fluids, and expels roundworms?
    a. Shi Jun Zi
    b. Wu Bei Zi
    c. Wu Wei Zi
    d. Wu Mei

993. What is Wu Wei Zi used to treat?
    a. Chronic cough caused by Deficient Lung
    b. Coughing caused by Lung Dry
    c. Coughing caused by Lung Heat
    d. Coughing caused by Lung Cold

994. Wu Bei Zi does *not* perform which of the following functions?
    a. Contain the leakage of the Lungs and clear Heat
    b. Bind up the Intestines
    c. Preserve and restrain
    d. Hold in urine

995. Which herb contains the leakage of the Lungs, stops coughing and wheezing, binds up the Essence, inhibits sweating, and quiets the Spirit?
    a. Wu Bei Zi
    b. Bai Zi Ren
    c. Suan Zao Ren
    d. Wu Wei Zi

996. Which herb clears Heat, dries Damp, binds up the Intestines, stops bleeding, and kills parasites?
    a. Qian Shi
    b. Huang Bai
    c. Ku Shen
    d. Chun Pi

997. Which herb treats chronic cough, wheezing caused by Deficient Lungs, and loss of voice?
    a. Wu Mei
    b. Wu Bei Zi
    c. Wu Wei Zi
    d. He Zi

998. Which herb treats chronic diarrhea, rectal prolapse, and dysenteric disorders?
    a. Rou Dou Kou
    b. Wu Wei Zi
    c. Bai Zhu
    d. He Zi

999. Which herb warms the Middle Energizer, moves the Qi, binds up the Intestines, and stops diarrhea?
    a. He Zi
    b. Rou Dou Kou
    c. Chun Pi
    d. Cao Gua

1000. Which herb alleviates pain, contains the leakage of the Lungs, and binds up the Intestines?
   a. Wu Wi Zi
   b. He Zi
   c. Ying Su Ke
   d. Mu Xiang

1001. Which herb tonifies the Spleen, stops diarrhea, tonifies the Kidneys, and stabilizes the Essence?
   a. Jin Ying Zi
   b. Shan Yu Rou
   c. Bai Zhu
   d. Lian Zi

1002. Which herb tonifies the Spleen, expels Damp, stabilizes the Kidneys, and retains the Essence?
   a. Jin Ying Zi
   b. He Zi
   c. Sang Piao Xioa
   d. Qian Shi

1003. Which herb treats impotence caused by Deficient Yin of the Liver and Kidneys?
   a. Ba Ji Tian
   b. Nu Zhen Zi
   c. Shan Yu Rou
   d. Shu Di Huang

1004. Which herb treats spermatorrhea, excessive urination, and excessive sweating?
   a. Yi Zhi Ren
   b. Fu Pen Zi
   c. Shan Yu Rou
   d. Jin Ying Zi

1005. Which herb tonifies the Kidneys, assists the Yang, retains Essence, and restrains urine?
   a. Bai Guo
   b. Shan Yu Rou
   c. Wu Wei Zi
   d. Sang Piao Xiao

1006. Hai Piao Xiao does *not* perform which of the following functions?
   a. Control acidity and alleviate pain
   b. Retain Essence
   c. Resolve Damp and promote healing
   d. Stop sweating

1007. Which three herbs each bind up the Intestines and stop diarrhea?
   a. He Zi, Wu Wei Zi, and Fu Pen Zi
   b. He Zi, Chi Shi Zhi, and Rou Dou Kou
   c. He Zi, Wu Mei, and Shan Zhu Yu
   d. He Zi, Wu Bei Zi, and Qian Shi

1008. Which two herbs each astringe and stop sweating?
   a. Wu Wei Zi and Jin Ying Zi
   b. Wu Wei Zi and Wu Mei
   c. Wu Wei Zi and Ma Huang Gen
   d. Wu Wei Zi and Shi Liu Pi

1009. Which two herbs each bind up the Intestines, stop diarrhea, astringe, and stop bleeding?
    a. Chi Shi Zhi and Wu Wei Zi
    b. Hi Zi and Wu Bei Zi
    c. Chi Shi Zhi and Wu Mei
    d. Chi Shi Zhi and Rou Dou Kou

1010. Which two herbs each generate fluids and alleviate thirst?
    a. Wu Wei Zi and Wu Bei Zi
    b. Wu Wei Zi and Liou Zi
    c. Wu Wei Zi and Wu Mei
    d. Wu Wei Zi and Shan Yu Rou

1011. Chun Pi and Shi Liu Pi each perform which of the following functions?
    a. Clear Heat and dry Damp
    b. Promote urination and expel swelling
    c. Expel Phlegm and stop wheezing
    d. Bind up the Intestines and stop diarrhea

1012. Wu Wei Zi and Wu Bei Zi each perform which of the following functions?
    a. Tonify Qi and generate fluids
    b. Clear Lung Fire
    c. Quiet the Spirit and calm the Heart
    d. Contain the leakage of the Lungs and inhibit sweating

1013. Which two herbs each tonify the Spleen and Kidneys and stabilize Essence?
    a. Lian Zi and Wu Mei
    b. Lian Zi and Fu Pen Zi
    c. Lian Zi and Qian Shi
    d. Lian Zi and Fu Xiao Ma

1014. Which of the following would you treat with formulas that stabilize and bind?
    a. Sweating caused by Heat
    b. Metrorrhagia caused by Blood Heat
    c. Chronic cough caused by Deficient Lung
    d. Diarrhea caused by food stagnation

1015. Yu Ping Feng San does *not* contain which of the following?
    a. Huang Qi
    b. Fu Xiao Mai
    c. Bai Zhu
    d. Fang Feng

1016. Yu Ping Feng San is *not* indicated for which of the following?
    a. Spontaneous sweating caused by superficial Deficiency
    b. Aversion to drafts
    c. A shiny pale complexion
    d. Fever caused by Yin deficiency

1017. Yu Ping Feng San does *not* perform which of the following functions?
    a. Enrich the Yang
    b. Augment the Qi
    c. Stop sweating
    d. Stabilize the Exterior

1018. Mu Li San does *not* contain which of the following?
   a. Gan Cao
   b. Huang Qi
   c. Mu Li
   d. Ma Huang Gen

1019. Which formula would you select to stabilize the Exterior and inhibit sweating?
   a. Dang Gui Liu Huang Tang
   b. Gui Zhi Tang
   c. Gui Zhi Jia Long Gu Mu Li Tang
   d. Mu Li San

1020. In which of the formulas below does Huang Qi *not* serve as the chief (monarch or *jun*) component?
   a. Bu Zhong Yi Qi Tang
   b. Dang Gui Bu Xue Tang
   c. Gui Pi Tang
   d. Mu Li San

1021. Which formula treats the following pattern: spontaneous sweating that worsens at night, palpitations, shortness of breath, irritability, debility, lethargy, pale red tongue, thin-frail pulse?
   a. Gui Zhi Tang
   b. Yu Ping Fang San
   c. Qing Hao Bie Jia Tang
   d. Mu Li San

1022. Which statement regarding the herbs in Mu Li San is *false*?
   a. Mu Li is used to benefit the Yin, anchor the floating Yang, inhibit sweating, and relieve irritability
   b. Huang Qi is used to tonify the Qi, stabilize the Exterior, and inhibit sweating
   c. Ma Huang Gen is used to restrain sweating
   d. Huang Qi and Fu Xiao Mai are used to tonify the Qi of the Lungs and Spleen

1023. Which formula preserves the Lungs, stops coughing, augments the Qi, and nourishes the Yin?
   a. Sheng Mai San
   b. Ren Shen Hu Tao Tang
   c. Bai He Gu Jing Tang
   d. Jiu Xian San

1024. Jiu Xian San is *not* indicated for which of the following?
   a. Chronic, unremitting cough
   b. Spontaneous sweating
   c. Abundant expectoration
   d. A deficient, rapid pulse

1025. Which pathogenesis is *not* associated with ailments treated with Jiu Xian San?
   a. Lung Qi deficiency
   b. Lung Yin deficiency
   c. Deficiency of the Lungs and Kidneys
   d. Asthenic fever of the Interior

1026. Zhen Ren Yang Zang Tang does *not* contain which of the following?
   a. Fu Ling and Yi Yi Ren
   b. Ren Shen, Bai Zhu, and Dang Gui
   c. Rou Gui, Rou Dou Kou, and Gan Cao
   d. He Zi, Ying Su Ke, Bai Shao, and Mu Xiang

1027. Zhen Ren Yang Zang Tang does *not* perform which of the following functions?
   a. Restrain leakage from the Intestines and stop diarrhea
   b. Warm the Middle Energizer
   c. Tonify the spleen and Kidneys
   d. Promote the movement of Qi

1028. Zhen Ren Yang Zang Tang is *not* indicated for which of the following?
   a. Chronic diarrhea
   b. Abdominal pain that responds favorably to local pressure or warmth
   c. Epigastric distending pain
   d. Reduced appetite and prolapsed rectum

1029. What is the pathogenesis of the type of diarrhea you would treat with Zhen Ren Yang Zang Tang?
   a. The spleen and Kidneys are unable to restrain leakage from the intestine caused by Deficiency-Cold
   b. Cold in the spleen caused by deficiency of Kidney Yang
   c. The spleen and Stomach are unable to transport caused by Deficiency-Cold
   d. None of the above

1030. What would *not* be a recommended adaptation of Zhen Ren Yang Zang Tang?
   a. For chronic diarrhea and incontinence, add Bu Gu Zhi
   b. For heavy abdominal pain, double the dosage of Bai Shao
   c. For general debility, lethargy, and reduced appetite, add Ji Nei Jin and Shan Zha
   d. For prolapsed rectum and severe diarrhea, add Pao Fu Zi

1031. Which formula would you select to treat a case of Deficient Yang of the Spleen and Kidneys that involves daily occurrences of diarrhea just before sunrise?
   a. Zhen Ren Yang Zang Tang
   b. Tao Hua Tang
   c. Si Shen Wan
   d. Li Zhong Wan

1032. Si Shen Wan does *not* contain which of the following?
   a. Bu Gu Zhi
   b. Xiao Hui Xiang
   c. Wu Zhu Yu
   d. Rou Dou Kou and Wu Wei Zi

1033. Si Shen Wan does *not* perform which of the following functions?
   a. Warm and tonify the Spleen and Kidneys
   b. Transform Damp Cold
   c. Bind up the Intestines
   d. Stop diarrhea

1034. Bu Gu Zhi performs which of the following functions in Si Shen Wan?
   a. Warm the Spleen and Stomach, bind up the Intestines, and stop diarrhea
   b. Warm and tonify Kidney Yang, bind up the Intestines, and stop diarrhea
   c. Tonify the gate of vitality, and warm and nourish Spleen Yang
   d. None of the above

1035. Which herb would you add to Si Shen Wan to treat a case of diarrhea that occurs regularly just before sunrise and involves chronic prolapse of the rectum?
   a. Fu Zi
   b. Huang Qi and Sheng Ma
   c. Rou Gui
   d. Chai Hu and Xi Xin

1036. Tao Hua Tang does *not* contain which of the following?
    a. Sheng Jiang
    b. Chi Shi Zhi
    c. Gan Jiang
    d. Gen Mi

1037. Which formula would you select to treat this chronic dysentery pattern: dark blood and pus in the stool, abdominal pain that responds favorably to local pressure or warmth, pale tongue, slow-frail or faint-thin pulse?
    a. Li Zhong Wan
    b. Huang Tu Tang
    c. Tao Hua Tang
    d. Huai Hua San

1038. Jin Suo Gu Jing Wan does *not* contain which of the following?
    a. Sang Piao Xiao and Wu Wei Zi
    b. Qian Shi and Lian Xu
    c. Sha Yuan Ji Li and Duan Mu Li
    d. Long Gu and Lian Rou

1039. Which herb serves as the chief (monarch or *jun*) component in Jin Suo Gu Jing Wan?
    a. Long Gu
    b. Qian Shi
    c. Lian Xu
    d. None of the above

1040. Jin Suo Gu Jing Wan is *not* indicated for which of the following?
    a. Hectic fever and night sweating
    b. Chronic spermatorrhea and impotence
    c. Fatigue and weakness accompanied by sore and weak limbs
    d. Lower back pain with tinnitus

1041. Which formula regulates and tonifies the Heart and Kidneys, stabilizes Essence, and stops leakage?
    a. Jin Suo Gu Jing Wan
    b. Suo Quan Wan
    c. Tian Wang Bu Xin Dan
    d. Sang Piao Xiao San

1042. Which herb is *not* part of the formula for Suo Quan Wan?
    a. Gou Ji
    b. Shan Yao
    c. Wu Yao
    d. Yi Zhi Ren

1043. Which formula treats frequent, clear, prolonged urination caused by Deficiency-Cold of the Kidneys?
    a. Sang Piao Xiao San
    b. Jin Suo Gu Jing Wan
    c. Shui Lu Er Xian Dan
    d. Suo Quan Wan

1044. Which formula would you select to treat this pattern: frequent urination, spermatorrhea, disorientation, forgetfulness, pale tongue?
    a. Suo Quan Wan
    b. Jin Suo Gu Jing Wan
    c. Shui Lu Er Xian Dan
    d. Sang Piao Xiao San

1045. Gu Jing Wan does *not* contain which of the following?
   a. Bie Jia and Nu Zhen Zi
   b. Gui Ban and Bai Shao
   c. Huang Bai and Huang Qin
   d. Chun Gen Pi and Xiang Fu

1046. Gu Jing Wan does *not* perform which of the following functions?
   a. Tonify the Spleen Qi
   b. Enrich the Yin and clear Heat
   c. Stop bleeding
   d. Stabilize the menses

1047. Which formula *best* treats Deficient Spleen that leads to the inability of the Spleen to govern Blood, and also treats instability of the Chong meridian leading to profuse menstrual bleeding?
   a. Gui Pi Wan
   b. Wen Jing Tang
   c. Bu Zhong Yi Qi Tang
   d. Gu Chong Tang

1048. Which formula would you select to treat this pattern: continuous uterine bleeding caused by Cold that results from Deficiency of the Chong and Ren channels and Blood Stasis in the Lower Energizer?
   a. Gu Jing Wan
   b. Gu Chong Tang
   c. Zhen Ling Dan
   d. None of the above

1049. Which herbs in Zhen Ling Dan are used to invigorate the Blood?
   a. Ru Xiang, Mo Yao, and Tao Ren
   b. Ru Xiang, Mo Yao, and Chi Shao
   c. Ru Xiang, Mo Yao, and Hong Hua
   d. Ru Xiang, Mo Yao, and Wu Ling Zhi

1050. Wan Dai Tang does *not* contain which of the following?
   a. Huang Qi, Long Gu, and Dang Gui
   b. Bai Zhu, Shan Yao, and Ren Shen
   c. Cang Zhu, Chen Pi, and Che Qian Zi
   d. Bai Shao, Chai Hu, Jie Su Tan, and Gan Cao

1051. Wan Dai Tang does *not* perform which of the following functions?
   a. Tonify the Qi and clear Heat
   b. Tonify the Middle Energizer
   c. Strengthen the Spleen and transform Damp
   d. Stop vaginal discharge

1052. Which pattern would you treat with Qing Dai Tang?
   a. Deficient Spleen, continuous vaginal discharge that is thin and clear or red
   b. Deficient Spleen, continuous vaginal discharge, Damp-Heat
   c. Deficient Kidney Yang, inability of the Dai meridian to control, continuous vaginal discharge
   d. Deficient Kidney Qi, inability of the Ren meridian to stabilize, continuous vaginal discharge

1053. Wan Dai Tang is *not* indicated for which of the following?
   a. Profuse vaginal discharge that is white or pale yellow in color and has a thin consistency
   b. Pale complexion
   c. Loose stool, fatigue, lethargy
   d. Thin-wiry pulse

1054. Zhu Sha does *not* perform which of the following functions?
    a. Nourish the Heart and calm the Spirit
    b. Clear Heat
    c. Relieve toxicity
    d. Sedate the Heart and calm the Spirit

1055. Which of the following indicates the use of Zhu Sha?
    a. Deficient Heart Blood with disturbed Spirit
    b. Deficient Heart Qi
    c. Excessive Heart Fire
    d. Imbalance between Heart Yang and Kidney Yin

1056. Ci Shi does *not* perform which of the following functions?
    a. Anchor and calm the Spirit
    b. Clear the Heart and calm the Spirit
    c. Improve hearing and vision
    d. Aid in grasping the Qi and in the treatment of asthma

1057. Which herb clears Heat, relieves toxicity, sedates the Heart, and calms the Spirit?
    a. Ci Shi
    b. Long Gu
    c. Hu Po
    d. Zhu Sha

1058. Which of the following indicates Ci Shi?
    a. Coughing or asthma caused by inhibited Lung Qi
    b. Deficiency coughing caused by insufficiency of Lung Qi
    c. Chronic asthma caused by inability of the Kidneys to grasp Qi
    d. None of the above

1059. Which herb arrests tremors, calms the Spirit, invigorates the Blood, dissipates stasis, promotes urination, and reduces swelling?
    a. Ci Shi
    b. Hua Rai Shi
    c. Shi Wei
    d. Hu Po

1060. Which of the following indicates the use of Hu Po?
    a. Stranguria caused by disorder of Qi
    b. Stranguria complicated by hematuria
    c. Stranguria caused by urinary stone
    d. Stranguria caused by Heat evil

1061. Which herb treats palpitations, insomnia, irritability, anxiety, dreaminess, amnesia, and hyperhidrosis?
    a. Zhu Sha
    b. Bai Zi Ren
    c. Suan Zao Ren
    d. Yuan Zhi

1062. Which herb nourishes the Heart, calms the Spirit, moistens the Intestines, and unblocks the bowels?
    a. Yuan Zhi
    b. Bai Zi Ren
    c. Suan Zao Ren
    d. Long Gu

1063. Which herb astringes sweating, nourishes the Heart, and calms the Spirit?
    a. Long Gu
    b. Ma Huang Gen
    c. Suan Zao Ren
    d. Mu Li

1064. Which herb treats Phlegm enveloping the orifices of the Heart that is manifested by emotional and mental disorientation or seizures?
    a. Suan Zao Ren
    b. Bai Zi Ren
    c. Hu Po
    d. Yuan Zhi

1065. Which herb quiets the Heart, calms the Spirit, expels Phlegm, clears the orifices, reduces abscesses, and dissipates swelling?
    a. He Huan Pi
    b. Yu Jin
    c. Yuan Zhi
    d. Shi Chang Pu

1066. He Huan Pi does *not* perform which of the following functions?
    a. Promote urination and dissipate swelling
    b. Calm the Spirit
    c. Relieve constraint
    d. Invigorate the Blood and dissipate swelling

1067. Which herb functions like Long Gu, yet also benefits the Yin, softens hardness, and dissipates nodules?
    a. Ci Shi
    b. Mu Li
    c. Shi Jue Ming
    d. Zhu Sha

1068. Which herb is *not* used to sedate the Heart and calm the Spirit?
    a. Zhu Sha
    b. Zhen Zhu
    c. Suan Zao Ren
    d. Zi Shi Ying

1069. How is Hu Po prepared?
    a. Cooked before other ingredients
    b. Cooked after other ingredients
    c. Taken in powder or pill form, not in decoction
    d. None of the above

1070. Zhu Sha An Shen Wan does *not* contain which of the following?
    a. Fu Shen
    b. Zhu Sha
    c. Huang Lian and Dang Gui
    d. Sheng Di Huang and Zhi Gan Cao

1071. Which formula contains Shu Di Huang and Chen Xiang
    a. Tian Wang Bu Xin Dan
    b. Ci Zhu Wan
    c. Zhu Sha An Shen Wan
    d. Zhen Zhu Mu Wan

1072. Which formula would you select to treat this pattern: irritability, restless sleep, occasional palpitations, anxiety, dizziness, thin-wiry pulse?
    a. Ci Zhu Wan
    b. Zhu Sha An Shen Wan
    c. Zhen Zhu Mu Wan
    d. Sheng Tie Luo Yin

1073. Which formula treats the following pattern: insomnia, continuous palpitations, a hot irritable sensation in the chest, red tongue, thin-rapid pulse?
    a. Tian Wang Bu Xin Dan
    b. Gui Pi Tang
    c. Ci Zhu Wan
    d. Zhu Sha An Shen Wan

1074. Which formula sedates the Heart, calms the Spirit, drains Fire, and nourishes the Yin?
    a. Zhen Zhu Mu Wan
    b. Tian Wang Bu Xin Dan
    c. Gan Mai Da Zao Tang
    d. Zhu Sha An Shen Wan

1075. Which statement about the herbs in Zhu Sha An Shen Wan is false?
    a. Zhu Sha nourishes Kidney Yin to calm the Spirit
    b. Huang Lian clears the Heart to relieve irritability
    c. Dang Gui nourishes the Blood
    d. Sheng Di Huang nourishes Yin, and in combination with Dang Gui drains Fire and generates Blood

1076. Ci Zhu Wan does *not* contain which of the following?
    a. Zhi Gan Cao
    b. Ci Shi
    c. Zhu Sha
    d. Shen Qu

1077. Ci Zhu Wan does *not* perform which of the following functions?
    a. Heavily sedate and calm the Spirit
    b. Nourish Yin and Blood
    c. Weigh down the Yang
    d. Improve vision and hearing

1078. Suan Zao Ren Tang does *not* contain which of the following?
    a. Fu Ling
    b. Yuan Zhi
    c. Suan Zao Ren and Zhi Mu
    d. Chuan Xiong and Gan Cao

1079. Suan Zao Ren Tang does *not* perform which of the following functions?
    a. Nourish the Blood and calm the Spirit
    b. Sedate the Heart and calm the Spirit
    c. Clear Heat
    d. Eliminate irritability

1080. Which of the following indicates the use of Suan Zao Ren Tang?
    a. Insomnia caused by excessive Heart Fire flaming upwards
    b. Insomnia caused by imbalance between Heart Yang and Kidney Yin
    c. Irritability, with inability to sleep caused by Deficient Liver Blood
    d. None of the above

1081. Which statement about the herbs in Suan Zao Ren Tang is false?
    a. Suan Zao Ren nourishes the Liver and Heart Blood, and calms the Spirit
    b. Chuan Xiong regulates the Liver Blood
    c. Fu Ling calms the Spirit and tonifies the Spleen
    d. Zhi Mu clears Heat and quells Fire

1082. What are the "three Shens" in Tian Wang Bu Xin Dang?
    a. Ren Shen, Dan Shen, and Xuan Shen
    b. Ren Shen, Sha Shen, and Hai Er Shen
    c. Ren Shen, Sha Shen, and Dang Shen
    d. Ren Shen, Sha Shen, and Xi Yang Shen

1083. Tian Wang Bu Xing Dan does *not* perform which of the following functions?
    a. Clear Heat and eliminate irritability
    b. Tonify the Heart and calm the Spirit
    c. Enrich the Yin
    d. Nourish the Blood

1084. Which formula would you select to treat this pattern: irritability, palpitations, very restless sleep, nocturnal emissions, forgetfulness, dry stool, red tongue with little fur, thin-rapid pulse?
    a. Gui Pi Tang
    b. Suan Zao Ren Tang
    c. Zhi Gan Cao Tang
    d. Tian Wang Bu Xin Dan

1085. Which formula would you select to treat this pattern: hysteria, disorientation, frequent attacks of melancholy and crying spells, inability to control oneself, restless sleep, frequent bouts of yawning, red tongue with little fur, thin-rapid pulse?
    a. Gui Pi Tang
    b. Suan Zao Ren Tang
    c. Wen Pi Tang
    d. Gan Mai Da Zao Tang

1086. Which formula nourishes the Heart, calms the Spirit, and harmonizes the Middle Energizer?
    a. Bai Zi Yang Xin Wan
    b. Gan Mai Da Zao Tang
    c. Suan Zao Ren Tang
    d. Gui Pi Tang

1087. Which herb opens the orifices intensely, revives the Spirit, invigorates the Blood, and dissipates clumps?
    a. Shi Chang Pu
    b. Bing Pian
    c. Yuan Zhi
    d. She Xiang

1088. Bing Pian does *not* perform which of the following functions?
    a. Invigorate the Blood and dissipate clumps
    b. Aromatically open the orifices and revives the Spirit
    c. Clear Heat and alleviate pain
    d. Dissipate nodules

1089. Which herb treats Heat entering the Pericardium and cases where either a dead fetus or the placenta after childbirth has failed to descend?
    a. Su He Xiang
    b. Niu Xi
    c. Tian Hua Fen
    d. She Xiang

1090. Which herb treats throat pain and swelling, scabies, and photophobia or excessive tearing?
    a. She Xiang
    b. Zhu Sha
    c. Jue Ming Zi
    d. Bing Pian

1091. Which herb treats coma caused by Cold disorders?
    a. She Xiang
    b. Bing Pian
    c. Su He Xiang
    d. Shi Chang Pu

1092. Which herb treats both Cold and Heat disorders?
    a. Bing Pian
    b. Niu Huang
    c. Su He Xiang
    d. She Xiang

1093. Which herb treats traumatic injury, pain in the Heart or abdomen, and coronary artery disease?
    a. Tao Ren
    b. Wu Ling Zhi
    c. She Xiang
    d. Nui Huang

1094. Which herb opens the orifices, quiets the Spirit, transforms turbid Damp, and harmonizes the Stomach?
    a. Yuan Zhi
    b. Sha Ren
    c. Bing Pian
    d. Shi Chang Pu

1095. Which herb treats Damp-Phlegm that veils the sensory orifices and causes deafness, dizziness, coma, seizures, or stupor?
    a. Shi Chang Pu
    b. Bing Pian
    c. Yu Jin
    d. Bai Zi Ren

1096. Which portion of Su He Xiang is used medicinally?
    a. The flower bud
    b. The pollen
    c. The seed
    d. The styrax

1097. What is the method of preparation for Su He Xiang?
    a. Wrapped in cloth during decoction
    b. Added to the decoction near the end
    c. Added to the decoction at the beginning
    d. None of the above

1098. Shi Chang Pu does *not* perform which of the following functions?
    a. Open the orifices and vaporizes Phlegm
    b. Transform Damp
    c. Promote urination
    d. Harmonize the Middle Energizer

1099. Which herbs are the "four Huang" in An Gong Niu Huang Wan?
    a. Niu Huang, Huang Qin, Huang Bai, and Huang Lian
    b. Niu Huang, Huang Qin, Huang Bai, and Da Huang
    c. Niu Huang, Huang Qin, Huang Bai, and Xiong Huang
    d. Niu Huang, Huang Qin, Huang Lian, and Xiong Huang

1100. An Gong Niu Huang Wan does *not* perform which of the following functions?
    a. Clear Heat and relieve toxicity
    b. Dislodge Phlegm
    c. Open the orifices
    d. Promote the circulation of Qi to relieve pain

1101. Which statement about An Gong Niu Huang Wan is false?
    a. If there is an Excess pulse, take with a decoction of Jin Yin Hua and Bo He
    b. If there is a deficient pulse, take with a decoction of Ren Shen
    c. If there is an exhausted pulse, take with a decoction of Ren Shen and Fu Zi
    d. Children should take one half of the adult dose

1102. Which of the following serve as the chief (monarch or *jun*) component of An Gong Niu Huang Wan?
    a. Niu Huang and Huang Lian
    b. Niu Huang and Bing Pian
    c. Niu Huang and She Xiang
    d. Niu Huang and Zhen Zhu

1103. Niu Huang Qin Xin Wan does *not* perform which of the following functions?
    a. Clear Heat and relieve toxicity
    b. Open the orifices
    c. Transform Phlegm
    d. Calm the Spirit

1104. Zi Xue Dan performs which of the following functions?
    a. Clear the Heart and relieve toxicity
    b. Dislodge Phlegm and open the orifices
    c. Control spasms and convulsions and open the orifices
    d. Transform turbidity and open the orifices

1105. Which formula would you select to treat this pattern: coma, delirious speech, copious sputum with labored and raspy breathing, fever, irritability, red tongue with foul and greasy yellow fur?
    a. An Gong Niu Huang Wan
    b. Zi Xue Dan
    c. Zhi Bao Dan
    d. Niu Huang Qing Xin Wan

1106. What is the proper dosage of Zi Xue Dan?
    a. Take 0.5–1.0 grams once day
    b. Take 4.0–6.0 grams once a day
    c. Take 6.0–10.0 grams once a day
    d. Take 1.5–3.0 grams one to two times a day

1107. Zi Xue Dan is *not* indicated for which of the following?
    a. High fever, irritability, delirium, and impaired consciousness
    b. Muscle twitches, spasms, convulsions, thirst, and parched lips
    c. Fever and dyspnea
    d. Dark urine, childhood convulsions, and severe constipation

1108. What treatment is achieved by taking Zhi Bao Dan with a decoction of Ren Shen?
   a. Promote fluids and stop thirst
   b. Tonify the Spleen and nourish the Lungs
   c. Supplement Qi and restore Yang
   d. Supplement Qi and support healthy energy

1109. Which formula would you select to treat a one-and-a-half-years-old boy who has suffered for three days from high fever, dyspnea, mucus in the throat, irritability, impaired consciousness, night crying, and vomiting of milk?
   a. Zi Xue Dan
   b. An Gong Niu Huang Wan
   c. Zhi Bao Dan
   d. Hiu Chun Dan

1110. Su He Xiang Wan does *not* contain which of the following?
   a. Su He Xiang and An Xi Xiang
   b. Xiang Ru and Jiang Xiang
   c. She Xiang, Tan Xiang, and Mu Xiang
   d. Chen Xiang, Ru Xiang, and Xiang Fu

1111. Su He Xiang Wan does *not* perform which of the following functions?
   a. Transform Phlegm and relieve toxicity
   b. Aromatically open the orifices
   c. Promote the movement of Qi
   d. Alleviate pain

1112. Su He Xiang Wan is *not* indicated for which of the following?
   a. Measles, dyspnea in children, fever, coma
   b. Sudden collapse, loss of consciousness, a clenched jaw
   c. Fullness, pain, and a sensation of Cold in the chest and abdomen, sudden coma
   d. An urge to vomit and defecate, sudden coma

1113. What are the important symptoms treated by Su He Xiang Wan?
   a. Clenched jaw, turbid Phlegm veiling the orifices, coma
   b. Pale or purple complexion
   c. Open mouth and Cold extremities
   d. A submerged, Excess pulse

1114. Ling Yang Jiao enters which meridians?
   a. Spleen and Stomach
   b. Lung and Gallbladder
   c. Kidney and Spleen
   d. Liver and Heart

1115. Which herb clears Liver Heat, extinguishes Wind, calms the Liver, and anchors the Yang?
   a. Niu Huang
   b. Shi Jue Ming
   c. Xia Ku Cao
   d. Ling Yang Jiao

1116. How is Ling Yang Jiao prepared in decoction?
   a. Cooked with the other herbs
   b. Cooked after the other herbs
   c. Cooked separately from the other herbs
   d. Wrapped in cheese cloth

1117. Which herb drains Fire, causes the Yang to descend, and improves vision?
    a. Chi Shao
    b. Xia Ku Cao
    c. Shi Jue Ming
    d. Mu Zei

1118. Which herb treats high fever, Wind syndrome caused by dominant Heat evil, and hand or foot spasms?
    a. Huang Lian
    b. Shi Gao
    c. Ling Yang Jiao
    d. Mu Li

1119. What is the primary visual problem treated with Shi Jue Ming?
    a. Liver Heat leading to red eyes
    b. Blurring of the vision caused by Deficient Blood
    c. Itching of the eyes caused by Wind-Heat evil
    d. Dryness and an uneasy feeling of the eyes caused by Deficient Yin

1120. Which herb drains Liver Heat and pacifies Liver Yang?
    a. Tian Ma
    b. Bai Ji Li
    c. Mu Li
    d. Gou Teng

1121. What condition is associated with the Wind and spasms that Gou Teng treats?
    a. Tetanus
    b. Hemiplegia
    c. Deviation of the eye and mouth
    d. Tremors, seizure, and eclampsia

1122. What is the proper method of decoction for Gou Teng?
    a. Decoct before the other herbs
    b. Decoct after the other herbs
    c. Decoct wrapped in cheese cloth
    d. Decoct separately from the other herbs

1123. Which herb clears Heat, pacifies the Liver, extinguishes Wind, and alleviates spasms?
    a. Xia Ku Cao
    b. Ju Hua
    c. Gou Teng
    d. Bai Ji Li

1124. Which herb extinguishes endogenous Wind evil and expels exogenous Wind evil?
    a. Ling Yang Jiao
    b. Gou Teng
    c. Wu Gong
    d. Di Long

1125. Which herb calms the Liver, anchors the Yang, and is known for extinguishing Wind and controlling spasms and tremors?
    a. Bai Ji Li
    b. Tian Ma
    c. Di Long
    d. Dai Zhe Shi

1126. Which herb treats infantile convulsions and tremors caused by Heat or Cold patterns?
    a. Tian Ma
    b. Tian Nan Xing
    c. Di Long
    d. Chan Tui

1127. Which herb treats Liver-Wind stirring inside caused by Excess Liver Yang?
    a. Chan Tui
    b. Jue Ming Zi
    c. Jiang Can
    d. Tian Ma

1128. Which herb disperses depressed Liver Qi and calms the Liver?
    a. Bai Ji Li
    b. Yu Jin
    c. Jue Ming Zi
    d. Chai Hu

1129. Which herb extinguishes Wind, stops tremors, and has sweet and neutral properties?
    a. Gou Teng
    b. Bai Ji Li
    c. Ling Yang Jiao
    d. Tian Ma

1130. Which herb would you select to treat Wind-stroke syndrome with deviation of the eye and mouth?
    a. Niu Huang
    b. Bai Ji Li
    c. Ling Yang Jiao
    d. Quan Xie

1131. Which herb is often used with Wu Gong to treat tetanus convulsions and severe seizures?
    a. Niu Huang
    b. Bai Ji Li
    c. Quan Xie
    d. Shi Jue Ming

1132. Which of the following is another name for Jiang Can?
    a. Bai Zu
    b. Quan Chong
    c. Tian Chong
    d. Qiu Yin

1133. Which herb is *not* poisonous?
    a. Quan Xie
    b. Wu Gong
    c. Jiang Can
    d. Ban Mao

1134. Which herb drains Heat, extinguishes Wind, calms wheezing, unblocks the meridians and collaterals, and promotes urination?
    a. Jiang Can
    b. Wu Gong
    c. Quan Xie
    d. Di Long

1135. Which herb extinguishes Wind, stops spasms and convulsions, and transforms Phlegm?
    a. Tian Ma
    b. Gou Teng
    c. Jiang Can
    d. Yuan Zhi

1136. Which two herbs each calm the Liver, anchor the Yang, and improve vision?
    a. Mu Zei and Xia Ku Cao
    b. Bai Ji Li and Jue Ming Zi
    c. Ling Yang Jiao and Shi Jue Ming
    d. Mu Li and Long Gu

1137. Which herb strongly directs rebellious Qi downward, calms the Liver, and anchors the floating Yang?
    a. Ci Shi
    b. Long Gu
    c. Zhan Zhu
    d. Dai Zhe Shi

1138. Which two herbs each extinguish Wind, stop tremors, relieve toxins, and dissipate nodules?
    a. Wu Gong and Qian Xie
    b. Di Long and Jiang Can
    c. Ling Yang Jiao and Zhen Zhu
    d. Bai Ji Li and Zhen Zhu

1139. Which two herbs each treat obstinate migraines and arthralgia syndrome?
    a. Jiang Can and Gou Teng
    b. Wu Gong and Quan Xie
    c. Tian Ma and Du Huo
    d. Qin Jiao and Qiang Huo

1140. Jiang Can and Bai Ji Li each perform which of the following functions?
    a. Extinguish Wind and stop convulsions, and expel Wind and improve vision
    b. Extinguish Wind and stop convulsions, and relieve toxin and dissipate nodules
    c. Calm the Liver and anchor the Yang, and transform Phlegm and dissipate nodules
    d. Dispel Wind and stop itching

1141. Which two herbs each extinguish Wind, stop convulsions, unblock the collaterals, and stop pain?
    a. Wu Gong and Quan Xie
    b. Shi Jue Ming and Bai Ji Li
    c. Gou Teng and Luo Shi Teng
    d. Mu Gua and Du Huo

1142. Which herb calms the Liver, extinguishes Wind, clears Heat, relieves toxins, clears the Liver, and improves the vision?
    a. Gou Teng
    b. Ling Yang Jiao
    c. Shi Jue Ming
    d. Xia Ku Cao

1143. Which herb calms the Liver, anchors the Yang, clears the Liver, and improves the vision?
    a. Di Long
    b. Xia Ku Cao
    c. Jue Ming Zi
    d. Zhen Zhu Mu

1144. Which herb calms the Liver, anchors the Yang, softens hardness, dissipates nodules, and astringes?
    a. Di Long
    b. Shi Jue Ming
    c. Long Gu
    d. Mu Li

1145. Which herb extinguishes Wind, stops convulsions, attacks toxins, and dissipates nodules?
    a. Tu Bie Chong
    b. Shi Chang Pu
    c. Wu Gong
    d. Ban Mao

1146. Da Qin Jiao Tang does *not* perform which of the following functions?
    a. Expel Wind
    b. Clear Heat
    c. Nourish and invigorate the Blood
    d. Alleviate pain and itching

1147. Which formula would you select to treat this pattern: eyes and mouth awry, difficulty in using the tongue, unable to talk, experiences numbness and lack of sensation in the head and feet?
    a. Xiao Feng San
    b. Ye Zhen San
    c. Xiao Huo Luo Dan
    d. None of the above

1148. Which herbs in Xian Feng San are used to expel Wind and release the Exterior?
    a. Jing Jie, Fang Feng, Niu Bang Zi, and Chan Tui
    b. Jing Jie, Fang Feng, Niu Bang Zi, and Sang Ye
    c. Jing Jie, Fang Feng, Bo He, and Sang Ye
    d. Jing Jie, Fang Feng, Ge Gen, and Dan Dou Chi

1149. Xiao Feng San does *not* perform which of the following functions?
    a. Disperse Wind
    b. Detoxify
    c. Eliminate Damp
    d. Clear Heat and nourish the Blood

1150. Chuan Xiong Cha Tiao San does *not* contain which of the following?
    a. Bo He and Chuan Xiong
    b. Dang Gui and Sheng Di Huang
    c. Qiang Huo, Xi Xin and Jing Jie
    d. Fang Feng and Gan Cao

1151. Chuan Xiong Cha Tiao San performs which of the following functions?
    a. Expel Cold and alleviate pain
    b. Disperse Wind and alleviate pain
    c. Nourish the Blood and alleviate pain
    d. Unblock the collaterals and alleviate pain

1152. Chuan Xiong Cha Tiao San should *not* be used to treat which of the following?
    a. Migraine
    b. Parietal headache
    c. Ascendant Liver Yang headache
    d. A floating pulse

1153. Which formula would you select to treat this pattern: weepy, itchy, red skin lesions over a large part of the body, white or yellow tongue fur, floating-rapid-forceful pulse?
    a. Ma Xing Yi Gan Tang
    b. Wu Pi San
    c. Xiao Feng San
    d. Qiang Huo Sheng Shi Tang

1154. Qian Zheng San does *not* contain which of the following?
    a. Fu Zi
    b. Bai Fu Zi
    c. Jiang Can
    d. Quan Xie

1155. Qian Zheng San performs which of the following functions?
    a. Dispel Wind, unblock the collaterals, and stop pain
    b. Dispel Wind, transform Damp, and stop pain
    c. Dispel Wind, transform Phlegm, and stop pain
    d. Dispel Wind, transform Phlegm, and stop spasms

1156. Yu Zhen San does *not* contain which of the following?
    a. Bai Fu Zi and Tian Nan Xing
    b. Quan Xie and Gou Teng
    c. Qiang Huo and Bai Zhi
    d. Fang Feng and Tian Ma

1157. Yu Zhen San does *not* perform which of the following functions?
    a. Dispel Wind
    b. Transform Phlegm
    c. Invigorate the Blood and stop pain
    d. Relieve spasms and stop pain

1158. Xiao Huo Luo Dan does *not* contain which of the following?
    a. Cao Wu
    b. Bai Fu Zi
    c. Chuan Wu and Tian Nan Xing
    d. Mo Yao, Ru Xiang, and Di Long

1159. Xiao Huo Luo Dan does *not* perform which of the following functions?
    a. Expel Wind and dispel Damp
    b. Transform Phlegm and unblock the collaterals
    c. Invigorate the Blood and stop pain
    d. Reduce swelling and stop pain

1160. Which formula would you select to treat stiffness and spasms of the jaw, clenched mouth, deviation of the eyes, and rigidity of the entire body to the point of opisthotonos?
    a. Qian Zheng San
    b. Xiao Huo Luo Dan
    c. Da Qin Jia Tang
    d. Yu Zhen San

1161. Which formula would you select to treat chronic pain, weakness and numbness, fixed or migrating pain in the bones and joints with reduced range of motion caused by Wind-Damp-Cold evil obstructing the meridians?
    a. Qing Huo Sheng Shi Tang
    b. Dan Dou Qu Hui Tang
    c. Xiao Huo Luo Dan
    d. Du Huo Ji Sheng Tang

1162. Ling Jiao Gou Teng Tang does *not* contain which of the following?
    a. Sheng Di Huang, Bai Shao, and Zhu Ru
    b. Ling Yang Jiao, Gou Teng, and Fu Shen
    c. Sang Ye, Ju Hua, and Chuan Bei Mu
    d. Tian Nan Xing, Chuan Xiong, and Chi Shao

1163. Ling Jiao Gou Teng Tang does *not* perform which of the following functions?
    a. Cool the Liver and extinguish Wind
    b. Clear Heat and nourish the Yin
    c. Increase the fluids
    d. Relax the sinews

1164. Which formula is *not* used to treat Liver Fire?
    a. Zhen Gan Xi Feng Tang
    b. Long Dan Xie Gan Tang
    c. Zuo Jin Wan
    d. Dang Gui Long Hui Wan

1165. What is the pathogenesis of the syndrome for which Zhen Gan Xi Feng Tang is the indicated treatment?
    a. Excess Liver Yang with abnormal rising of Liver Qi
    b. Dominant Fire of the Liver meridian
    c. Deficient Yin of the Liver and Kidneys with ascendant Liver Yang causing the Qi and Blood to rebel
    d. Wind syndrome resulting from domination of Heat evil causing injury to the Yin

1166. Which formula would you select to treat this pattern: persistent high fever, irritability, restlessness, twitching and spasms of the extremities with possible impairment or loss of consciousness, deep red and dry tongue, wiry-rapid pulse?
    a. Zi Xue Dan
    b. Zhi Bao Dan
    c. Tian Ma Gou Teng Yin
    d. Ling Jiao Gou Teng Tang

1167. What are the characteristics of the pulse of a patient for whom Zhen Gan Xi Feng Tang is indicated?
    a. Wiry and rapid
    b. Wiry and thin
    c. Wiry, rapid, and forceful
    d. Wiry, long, and forceful

1168. Tian Ma Gou Teng Yin, Ling Jiao Gou Teng Tang and Jian Ling Tang are all used to treat Deficient Liver and Kidneys, with Liver Yang ascending and causing dizziness and vertigo. What is the particular function of Jian Ling Tang?
    a. Sedate and extinguish Liver Wind, enrich the Yin, and calm the Spirit
    b. Sedate and extinguish Liver Wind, unblock the collaterals, and stop pain
    c. Sedate and extinguish Liver Wind, enrich the Yin, and anchor the Yang
    d. Sedate and extinguish Liver Wind, clear Heat, and invigorate the Blood

1169. Which formula calms the Liver, extinguishes Wind, clears Heat, invigorates the Blood, and tonifies the Liver and Kidneys?
   a. Da Ding Feng Zhu
   b. Di Huang Yin Zi
   c. San Jia Fu Mai Tang
   d. Tian Ma Gou Teng Yin

1170. Which of the following indicates the use of Tian Ma Gou Tang Yin?
   a. Ascendant Liver Yang causing dizziness, vertigo and insomnia
   b. Heat excess in the Liver meridian causing dizziness, vertigo and insomnia
   c. Floating up of the asthenic Yang causing dizziness, vertigo and insomnia
   d. None of the above

1171. E Jiao Ji Zi Huang Tang does *not* perform which of the following functions?
   a. Soften the Liver and extinguish Wind
   b. Cool the Liver and extinguish Wind
   c. Enrich the Yin
   d. Nourish the Blood

1172. E Jiao Ji Zi Huang Tang is *not* indicated for which of the following?
   a. Rigid extremities
   b. Muscle spasms and twitches in the extremities
   c. Dizziness and vertigo
   d. Deviation of the eye and mouth

1173. Da Ding Feng Zhu performs which of the following functions?
   a. Calm the Liver and extinguish Wind
   b. Cool the Liver and extinguish Wind
   c. Nourish the Yin and extinguish Wind
   d. Soften the Liver and extinguish Wind

1174. Which herbs in Di Huang Yin Zi tonify the Kidney Yang?
   a. Fu Zi, Ba Ji Tian, Rou Gui and Bu Gu Zhi
   b. Fu Zi, Ba Ji Tian, Rou Gui and Xian Mao
   c. Fu Zi, Ba Ji Tian, Rou Gui and Suo Yang
   d. Fu Zi, Ba Ji Tian, Rou Gui and Rou Cong Rong

1175. Which formula would you select to treat a patient with long-standing retention of pathogenic Heat from a warm febrile disease with symptoms of weariness, muscle spasms with alternating flexion and extension of the extremities, deficient pulse, deep red tongue, slight tongue fur, and frequent appearance that the patient is about to go into shock?
   a. E Jiao Ji Zi Huang Tang
   b. Ling Jiao Gou Teng Tang
   c. Di Huang Yin Zi
   d. Da Ding Feng Zhu

1176. Di Huang Yin Zi does *not* perform which of the following functions?
   a. Enrich Kidney Yin
   b. Warm and tonify Kidney Yang
   c. Nourish the Heart and calm the Spirit
   d. Open the orifices and transform Phlegm

1177. Di Huang Yin Zi is *not* indicated for which of the following?
   a. Stiffness of the tongue with an inability to speak
   b. Disability or paralysis of the lower extremities
   c. Dizziness and vertigo
   d. A dry mouth with an absence of thirst

1178. When should a patient take herbs that expel parasites?
   a. Before eating
   b. After eating
   c. Before sleeping
   d. On an empty Stomach

1179. Which herb is sweet and tasty, has no trace of bitterness, and is used to treat roundworms?
   a. Bing Lang
   b. Lei Wan
   c. Shi Jun Zi
   d. Nan Gua Zi

1180. What is a common result of an overdoes of Shi Jun Zi?
   a. Diarrhea
   b. Hiccoughs, vomiting, and dizziness
   c. Constipation
   d. Jaundice

1181. Which herb treats fasciolopsis, pinworm, and roundworms?
   a. Shi Jin Zi
   b. Nan Gua Zi
   c. Bing Lang
   d. Ku Lian Gen Pi

1182. Which herb promotes the movement of Qi, promotes urination, and kills parasites?
   a. Lei Wan
   b. Nan Gua Zi
   c. Fei Zi
   d. Bing Lang

1183. What type of parasite is Bing Lang best suited to kill?
   a. Fasciolopsis
   b. Pinworm
   c. Roundworms
   d. Tapeworm

1184. What is the method of preparation of Lei Wan?
   a. Decocted before other herbs
   b. Decocted longer than other herbs
   c. Wrapped in cloth during decoction
   d. Prepared as either a pill or as powder

1185. Which herb prevents influenza, treats epidemic encephalitis and mumps, stops bleeding, and kills parasites?
   a. Guan Zhong
   b. Bing Lang
   c. Jin Yin Hua
   d. Ban Lan Gen

1186. Which herb is used fresh to clear Heat and relieve Fire toxicity, and is carbonized to stop bleeding?
   a. Ku Lian Gen Pi
   b. Bing Lang
   c. Lei Wan
   d. Guan Zhong

1187. Which two herbs are each used to kill tapeworms?
    a. Shi Jun Zi, Ku Lian Gen Pi
    b. Bing Lang, Nan Gua Zi
    c. Ku Lian Pi, Nan Gua Zi
    d. Shi Jun Zi, Nan Gua Zi

1188. Wu Yi performs which of the following functions?
    a. Kill parasites and move the Qi
    b. Kill parasites and cool the Blood
    c. Kill parasites and relieve childhood nutritional impairment
    d. Kill parasites and stop bleeding

1189. He Shi performs which of the following functions?
    a. Drain downward
    b. Transform Phlegm
    c. Promote the movement of Qi
    d. Kill parasites

1190. Which herb kills parasites and relieves childhood nutritional impairment?
    a. Shi Jun Zi
    b. Lei Wan
    c. Lai Fu Zi
    d. Niu Bang Zi

1191. Which herb is used in therapy for uterine bleeding?
    a. Shi Jin Zi
    b. Bing Lang
    c. Ku Lian Pi
    d. Guan Zhong

1192. Guan Zhong does *not* perform which of the following functions?
    a. Clear Heat and relieve toxicity
    b. Kill parasites
    c. Promote urination
    d. Stop bleeding

1193. Which herb kills parasites?
    a. Wu Bei Zi
    b. Niu Bang Zi
    c. Bai Jie Zi
    d. Nan Gua Zi

1194. Which herb kills parasites, reduces stagnation, and drives out water?
    a. Shi Jun Zi
    b. Shi Liu Pi
    c. Qian Niu Zi
    d. Lei Wan

1195. Which herb moistens the Lungs and kills parasites?
    a. Shi Liu Pi
    b. Lei Wan
    c. Fei Zi
    d. Nan Gua Zi

1196. Which herb moistens the Lungs, stops coughing, expels parasites, and kills lice?
    a. Fei Zi
    b. He Shi
    c. Guan Zhong
    d. Bai Bu

1197. Which herb kills roundworms and could be used to treat tinea infection?
    a. Shi Jun Zi
    b. Fei Zi
    c. Ku Lian Gen Pi
    d. Lei Wan

1198. Formulas that expel parasites fall under which of the eight methods of treatment?
    a. Therapy for dispersing the stagnation of evils
    b. Therapy for inducing vomiting
    c. Therapy for invigoration
    d. Therapy for purgation

1199. What is *not* a caution for formulas that expel parasites?
    a. Avoid greasy and rich foods during treatment; take medicine on an empty stomach
    b. Some of these formulas have toxic properties, and their dosage should be carefully monitored
    c. Use cautiously for old aged, weak and pregnant patients
    d. Herbs that expel parasites must be taken with herbs that regulate the Qi

1200. Wu Mei Wan does *not* contain which of the following?
    a. Bing Lang, Chuan Lian Zi and Wu Yao
    b. Wu Mei, Chuan Jiao and Xi Xin
    c. Huang Lian, Haung Bai and Gan Jiang
    d. Fu Zi, Gui Zhi, Ren Shen and Dang Gui

1201. Which formula contains both Huang Lian and Fu Zi?
    a. Huang Lian Tang
    b. Wu Mei Wan
    c. Ban Xia Xie Xin Tang
    d. Wen Pi Tang

1202. Which statement is *not* true of Wu Mei Wan?
    a. It can be used to treat both Heat and Cold syndromes
    b. It has the properties of acrid, bitter and sour
    c. It is mainly used to kill parasites
    d. It is used to treat both evil and healthy energy

1203. Wu Mei Wan is *not* indicated for which of the following?
    a. Chronic dysentery
    b. Irritability, vomiting, and pain in the abdomen
    c. Vomiting of roundworms after eating
    d. Fullness of the upper abdomen

1204. Li Zhong An Hui Tang is *not* indicated for which of the following?
    a. Loose stools and clear and profuse urine
    b. Abdominal pain and borborygmus
    c. Feeling of cold in the extremities
    d. Shortness of breath and dizziness

1205. Lian Mei An Hui Tang performs which of the following functions?
   a. Warm the organs and calm roundworms
   b. Clear Heat and calm roundworms
   c. Stop pain and calm roundworms
   d. Kill parasites and stop pain

1206. Fei Er Wan does *not* contain which of the following?
   a. Ye Ming Sha and Cao Dou Kou
   b. Shen Qu and Huang Lian
   c. Rou Dou Kou and Shi Jun Zi
   d. Mai Ya, Bing Lang and Mu Xiang

1207. Which formula kills parasites, reduces accumulation, strengthens the Spleen, and clears Heat?
   a. Fei Er Wan
   b. Wu Mei Wan
   c. Hua Chong Wan
   d. Bu Dai Wan

1208. Bu Dai Wan can be created by adapting Si Jun Zi Tang in which of the following ways?
   a. Add Shi Jun Zi, Ye Ming Sha, Wu Yi, and Liu Hui
   b. Add Fei Zi and He Shi
   c. Add Lei Wan and Ku Lian Gen Pi
   d. Add Bing Lang, Guan Zhong, and Nan Gua Zi

1209. Fei Er Wan and Bu Dai Wan treat parasitic infestations. What else does Bu Dai Wan treat?
   a. Deficient Spleen and Stomach
   b. Food stagnation in the Middle Energizer
   c. Stasis of Damp evil and accumulation of Heat evil
   d. Spleen evil stagnating in the Middle Energizer

1210. Hua Chong Wan does *not* contain which of the following?
   a. Lei Wan
   b. He Shi
   c. Bing Lang
   d. Ku Lian Pi and Ming Fan

1211. Which formula would you select to treat a patient with intestinal parasites who has intermittent attacks of intense abdominal pain that move up and down, and who vomits up clear fluids or parasites?
   a. Fei Er Wan
   b. Wu Mei Wan
   c. Bu Dai Wan
   d. Hua Chong Wan

1212. Which herb checks malarial conditions and induces vomiting to expel Phlegm?
   a. Qing Hao
   b. Cao Guo
   c. Chang Shan
   d. She Chuang Zi

1213. Which formula treats parasitic infestations, abdominal pain and distention, indigestion, emaciation, feverishness, foul-smelling breath, and loose stools?
   a. Huan Chong Wan
   b. Wu Mei Wan
   c. Fei Er Wan
   d. Bu Dai Wan

1214. What is *not* an alternate name for Bing Pian?
 a. Long Nao Xiang
 b. Mei Pian
 c. Ai Pian
 d. Chao Nao

1215. Which herb is taken internally to tonify and unblock the bowels, and is used topically to kill parasites and stop itching?
 a. Niu Huang
 b. Ming Fan
 c. Xiong Huang
 d. Liu Huang

1216. Which herb is used topically to treat scabies, ringworm, Yin furuncles, and Damp festering carbuncles, and is taken internally to treat Deficient Kidney Yang and constipation caused by Cold in the Kidneys?
 a. Ming Fan
 b. Xiong Huang
 c. Peng Sha
 d. Liu Huang

1217. Which herb is used topically to relieve toxicity and kill parasites, and is taken internally to expel water and unblock the bowels?
 a. Xiong Huang
 b. Qing Fen
 c. Da Feng Zi
 d. Shang Lu

1218. Which herb is used topically to clear Heat and relieve toxicity, and is taken internally to clear the Lungs and transform Phlegm?
 a. Shi Gao
 b. Mang Xian
 c. Zhang Nao
 d. Peng Sha

1219. Which herb brightens the eyes, removes superficial visual obstructions, dries Damp, and generates flesh?
 a. Shi Gao
 b. Hua Shi
 c. Bing Pian
 d. Lu Gan Shi

1220. Which herb is used both topically and internally to stop pain?
 a. Rou Gui.
 b. Gao Liang Jiang
 c. Lu Gan Shi
 d. Chan Su

1221. Which herb relieves toxicity, reduces swelling, alleviates pain, and opens the orifices?
 a. Lu Feng Fang
 b. Ban Mao
 c. Chan Su
 d. Yu Jin

1222. Which herb attacks toxins, wears away sores, breaks up Blood stasis, and disperses clumps?
 a. Ma Qian Zi
 b. Da Feng Zi
 c. Ban Mao
 d. Lu Feng Fang

1223. What is an alternate name for Ma Qian Zi?
   a. Bai Jiang Can
   b. She Chuang Zi
   c. Mu Bie Zi
   d. Fan Mu Bie

1224. Which herb treats abscesses, sores, swelling, and pain caused by Wind trauma, and treats Wind-Damp pain obstruction, paresthesia, or spasms?
   a. She Chuang Zi
   b. Ma Qian Zi
   c. Lu Feng Fang
   d. Jiang Huang

1225. Ma Qian Zi does *not* perform which of the following functions?
   a. Dry Damp and stop itching
   b. Unblock the meridians
   c. Disperse clumps and reduce swelling
   d. Alleviate pain

1226. Which herb dispels Wind, dries Damp, kills parasites, warms the Kidneys, fortifies the Yang, and disperses Cold?
   a. Da Feng Zi
   b. Liu Huang
   c. Mu Bie Zi
   d. She Chuang Zi

1227. Shi Liu Pi does *not* perform which of the following functions?
   a. Expel Phlegm and stop wheezing
   b. Bind up the Intestines
   c. Stop diarrhea
   d. Kill parasites

1228. Xiong Huang performs which of the following functions?
   a. Relieve toxicity and reduce swelling
   b. Relieve toxicity and generate flesh
   c. Relieve toxicity and kill parasites
   d. Absorb fluids and stop bleeding

1229. Which herb expels toxins, stops itching, is astringent, and generates flesh?
   a. Qing Fen
   b. Xiong Huang
   c. Qian Dan
   d. Liu Huang

1230. Which herb is used topically to dry Damp and stop itching, and used internally to stop diarrhea?
   a. Xiong Huang
   b. Liu Huang
   c. Peng Sha
   d. Ming Fan

1231. Da Suan does *not* perform which of the following functions?
   a. Kill parasites
   b. Relieve toxicity
   c. Relieve food poisoning
   d. Generate flesh

1232. Which herb is used topically to attack toxins and wear away sores, and internally to treat congealed Blood?
    a. Da Suan
    b. Ming Fan
    c. Ban Mao
    d. Shan Ci Gu

1233. Ming Fan does *not* perform which of the following functions?
    a. Relieve toxicity and kill parasites
    b. Clear Heat and expel Phlegm
    c. Stop bleeding, diarrhea and itching
    d. Nourish the Blood and stop spasms

1234. Liu Huang does *not* perform which of the following functions?
    a. Unblock the bowels
    b. Invigorate the Blood
    c. Strengthen the Yang
    d. Kill parasites and stop itching

1235. Shan Ci Gu is *not* indicated for which of the following?
    a. Scrofula
    b. Toxic swelling
    c. Heat pattern carbuncle
    d. Wind rash

1236. Xian Fang Huo Ming Yin does *not* contain which of the following?
    a. Jin Yin Hua, Gan Cao, Zhe Bei Mu and Tian Hua Fen
    b. Dang Gui, Chi Shao, Ru Xiang and Mo Yao
    c. Fang Feng, Bai Zhi, Chuang Shan Jia and Zao Jiao Ci
    d. Chuan Xiong, Dan Shen, Ze Lan and Niu Xi

1237. Xian Fang Hiu Ming Yin does *not* perform which of the following functions?
    a. Clear Heat and relieve Fire toxin
    b. Reduce swelling and promote the discharge of pus
    c. Expel Wind and alleviate pain
    d. Invigorate the Blood and alleviate pain

1238. Wu Wei Xiao Du Yin does *not* contain which of the following?
    a. Jin Yin Hua
    b. Lian Qiao
    c. Pu Gong Ying and Zi Hua Di Ding
    d. Ye Ju Hua and Zi Bei Tian Kwei

1239. Wu Wei Xiao Du Yin does *not* perform which of the following functions?
    a. Clear Heat and relieve toxicity
    b. Invigorate the Blood and stop pain
    c. Cool the Blood
    d. Reduce swelling

1240. Which formula treats early stage sores and carbuncles (red, swollen, hot and painful skin lesions), where the patient has fever, mild chills, thin yellow tongue fur, and a rapid, forceful pulse?
    a. Wu Wei Xiao Du Yin
    b. Ren Shen Bai Du Yin
    c. Si Miao Yong An Tang
    d. Xian Fang Huo Ming Yin

1241. Hai Zao Yu Hu Tang does *not* perform which of the following functions?
    a. Transform Phlegm and soften hard masses
    b. Invigorate the Blood and transform Blood stasis
    c. Reduce nodules
    d. Dissipate goiters

1242. Si Miao Yong An Tang does *not* contain which of the following?
    a. Jin Yin Hua
    b. Mu Dan Pi
    c. Xuan Shen
    d. Dang Gui and Gan Cao

1243. Which formula clears Heat and relieves toxicity, invigorates the Blood, and alleviates pain?
    a. Wu Wei Xiao Du Yin
    b. Xi Huang Wan
    c. Si Miao Yong An Tang
    d. None of the above

1244. Which statement is *not* true of the type of gangrene that is treated with Si Miao Yong An Tang?
    a. It is dark red in appearance, slightly swollen, and generates a feeling of burning heat
    b. It is extremely painful
    c. There is a rotten smell to the lesion with copious discharge
    d. The patient has a purple tongue and a slippery pulse

1245. Which of the following represents the "Xi Huang" in Xi Huang Wan?
    a. Xi Jiao and Da Huang
    b. Xi Jiao and Niu Huang
    c. Xi Jiao and Huang Lian
    d. Niu Huang

1246. Xi Huang Wan does *not* contain which of the following?
    a. Xi Jiao
    b. Niu Huang
    c. Shi Xiang
    d. Ru Xiang, Mo Yao and Rice

1247. Xi Huang Wan is *not* indicated for which of the following?
    a. Mastocarcinoma
    b. Scrofula and multiple abscesses
    c. Lung carbuncles and subcutaneous nodules
    d. Diphtheria

1248. Which formula would you select to treat a serious case of furuncles accompanied by a red tongue with yellow fur and a rapid pulse?
    a. Xian Fang Huo Ming Yin
    b. Si Miao Yong An Tang
    c. Wu Wei Xiao Du Yin
    d. Liu Shen Wan

1249. Which formula treats indurated goiters that are rock-like in hardness, immobile, and cause no change in the color of the skin?
    a. Xi Huang Wan
    b. Wu Wei Xiao Du Yin
    c. Hai Zao Yu Hu Tang
    d. None of the above

1250. Which choice contains at least one herb that is *not* part of the formula for Tou Nong San?
   a. Dang Gui
   b. Chi Shao
   c. Chuan Xiong and Huang Qi
   d. Chuan Shan Jia and Zao Jioa Ci

1251. Tou Nong San is *not* indicated for which of the following?
   a. Chronic abscesses without heads that produce pus
   b. Chronic abscesses that are not readily perforated to discharge the pus
   c. Chronic abscesses that have produced pus which is seeping out
   d. Chronic abscess that are painful, swollen and hot

1252. What is the correct dosage of Ma Huang in Yang He Tang?
   a. 10 grams
   b. 6 ggrams
   c. 4 grams
   d. 1.5 grams

1253. Which formula is *not* used to clear Heat and relieve toxins?
   a. Tou Nong San
   b. Si Miao Yong An Tang
   c. Xian Fang Huo Ming Yin
   d. Wu Wei Xiao Du Yin

1254. Yang He Tang does *not* perform which of the following functions?
   a. Dispel Damp
   b. Warm the Yang
   c. Tonify the Blood
   d. Disperse Cold and unblock areas of stagnation

1255. Which formula treats localized painful swellings without heads, no feeling of local Heat, no change in the color of the skin, where the patient has no thirst, a pale tongue and a deep, thin pulse?
   a. Yang He Tang
   b. Si Miao Yong An Tang
   c. Tou Nong San
   d. Xian Fang Huo Ming Yin

1256. Wei Jing Tang does *not* contain which of the following?
   a. Wei Jing
   b. Gua Lou Ren
   c. Yi Yi Ren
   d. Dong Gua Ren and Tao Ren

1257. Da Huang Mu Dan Tang does *not* contain which of the following?
   a. Da Huang and Mu Dan Pi
   b. Tao Ren
   c. Dong Gua Ren
   d. Xing Ren

1258. Which formula would you select to treat this pattern: cough with foul-smelling sputum, slight fever, mild chest pain, dry and scaly skin, red tongue with yellow fur, slippery-rapid pulse?
   a. Qing Qi Hua Tan Wan
   b. Ma Xing Shi Gan Tang
   c. Wen Dan Tang
   d. Wei Jing Tang

1259. Da Huang Mu Dan Tang does *not* perform which of the following functions?
    a. Clear Heat and eliminate Phlegm
    b. Clear Heat and break up Blood stasis
    c. Disperse clumping
    d. Reduce swelling

1260. Yi Yi Fu Zi Bai Jiang San performs which of the following functions?
    a. Expel pus and alleviate pain
    b. Expel pus and reduce swelling
    c. Expel pus and break up Blood stasis
    d. Reduce swelling and disperse clumping

1261. Yi Yi Fu Zi Bai Jiang San is *not* indicated for which of the following?
    a. No fever
    b. Scaly skin
    c. Diarrhea with Blood and pus
    d. Taut skin around the abdomen that is soft to the touch

1262. Which formula would you select to treat this pattern: lower abdominal distention and pain on the right side that increases with pressure and is tender afterwards, a tendency to guard the abdominal musculature, pain in the groin relieved by flexing the hip and knee and intensified by extending the hip, normal urination, intermittent fever followed by chills and sweating, thin greasy yellow tongue fur?
    a. Da Cheng Qi Tang
    b. Fu Fang Da Cheng Qi Tang
    c. Yi Yi Fu Zi Bai Jiang San
    d. Da Huang Mu Dan Tang

1263. Yi Yi Ren Tang does *not* contain which of the following?
    a. Yi Yi Ren
    b. Tian Hua Fen
    c. Mu Dan Pi
    d. Gua Lou Ren and Tao Ren

1264. Emetic formulas are *not* indicated for which of the following?
    a. Food stagnation in the Stomach
    b. Toxins in the Stomach
    c. Fullness and distention of the upper abdomen caused by accumulation; chills and fever
    d. Apoplexy caused by accumulation of Phlegm

1265. Which formula would you select to treat this pattern: firm areas of focal distention in the chest, vexation caused by food stagnation in the Stomach, difficult breathing caused by a sensation of Qi rushing into the throat, slightly floating pulse at the distal position?
    a. Sheng Jiang Xie Xin Tang
    b. Xie Xin Tang
    c. Gua Di San
    d. Xuan Fu Dai Zhe Tang

1266. Which two herbs each treat Deficient Yang of the Spleen and Kidneys and edema caused by stagnation of fluids or Damp?
    a. Gan Jiang and Gan Cao
    b. Ren Shen and Gan Cao
    c. Ren Shen and Bai Zhu
    d. Fu Zi and Fu Ling

1267. Ju Hua, Long Dan Cao, and Mu Dan Pi each perform which of the following functions?
   a. Disperse Wind and clear Heat
   b. Clear Heat, cool the Blood, and relieve toxicity
   c. Drain Damp-Heat from the Liver and Gallbladder
   d. None of the above

1268. Which herb would you use with Gui Zhi to treat this pattern: Exterior Wind-Cold, sweating, intolerance to Wind, floating-moderate pulse?
   a. Huang Qi
   b. Fang Feng
   c. Bai Zhu
   d. Bai Shao

1269. Which of the following are treated by Huo Xiang, Pei Lan, and Xiang Ru?
   a. Wind-Cold Exterior syndrome
   b. Externally contracted patterns of Summer-Heat
   c. Edema and dysuria
   d. Vomiting

1270. Which pair of herbs represent different portions of the same plant?
   a. Chuan Wu and Cao Wu
   b. Jiang Huang and Sheng Jiang
   c. Ou Jie and Lian Zi
   d. Sang Ji Shang and Sang Zhi

1271. Sang Ji Sheng and Du Zhong each perform which of the following functions?
   a. Tonify the Liver and Kidneys and promote urination
   b. Invigorate the Blood and tonify the Liver and Kidneys
   c. Calm the fetus and tonify the Liver and Kidneys
   d. Calm the fetus and stop diarrhea

1272. Which herb is used with Da Huang to treat constipation caused by Cold?
   a. Dang Shen
   b. Dang Gui
   c. Fu Zi
   d. Bai Zhu

1273. Huang Lian, Sheng Jiang, and Wu Zhu Yu each perform which of the following functions?
   a. Clear Heat
   b. Expel Cold
   c. Stop vomiting
   d. Stop diarrhea

1274. Which two herbs are used with Xiang Fu to treat hypochondriac pain caused by constrained Liver Qi?
   a. Mu Xiang and Wu Yao
   b. Chai Hu and Bai Shao
   c. Fo Shou and Wu Yao
   d. Gan Jiang and Gao Liang Jiang

1275. Which syndrome is treated by Bai Zhi, Qing Huo, Xi Xin, and Chuan Xiong?
   a. Headache caused by Wind-Cold
   b. Headache caused by Wind-Heat
   c. Headache caused by Blood stasis
   d. Headache caused by Wind-Damp

1276. Which herb would you use with Huang Lian to treat abdominal pain caused by dysenteric disorders, with tenesmus and Blood and pus in the stool?
   a. Ge Gen
   b. Mu Xiang
   c. Huang Bai
   d. Rou Gui

1277. Which two herbs would you select to treat a patient with lack of appetite, loose stool, and tired limbs caused by insufficiency of Middle Energizer energy?
   a. Bai Zhu and Fu Ling
   b. Mu Xiang and Xiong Fu
   c. Rou Dou Kou and He Zi
   d. Huang Qi and Zhu Di

1278. Which two herbs would you select to treat irritability and insomnia caused by excessive Heart Fire?
   a. Long Gu and Mu Li
   b. Suan Zao Ren and Bai Zi Ren
   c. Huang Lian and E Jiao
   d. Zhen Zhu and Ye Jiao Teng

1279. Which three herbs would you select to treat hypochondriac pain caused by Stagnant Liver Qi and Blood?
   a. Chuan Xion, Chi Shao and Hong Hua
   b. Chuan Xiong, Chai Hu and Xiang Fu
   c. Chuan Xion, Tao Ren and Yi Mu Cao
   d. Chuan Xiong, Ze Lan and Dan Shen

1280. Which two herbs would you select to treat this pattern: severely Deficient Source Qi and sudden collapse of Yang Qi, cold extremities, sweating, weak breathing, faint pulse?
   a. Fu Zi and Huang Qi
   b. Fu Zi and Ren Shen
   c. Bai Zhu and Fu Zi
   d. Rou Gui and Fu Zi

1281. What ability of Ban Xia is strengthened by adding Sheng Jiang?
   a. Dry Damp
   b. Dissipate nodules
   c. Transform Phlegm
   d. Stop vomiting

1282. What are the special instructions for decocting Ling Yang Jiao, Xi Jiao, and Shan Ren Shen?
   a. Must be decocted before the other herbs
   b. Must be added to the decoction at the end
   c. Must be wrapped in cloth during decoction
   d. Must be decocted separately

1283. Which herbs are added to a decoction near the end of cooking?
   a. Sha Ren and Rou Gui
   b. Xi Xin and Fo Shou
   c. Ru Xiang and Yi Mu Cao
   d. Ding Xiang and Gao Liang Jiang

1284. Which two herbs each are decocted before the other herbs in a formula?
   a. Huang Jing and Bing Lang
   b. Guan Zhong and Ci Shi Zhi
   c. Sheng Shi Gao and Fu Zi
   d. Yin Guo and Shan Zha

1285. Bai Dou Kou and Rou Dou Kou each perform which of the following functions?
    a. Aromatically transform Damp
    b. Bind up the Intestines and stop diarrhea
    c. Warm the Middle Energizer and move the Qi
    d. Regulate the Qi and calm the fetus

1286. Fang Feng and Fang Ji each perform which of the following functions?
    a. Promote urination and reduce edema
    b. Release the Exterior and expel Wind
    c. Expel Wind-Damp
    d. Clear Damp-Heat from the Liver and Gallbladder

1287. Which two herbs each transform Phlegm and stop vomiting?
    a. Jie Geng and Xing Ren
    b. Xuan Fu Hua and Ban Xia
    c. Bai Jie Zi and Yin Guo
    d. Gua Lou and Qian Hu

1288. Mu Tong, Zhu Ye, Yu Jin, and Zhu Sha each perform which of the following functions?
    a. Clear Heart Fire
    b. Clear Heat and poisons
    c. Clear Liver Fire
    d. None of the above

1289. Long Gu and Mu Li each perform which of the following functions?
    a. Prevent leakage of fluids
    b. Soften hardness and dissipate nodules
    c. Benefit the Yin and anchor the floating Yang
    d. None of the above

1290. Dang Gui, Rou Cong Rong, and Gua Lou Ren each perform which of the following functions?
    a. Moisten the Lungs and stop coughing
    b. Tonify the Kidneys and fortify the Yang
    c. Moisten the Intestines and unblock the bowels
    d. None of the above

1291. Which two herbs each tonify the Blood, moisten the Intestines, and unblock the bowels?
    a. Shu Di and E Jiao
    b. He Shou Wu and Dang Gui
    c. Huang Ji and Suo Yang
    d. Long Yan Rou and Gou Qi Zi

1292. Which of the following indicates the use of Wu Wei Zi, Huang Qi, Tian Hua Fen, or Ge Gen?
    a. Spontaneous sweating
    b. Urinary frequency
    c. Diabetes
    d. Diarrhea caused by Damp-Heat

1293. Which of the following indicates the use of Jue Ming Zi, Xia Ku Cao, Sang Ye, or Qin Pi?
    a. Eye redness caused by Liver Fire
    b. Dysenteric disorder caused by Damp-Heat
    c. Externally contracted Wind-Heat
    d. Dry or infrequent stools or constipation

1294. Yuan Fu Hua and Dai Zhe Shi each perform which of the following functions?
   a. Cool the Blood and stop bleeding
   b. Redirect the Qi downwards
   c. Calm the Liver and anchor the floating Yang
   d. Clear Liver Heat

1295. Bai Bu and Bai He each perform which of the following functions?
   a. Moisten the Lungs and stop coughing
   b. Expel parasites and kill lice
   c. Clear Heart Fire and calm the Spirit
   d. None of the above

1296. Tian Nan Xing and Chan Tui each perform which of the following functions?
   a. Dry Damp and expel Phlegm
   b. Extinguish Wind and stop spasms
   c. Clear the eyes and remove superficial visual obstruction
   d. Reduce swelling and alleviate pain

1297. Pu Huang and Wu Ling Zhi each perform which of the following functions?
   a. Invigorate the Blood and stop bleeding
   b. Promote urination and stop bleeding
   c. Cool the Blood and stop bleeding
   d. None of the above

1298. Bai Mao Gen, Guan Zhong, Di Yu, and Han Lian Cao each perform which of the following functions?
   a. Clear Heat and promote urination
   b. Tonify and nourish the Liver and Kidneys
   c. Cool the Blood and stop bleeding
   d. Kill parasites

1299. Gan Cao, Guan Zhong, Ling Yang Jiao, and Sheng Ma each perform which of the following functions?
   a. Raise the Yang and lift the sunken Qi
   b. Clear Heat and relieve toxicity
   c. Cool the Blood and stop bleeding
   d. Calm the Liver and extinguish Wind

1300. Che Qian Zi and Jue Ming Zi each perform which of the following functions?
   a. Moisten the Intestines and unblock the bowels
   b. Promote urination and clear Heat
   c. Expel Phlegm and stop coughing
   d. Clear the Liver and benefit the eyes

1301. Which of the following indicates the use of Fu Ling, Bai Zhu, Yi Yi Ren, or Shan Yao?
   a. Diarrhea caused by deficiency of the Spleen
   b. Palpitations and insomnia
   c. Spermatorrhea and spontaneous sweating
   d. Frequent urination

1302. Fu Zi, Bu Gu Zhi, She Chuang Zi, and Ding Xiang each perform which of the following functions?
   a. Moisten the Intestines and unblock the bowels
   b. Warm/tonify the Kidneys and fortify the Yang
   c. Warm the Middle Energizer and stop vomiting
   d. Aid the Kidneys to grasp Qi

1303. Yuan Zhi, Chan Su, Niu Huang, and Zao Jiao each perform which of the following functions?
    a. Clear Heat and relieve toxicity
    b. Open the orifices
    c. Dispel Phlegm and stop coughing
    d. Calm the Spirit

1304. Which of the following indicates the use of Jie Geng, Yi Yi Ren, Yu Xing Cao, or Lu Gen?
    a. Lung abscesses and pain in the chest
    b. Wind-Heat coughing
    c. Diarrhea caused by Damp-Heat
    d. Damp leg Qi

1305. Which of the following indicates the use of Yin Chen Hao, Da Huang, Zhi Zi, and/or Huang Bai?
    a. Constipation and pain in the abdomen
    b. Jaundice caused by Damp-Heat
    c. Fire toxin generated sores
    d. Steaming bone disorder

1306. Qian Niu Zi, Bai Bu, Shi Liu Pi, and Chuan Lian Zi each perform which of the following functions?
    a. Drive out water
    b. Drive out Phlegm
    c. Stop diarrhea
    d. Expel parasites

1307. Which of the following indicates the use of Huang Bai, Qin Jiao, Mu Dan Pi, and/or Bie Jia?
    a. Wind-Damp painful obstruction
    b. Deficient Yin patterns with fever
    c. Frequent and profuse menstruation caused by Heat in the Blood
    d. None of the above

1308. Which of the following indicates the use of Xuan Shen, Mu Li, Jiang Can, and/or Zhe Bei Mu?
    a. Coughing with sputum that is difficult to expectorate
    b. Scrofula and goiter
    c. Dizziness from Liver Yang
    d. Palpitations with anxiety and insomnia

1309. Which of the following indicates the use of Mu Dan Pi, Da Huang, Yi Yi Ren, and/or Pu Gong Ying?
    a. Chronic low grade fevers
    b. Jaundice caused by Damp-Heat
    c. Intestinal abscesses and abdominal pain
    d. Bleeding caused by Heat in the Blood

1310. Sheng Ma, Chan Tui, Ge Gen, and Zi Cao each perform which of the following functions?
    a. Clear Heat and relieve toxicity
    b. Release Exterior Wind-Heat
    c. Raise the Yang
    d. Vent measles

1311. Chai Hu and Yin Chai Hu each perform which of the following functions?
    a. Release the Exterior and clear Heat
    b. Spread Liver Qi and relieve constraint
    c. Raise the Yang Qi
    d. None of the above

1312. Ju Hua, Bai Shao, Dai Zhe Shi, and Ci Shi each perform which of the following functions?
    a. Clear the Liver and the eyes
    b. Clear Heat and relieve toxicity
    c. Calm and curb Liver Yang
    d. None of the above

1313. Chai Hu, Qing Pi, Xiang Fu, and Bai Ji Li each perform which of the following functions?
    a. Calm and curb Liver Yang
    b. Spread Liver Qi and relieve constraint
    c. Expel Wind and stop itching
    d. Regulate menstruation and stop pain

1314. Which of the following indicates the use of Du Zhong, Sha Ren, Huang Qin, or Zi Su Ye?
    a. Externally contracted Wind Cold
    b. Restless fetus
    c. Diarrhea caused by Damp-Heat
    d. Damp distressing the Spleen and Stomach

1315. Shi Jue Ming and Jue Ming Zi each perform which of the following functions?
    a. Clear the Liver and benefit the eyes
    b. Calm and curb Liver Yang
    c. Moisten the Intestines and unblock the bowels
    d. Extinguish Wind and stop spasms

1316. Sang Ji Sheng and Gou Ji each perform which of the following functions?
    a. Tonify the Liver and Kidneys, strengthen the sinews and bones, and expel Wind-Damp
    b. Tonify the Liver and Kidneys, strengthen the sinews and bones, and calm the womb
    c. Tonify the Liver and Kidneys, strengthen the sinews and bones, and promote urination
    d. Tonify the Liver and Kidneys, strengthen the sinews and bones, and benefit the skin

1317. Hu Tao Ren and Su Zi each perform which of the following functions?
    a. Stop coughing
    b. Tonify the Kidneys
    c. Moisten the Intestines
    d. Alleviate pain

1318. Shan Yao, Qian Shi, and Bian Dou each perform which of the following functions?
    a. Clear Summer-Heat
    b. Strengthen the Spleen and stop diarrhea
    c. Nourish the Yin and Qi
    d. Stabilize the Kidneys and bind the Essence

1319. Ren Shen does *not* perform which of the following functions?
    a. Strongly tonify the basal Qi
    b. Benefit the Heart Qi and calm the Spirit
    c. Dry Damp and expel Cold
    d. Generate fluids and stop thirst

1320. Which herb is used to release the Exterior and disperse Cold, warm the Middle Energizer and stop vomiting, and warm the Lungs and stop coughing?
    a. Gan Jiang
    b. Jiang Ji
    c. Sheng Jiang
    d. Pao Jiang

1321. Which herb is warming, tonifies and invigorates the Blood, stops pain, and moistens the Intestines?
    a. Bai Shao
    b. Dang Gui
    c. E Jiao
    d. Shu Di Huang

1322. Which herb binds up the Intestines, stops diarrhea, warms the Middle Energizer, and moves Qi?
    a. Mu Xiang
    b. Bai Dou Kou
    c. Rou Dou Kou
    d. He Zi

1323. Which herb anchors the Yang and nourishes the Yin?
    a. Bie Jia
    b. Long Gu
    c. Bai Shao
    d. Dai Zhe Shi

1324. Which herb treats coma caused by Heat or Cold evil invading the body?
    a. Niu Huang
    b. She Xiang
    c. Su He Xiang
    d. Fu Zi

1325. Which herb is cooling, strongly directs rebellious Qi downward, calms the Liver, and anchors the floating Yang?
    a. Ci Shi
    b. Hua Rui Shi
    c. Dai Zhe Shi
    d. Gui Ban

1326. Which herb tonifies the Qi, nourishes the Yin, augments the three Yin, and stabilizes and binds?
    a. Bai Zhu
    b. Shan Yao
    c. Bai Bian Dou
    d. Yu Zhu

1327. Which herb is *not* to be used in the early stages of a warm febrile disease, or in cases of abdominal distention where there is thick greasy tongue fur?
    a. Yu Zhu
    b. Shi Hu
    c. Lu Gen
    d. Shi Gao

1328. Which herb warms the Kidneys, retains Essence, retains urine, warms the Spleen, increases appetite, and holds excessive salivation?
    a. Yi Zhi Ren
    b. Bu Gu Zhi
    c. Shan Yao
    d. Jin Ying Zi

1329. Which herb is used as a purgative to unblock the Intestines, and to clear the Liver and drain Fire?
    a. Lu Hui
    b. Huo Ma Ren
    c. Shang Lu
    d. Mang Xiao

1330. Which two herbs each treat Blood in the stool and bleeding hemorrhoids?
   a. Ai Ye and Xue Yu Tan
   b. Di Yu and Huai Jiao
   c. Zong Lu Tan and San Qi
   d. Bai Mao Gen and Fu Long Gen

1331. Which three herbs each treat coughing caused by Deficient Yin that yields bloody Phlegm?
   a. San Qi, Da Ji, and Ce Bai Ye
   b. Hua Rui Shi, Bai Mao Gen, and Zi Zhu Cao
   c. Qian Cao Gen, Ai Ye, and Fu Long Gan
   d. E Jiao, Bai Ji, and Bai Bu

1332. Which two herbs each invigorate the Blood, alleviate pain, reduce swelling, and generate flesh?
   a. Yu Jin and Jiang Huang
   b. Sang Leng and E Zhu
   c. Pu Huang and Wu Ling Zhi
   d. Ru Xiang and Mo Yao

1333. Which herb is used raw to treat chronic cough and loss of voice, and is used roasted to treat chronic diarrhea and dysenteric disorders?
   a. Rou Dou Kou
   b. Ge Gen
   c. Wu Mei
   d. He Zi

1334. Which herb is used raw to regulate stagnant Qi, and is used roasted to stop diarrhea?
   a. Ge Gen
   b. Wu Mei
   c. Rou Dou Kou
   d. Mu Xiang

1335. Which herb calms the Liver, anchors the Yang, and improves vision?
   a. Shi Jue Ming
   b. Mu Zei
   c. Jue Ming Zi
   d. Xia Ku Cao

1336. Which herb drains Liver Fire, clears Heat, and dries Damp?
   a. Mu Zei
   b. Xia Ku Cao
   c. Long Dan Cao
   d. Qing Xiang Zi

1337. Bo He does *not* perform which of the following functions?
   a. Clear the head and eyes and benefit the throat
   b. Vent rashes
   c. Promote Blood circulation
   d. Allow constrained Liver Qi to flow freely

1338. Which herb should be used cautiously during pregnancy, menstruation, or postpartum nursing?
   a. Zi Su Ye
   b. Da Huang
   c. Tong Cao
   d. Yu Li Ren

1339. Which herb cools and invigorates the Blood, and is most suitable for steaming bone disorder where there is absence of sweating?
   a. Che Shao
   b. Bai Wei
   c. Di Gu Pi
   d. Mu Dan Pi

1340. Which herb clears Heat, relieves toxicity, and dissipates nodules?
   a. Mai Men Dong
   b. Xuan Shen
   c. Shu Di Huang
   d. Gou Qi Zi

1341. Which herb has similar functions to Sheng Di Huang and also tonifies the three Yin and the Essence?
   a. Gou Qi Zi
   b. Shan Yao
   c. Mai Men Dong
   d. Shi Hu

1342. Which herb is particularly useful to expel Phlegm, clear the orifices, and dissipate swellings, and is also used to reduce abscesses and calm the Spirit?
   a. Suan Zao Ren
   b. Yuan Zhi
   c. Bai Zi Ren
   d. Dan Shen

1343. Which herb is used raw to moisten the Intestines, decrease inflammation, and treat malaria, and is used prepared to tonify and augment the Blood and extremities?
   a. Bing Lang
   b. He Shou Wu
   c. Qing Hao
   d. Chang Shan

1344. Which herb reduces Heat from Deficiency and treats childhood nutritional impairment?
   a. Huang Bai
   b. Yin Chai Hu
   c. Chai Hu
   d. Bai Wei

1345. Which herb clears Heat, promotes urination, drains Damp, expels Phlegm, and clears the eyes?
   a. Dong Kui Zi
   b. Che Qian Zi
   c. Fu Hai Shi
   d. Chuan Bei Mu

1346. Which herb clears Heat, promotes urination, drains Damp, and clears Summer-Heat?
   a. Hua Shi
   b. Qu Mai
   c. Yi Yi Ren
   d. Mu Tong

1347. Which herb treats seizure caused by Heat-Phlegm, frequently in combination with Yu Jin?
   a. Bai Zhu
   b. Bai Shao
   c. Bai Ji
   d. Ming Fan

1348. Which herb tonifies the Qi, stabilizes the Exterior, stops sweating, and dries Damp?
    a. Huang Qi
    b. Fang Feng
    c. Shan Yao
    d. Bai Zhu

1349. Which herb disperses Wind, clears Heat, vents rashes, stops spasms, and clears the eyes?
    a. Niu Huang
    b. Niu Bang Zi
    c. Ye Ju Hua
    d. Chan Tui

1350. Which herb tonifies the Kidneys and Liver, nourishes and tonifies the Essence and Blood, and stops bleeding?
    a. Gou Qi Zi
    b. Lu Rong
    c. Lu Jiao Shuang
    d. Lu Jiao Jiao

1351. Which herb tonifies the Liver and Kidneys, inhibits sweating, and supports that which has collapsed?
    a. Ren Shen
    b. Huang Qi
    c. Bai Zhu
    d. Shan Zhu Yu

1352. Which herb warms the Middle Energizer, rescues the devastated Yang, warms the Lungs, and transforms Phlegm?
    a. Rou Gui
    b. Xi Xin
    c. Fu Zi
    d. Gan Jiang

1353. Which herb is particularly useful to stop bleeding and vaginal discharge, and is also used to control acidity and alleviate pain?
    a. Fu Pen Zi
    b. Lian Zi
    c. Hua Rui Shi
    d. Hai Piao Xiao

1354. Which herb treats chronic diarrhea and dysentery caused by Cold from Deficiency, and treats distention in the epigastrium and abdomen?
    a. Ma Xiang
    b. He Zi
    c. Chi Shi Zhi
    d. Roasted Rou Dou Kou

1355. Which herb treats Deficient Spleen, constrained Liver Qi with symptoms of chest or flank pain, dizziness, vertigo, shortness of Qi, and prolapse?
    a. Xiang Fu
    b. Chai Hu
    c. Qing Pi
    d. Sheng Ma

1356. Which herb invigorates the Blood, promotes the movement of Qi, expels Wind, and treats headaches and many types of pain caused by Wind or Deficient Blood?
    a. Chuan Xiong
    b. Yu Jin
    c. Jiang Huang
    d. Gao Ben

1357. Which herb treats Wind-Heat common cold, vents measles, treats head sores, and is charred when used to treat uterine bleeding?
    a. Da Qing Ye
    b. Ban Lan Gen
    c. Zi Cao
    d. Guan Zhong

1358. Which herb opens the orifices, quiets the Spirit, transforms turbid Damp, and harmonizes the Stomach?
    a. Niu Huang
    b. Huo Xiang
    c. Shi Chang Pu
    d. Su He Xiang

1359. Which herb nourishes the Yin without cloying and retaining pathogenic influences, and is often used to treat externally contracted pathogens where there is Deficient Yin?
    a. Shi Hu
    b. Sha Shen
    c. Bai Wei
    d. Yu Zhu (Wei Rui)

1360. Which herb treats externally contracted Wind-Cold and tetanus?
    a. Fang Feng
    b. Xi Xin
    c. Quan Xie
    d. Wu Gong

1361. Which herb treats diarrhea before dawn caused by Deficient Yang?
    a. Wu Mei
    b. Roasted He Zi
    c. Bu Gu Zhi
    d. Yi Zhi Ren

1362. Which herb transforms Damp and releases Summer-Heat?
    a. Huang Bai
    b. Cang Zhu
    c. Pei Lan
    d. Qing Hao

1363. Which salty and cold herb treats cough caused by Lung Heat due to Liver Fire attacking the Lungs?
    a. Qian Hu
    b. Chuan Xin Lian
    c. Shan Dou Gen
    d. Qing Dai

1364. Which herb cools and invigorates the Blood, relieves toxicity, and vent rashes?
    a. Sheng Di Huang
    b. Mu Dan Pi
    c. Zi Cao
    d. Chi Shao

1365. Which herb clears Heat, relieves toxicity, cools the Blood, and reduces blotches?
   a. Pu Gong Ying
   b. Shan Ci Gu
   c. Tu Fu Ling
   d. Da Qing Ye

1366. Which herb treats headaches due to rising Liver Qi and treats Middle Energizer Cold due to Deficiency?
   a. Chuan Xiong
   b. Wu Zhu Yu
   c. Gao Ben
   d. Bai Zhi

1367. Which herb treats sinusitis, stuffy nose, nasal discharge, and headaches?
   a. Gao Ben
   b. Xi Xin
   c. Jing Jie
   d. Chuan Xiong

1368. Which herb treats muscular twitching of the extremities, rigidity and spasms of the entire body to the point of opisthotonos, trismus or convulsions, and is usually taken with Quan Xie?
   a. Long Gu
   b. Di Long
   c. Bai Ji Li
   d. None of the above

1369. Which herb should *not* be used in the early stages of a warm febrile disease or when a Damp-Warm disease has not yet changed to Dry?
   a. Shi Gao
   b. Zhi Mu
   c. Yu Zhu
   d. None of the above

1370. Which herb releases the Exterior, disperses Wind-Cold, and promotes the movement of stagnant Qi?
   a. Cang Zhu
   b. Qiang Huo
   c. Zi Su Ye
   d. None of the above

1371. Which herb tonifies the Kidneys, augments the Lungs, stops bleeding, and transforms Phlegm?
   a. Sha Shen
   b. Shan Yao
   c. Dong Chong Xia Cao
   d. None of the above

1372. Which herb disperses Cold, dries Damp, relieves constraint in the Liver meridian, redirects rebellious Qi downward, and alleviates pain?
   a. Xi Xin
   b. Chai Hu
   c. Wu Zhu Yu
   d. None of the above

1373. Which herb is used raw to invigorate the Blood, disperse Blood Stasis, alleviate pain, and is used dry-fried to stop bleeding?
   a. Wu Ling Zhi
   b. San Qi
   c. Chi Shao
   d. None of the above

1374. Which herb has functions similar to Hai Zao, and also reduces Phlegm, softens areas of hardness, and promotes urination?
    a. Bei Mu
    b. Kun Bu
    c. Xia Ku Cao
    d. None of the above

1375. Which herb redirect Qi downward, stops vomiting, reduces Phlegm, promotes urination?
    a. Dai Zhe Shi
    b. Huo Xiang
    c. Su Zi
    d. None of the above

1376. Which herb clears Liver Fire, dissipates nodules, and treats hypertension?
    a. Che Shao
    b. Xia Ku Cao
    c. Long Dan Cao
    d. None of the above

1377. Bai Bian Dou performs which of the following functions?
    a. Strengthen the Spleen and transform Damp
    b. Strengthen the Spleen and promote urination
    c. Calm the Spirit
    d. Nourish the Blood

1378. Which herb is *not* used for headache caused by sinusitis?
    a. Xin Yi Hua
    b. Xi Xin
    c. Bai Zhi
    d. Gui Zhi

1379. Which herb dissipates nodules, reduces masses, but can cause significant Liver damage and jaundice?
    a. Xia Ku Cao
    b. Kun Bu
    c. Hai Zao
    d. Huang Yao Zi

1380. Which function is *not* associated with sweet-flavored herbs?
    a. Tonify
    b. Expel Cold
    c. Moderate spasms
    d. Relieve toxicity

1381. Which function is *not* associated with acrid-flavored herbs?
    a. Release the Exterior
    b. Disperse
    c. Moisten and nourish
    d. Promote the movement of Qi

1382. Which function is *not* associated with bitter-flavored herbs?
    a. Drain
    b. Release the Exterior
    c. Dry
    d. Move downward

1383. Which herb does *not* dissipate nodules when used to treat scrofula?
   a. Bei Mu
   b. Lian Qiao
   c. Chuan Shan Jia
   d. Lei Wan

1384. Which herb does *not* kill roundworms and hookworms?
   a. Ku Lian Gen Pi
   b. Fei Zi
   c. Chuan Jiao
   d. Xian He Cao

1385. Which herb does *not* treat prematurely gray hair?
   a. He Shou Wu
   b. Ce Bai Ye
   c. Sang Shen
   d. Wu Yao

1386. Which herb does *not* treat toothache caused by Stomach-Fire?
   a. Huang Lian
   b. Zi Cao
   c. Shi Gao
   d. Tian Hua Fen

1387. Which herb dries Damp, but is *not* bitter-flavored?
   a. Mu Tong
   b. Ban Xia
   c. Huang Lian
   d. Hou Po

1388. Which herb does *not* treat redness, pain and swelling of the eyes caused by Liver Fire?
   a. Ju Hua
   b. Sang Ye
   c. Shi Jue Ming
   d. Shan Yu Rou

1389. Which herb does *not* treat night sweating caused by Deficient Yin?
   a. Bai Shao
   b. Bai Zhu
   c. Suan Zao Ren
   d. Bai Zi Ren

1390. Which herb does *not* promote lactation?
   a. Mu Tong
   b. Tong Cao
   c. Deng Xin Cao
   d. Wang Bu Liu Xing

1391. Which herb is *not* suitable for treating the early stages of externally contracted measles?
   a. Niu Bang Zi
   b. Huang Lian
   c. Lu Gen
   d. Chan Tui

1392. Which herb treats constipation caused by Dry in the Intestines?
   a. Lu Hui
   b. Fan Xie Ye
   c. Qian Niu Zi
   d. Dang Gui

1393. Which herb tonifies the Liver and Kidneys and stabilizes and binds?
   a. Shan Zhu Yu
   b. Gou Qi Zi
   c. Huang Jing
   d. He Zi

1394. Which herb does *not* treat Damp obstructing the Middle Energizer and causing epigastric distention, fullness, and pain?
   a. Chen Pi
   b. Cang Zhu
   c. Wu Ling Zhi
   d. Huo Xiang

1395. Which herb does *not* treat convulsions and seizures?
   a. Di Long
   b. Tian Ma
   c. Jue Ming Zi
   d. Gou Teng

1396. Which herb does *not* treat Damp-Cold painful obstruction?
   a. Chuan Wu
   b. Xi Xin
   c. Sang Zhi
   d. Cao Wu

1397. Which herb that releases the Exterior is used to invigorate the Blood and expel pus?
   a. Zi Su Ye
   b. Gui Zhi
   c. Bai Zhi
   d. Gao Ben

1398. Which herb cools the Blood, stops bleeding, clears Heat, and promotes urination?
   a. Ou Jie
   b. Ce Bai Ye
   c. Bai Mao Gen
   d. Mu Tong

1399. Which herb moistens the Lungs, clears the Heart, augments the Stomach, and generates fluids?
   a. Lu Gen
   b. Yu Zhu
   c. Sha Shen
   d. Mai Men Dong

1400. Which herb tonifies Qi, nourishes Yin, clears Fire, and generates fluids?
   a. Sha Shen
   b. Ren Shen
   c. Hai Er Shen
   d. Xi Yang Shen

1401. Which herb tonifies and augments the Heart and Spleen, nourishes the Blood, and calms the Spirit?
    a. Gou Qi Zi
    b. Dang Gui
    c. Da Zao
    d. Long Yan Rou

1402. Which herb invigorates the Blood, benefits the Gallbladders and reduces jaundice?
    a. Niu Xi
    b. San Qi
    c. Ru Xiang
    d. Yu Jin

1403. Which herb clears Heat, eliminates irritability, drains Damp-Heat, and cools the Blood?
    a. Huang Lian
    b. Lu Gen
    c. Zhi Zi
    d. Mu Dan Pi

1404. Which herb dispels Wind-Damp, relaxes the sinews, and clears Heat from Deficiency?
    a. Mu Gua
    b. Qin Jiao
    c. Hai Tong Pi
    d. Wu Jia Pi

1405. Which herb tonifies the Blood, stops bleeding, nourishes the Yin, and moistens the Lungs?
    a. Gou Qi Zi
    b. E Jiao
    c. Bai Shao
    d. Han Lian Cao

1406. Which herb treats ascending Liver Fire that causes red, painful, swollen eyes, headache, dizziness, scrofula, and lipoma?
    a. Xia Ku Cao
    b. Mu Zei
    c. Gu Jing Cao
    d. Chan Tui

1407. Which herb is frequently used with Shi Gao to treat dyspnea caused by externally contracted Heat obstructing the Lungs?
    a. Zhi Mu
    b. Huang Qin
    c. Ma Huang
    d. Zhi Zi

1408. Which herb clears Deficiency fevers and checks malarial disorders?
    a. Bai Wei
    b. Qing Hao
    c. Di Gu Pi
    d. Yin Chai Hu

1409. Which herb promotes urination, leaches out Damp, strengthens the Spleen, expels Wind-Damp, clears Heat, and expels pus?
    a. Mu Tong
    b. Fang Ji
    c. Fu Ling
    d. Yi Yi Ren

1410. Which herb treats edema that accompanies an Exterior pathogenic influence?
   a. Xi Xin
   b. Ban Xia
   c. Che Qian Zi
   d. Ma Huang

1411. Which herb does *not* treat internal movement of Liver-Wind?
   a. Bie Jia
   b. Gui Ban
   c. Gou Teng
   d. Long Yan Rou

1412. Which herb is used with Ge Jie to treat coughing and wheezing due to Deficient Lungs and Kidneys?
   a. Ma Huang
   b. Wu Wei Zi
   c. Su Zi
   d. Sheng Di Huang

1413. Which herb clears the Liver, benefit the eyes, moistens the Intestines, and unblocks the bowels?
   a. Jue Ming Zi
   b. Qing Xiang Zi
   c. Che Qian Zi
   d. Gu Jing Cao

1414. Which herb clears Heat and toxins, dissipates nodules, and expels externally contracted Wind-Heat?
   a. Tu Fu Ling
   b. Lian Qiao
   c. Jin Yin Hua
   d. Bo He

1415. Which herb releases Shaoyin meridian Wind-Cold that has caused Deficient Yang and a deep pulse?
   a. Fang Feng
   b. Xi Xin
   c. Du Huo
   d. Wu Zhu Yu

1416. Which formula would you select to treat this pattern: slight headache, aversion to cold, no sweating, cough with watery sputum, stuffy nose, dry throat, white tongue fur, wiry pulse?
   a. San Ao Tang
   b. Gui Zhi Tang
   c. Cong Chi Tang
   d. Xing Su San

1417. Which formula would you select to treat this pattern: moderate fever, dry hacking cough or one with scanty thick and sticky sputum, thirst, dry throat, floating-rapid pulse on the right side?
   a. Xing Su San
   b. Sang Ju Yin
   c. Sang Xing Tang
   d. Ma Xing Yi Gan Tang

1418. Which formula nourishes the Yin, moistens the Lungs, transforms Phlegm, and stops coughing?
   a. Qing Zao Jiu Fei Tang
   b. Sang Xing Tang
   c. Bei He Gu Jin Tang
   d. Zhi Sou San

1419. Which formula treats white throat *(bai hou)* or diphtherial disorders?
   a. Bei He Gu Jin Tang
   b. Yang Yin Qing Fei Tang
   c. Ren Shen Bai Du San
   d. Huang Lian Jie Du Tang

1420. Which formula contains Mai Men Dong, Ren Shen, Geng Mi, Da Zao, Gan Cao, and Ban Xia?
   a. Mai Men Dong Tang
   b. Yang Yin Qing Fei Tang
   c. Zhi Gan Cao Tang
   d. Sheng Mai San

1421. Which formula contains Xuan Shen, Mai Men Dong, and Sheng Di Huang?
   a. Yu Ye Tang
   b. Zeng Ye Tang
   c. Da Bu Yin Wan
   d. Yi Wei Tang

1422. Which formula treats constipation that recurs two to three days after treatment and is accompanied by a deep-weak-forceless pulse?
   a. Zhi Shi Dao Zhi Wan
   b. Tiao Wei Cheng Qi Tang
   c. Zeng Ye Tang
   d. Zeng Ye Cheng Qi Tang

1423. Which formula is used when the Qi is too weak to spread the fluids and Deficient Kidneys and Dry Stomach lead to diabetes?
   a. Zeng Ye Tang
   b. Yu Ye Tang
   c. Liu Wei Di Huang Wan
   d. Da Bu Yin Wan

1424. Which formula does *not* nourish Lung Yin?
   a. Zeng Ye Tang
   b. Bai He Gu Jin Tang
   c. Qing Zao Jiu Fei Tang
   d. Mai Men Dong Tang

1425. Which two herbs are *not* both used in Yang Yin Qing Fei Tang and in Bai He Gu Jin Tang?
   a. Sheng Di Huang and Mai Men Dong
   b. Mu Dan Pi and Shu Di Huang
   c. Xuan Shen and Bai Shao
   d. Bei Mu and Gan Cao

1426. Which formula does *not* contain Ren Shen and Wu Wei Zi?
   a. Hui Yang Jiu Ji Tang
   b. Sheng Mai San
   c. Tian Wang Bu Xin Dan
   d. Ding Zhi Wan

1427. Which formula would you select to treat this pattern: severe fever and chills, no sweating, aversion to cold, body aches, irritability, floating-tight pulse?
   a. Xiao Qing Long Tang
   b. Da Qing Long Tang
   c. Ma Huang Tang
   d. None of the above

1428. Which formula would you select to treat this pattern: fever, aversion to cold, no sweating, cough, wheezing, copious stringy sputum, body aches, floating edema, moist white tongue fur, floating pulse?
    a. Xiao Qing Long Tang
    b. Da Qing Long Tang
    c. Wu Ling San
    d. Ling Gui Zhu Gan Tang

1429. Which formula would you select to treat this pattern: headache, slight fever, aversion to cold, heavy chills, absence of sweating, cold extremities, fatigue with a constant desire to lie down, pallid complexion, weak voice, pale tongue with white fur, deep-forceless pulse?
    a. Jing Fang Bai Du San
    b. Zai Zao San
    c. Bu Zhong Yi Qi Tang
    d. Ren Shen Bai Du San

1430. Which formula would you select to treat this pattern: strong fever, mild chills, headache, stiff extremities, orbital and eye pain, dry nasal passages, irritability, insomnia, floating-slightly flooding pulse?
    a. Yue Ju Wan
    b. Chai Ge Jie Ji Tang
    c. Yin Qiao San
    d. Sang Xing Tang

1431. Which formula would you select to treat this pattern: high fever, aversion to cold, no sweating, stiff head and neck, sore extremities, focal distention and fullness of the chest, nasal congestion with sonorous breathing and abundant phlegm, greasy white tongue fur, floating-soft pulse?
    a. Chai Ge Jie Ji Tang
    b. Ren Shen Bai Du San
    c. Xian Fang Huo Ming Yin
    d. Zai Zao San

1432. Which formula would you select to treat this pattern: constipation, abdominal pain, cold extremities, wiry-deep pulse?
    a. Wen Pi Tang
    b. Da Jian Zhong Tang
    c. Li Zhong Tang
    d. Yang He Tang

1433. Which formula would you select to treat this pattern: abdominal pain, constipation, hypochondriac pain, low-grade fever, cold hands and feet, wiry-tight pulse?
    a. Wen Pi Tang
    b. Li Zhong Tang
    c. Si Ni San
    d. Da Huang Fu Zi Tang

1434. Which formula moistens the Intestines, unblocks the bowels, and moves the Qi?
    a. Ma Zi Ren Wan
    b. Zeng Ye Tang
    c. Wu Ren Wan
    d. Ji Chuan Jian

1435. Which formula promotes the movement of Qi and harshly drives out water?
    a. Zhou Che Wan
    b. Shi Zao Tang
    c. Tao He Cheng Qi Tang
    d. San Wu Bei Ji Wan

1436. Which formula contains Chai Hu, Huang Qin, Ban Xia, Sheng Jiang, Ren Shen, Zhi Gan Cao, and Da Zao?
   a. Da Chai Hu Tang
   b. Xiao Chai Hu Tang
   c. Xiao Yao San
   d. Chai Hu Gui Zhi Tang

1437. Xiao Chai Hu Tang is *not* indicated for which of the following?
   a. Irritability, heartburn, nausea, and vomiting
   b. Diarrhea
   c. Alternating fever and chills and a sensation of fullness in the chest and hypochondria
   d. A bitter or sour taste in the mouth and a dry throat

1438. Which formula clears Gallbladder Heat, expels Damp, harmonizes the Stomach, and transforms Phlegm?
   a. Wen Dan Tang
   b. Long Dan Xie Gan Tang
   c. Hao Qin Qing Dan Tang
   d. Gan Lu Xiao Du Dan

1439. Which formula consists of Chai Hu, Zhi Shi, Bai Shao and Zhi Gan Cao?
   a. Si Ni San
   b. Si Ni Tang
   c. Chai Ge Jie Ji Tang
   d. None of the above

1440. Which formula would you select to treat this pattern: mild chills alternating with pronounced fever, bitter taste in the mouth, stifling sensation in the chest, spitting up bitter or sour fluid or vomiting yellow brackish fluid, red tongue with greasy white fur, wiry-rapid pulse?
   a. Da Chai Hu Tang
   b. Hao Qin Qing Dan Tang
   c. Xiao Chai Hu Tang
   d. Xiao Yao San

1441. Si Ni San is *not* indicated for which of the following?
   a. Dysmenorrhea caused by Liver constraint with Qi Stagnation
   b. Pain in the abdomen caused by incoordination between the Liver and Spleen
   c. Diarrhea caused by incoordination between the Liver and Spleen
   d. Fullness in the chest and epigastrium caused by incoordination between the Liver and Spleen

1442. What is the pathogenesis of the syndrome treated by Si Ni San that involves cold fingers and toes?
   a. Cold evil entering the Interior
   b. Heat entering the Interior where it constrains the Yang Qi
   c. Deficient Kidney Yang
   d. Severe sweating

1443. Which of the following is *not* a proper modification of Si Ni San?
   a. If there is coughing, add Wu Wei Zi and Gan Jiang
   b. If there are palpitations, add Gui Zhi
   c. If there is urinary difficulty, add Fu Ling
   d. If there is diarrhea, add Bai Tou Weng

1444. Xiao Yao San does *not* contain which of the following?
   a. Chai Hu and Dang Gui
   b. Zhi Shi and Mu Dan Pi
   c. Bai Shao, Bai Zhu and Fu Ling
   d. Zhi Gan Cao, Wei Jiang and Bo He

1445. Xiao Yao San does *not* perform which of the following functions?
    a. Invigorate the Blood and alleviate pain
    b. Spread Liver Qi
    c. Strengthen the Spleen
    d. Nourish the Blood

1446. Which herb is added to Xiao Yao San to produce Hei Xiao Yao San?
    a. Sheng Di Huang
    b. Huang Qin
    c. Mu Dan Pi
    d. Zhi Zi

1447. Tong Xie Yao Fang does *not* contain which of the following?
    a. Bai Zhu
    b. Bai Shao
    c. Huang Lian
    d. Chen Pi and Fang Feng

1448. Which formula does *not* contain Ban Xia and Huang Qin?
    a. Tong Xie Yao Fang
    b. Da Chai Hu Tang
    c. Hao Qin Qing Dan Tang
    d. Ban Xia Xie Xin Tang

1449. Tong Xie Yao Fang is *not* indicated for which of the following?
    a. Borborygmus and diarrhea
    b. Abdominal pain
    c. A thin white tongue fur
    d. Retching and abnormal rising of Qi

1450. Ban Xia Xie Xin Tang does *not* contain which of the following?
    a. Ban Xia and Ren Shen
    b. Chai Hu and Zhi Zi
    c. Huang Qin and Huang Lian
    d. Gan Jiang, Gan Cao and Da Zao

1451. Ban Xia Xie Xin Tang does *not* perform which of the following functions?
    a. Drain Fire and relieve toxicity
    b. Harmonize the Stomach
    c. Direct rebellious Qi downward
    d. Disperse clumping and eliminate focal distention

1452. Which formula would you select to treat this pattern: borborygmus, abdominal pain, diarrhea, thin white tongue fur, wiry-moderate pulse?
    a. Si Ni San
    b. Ban Xia Xie Xin Tang
    c. Tong Xie Yao Fang
    d. Bai Du San

1453. Which formula would you select to treat this pattern: epigastric focal distention, fullness and tightness with very slight or no pain, dry heaves or vomiting, borborygmus with diarrhea, thin greasy yellow tongue fur, wiry-rapid pulse?
    a. Sheng Jiang Xie Xin Tang
    b. Huang Lian Tang
    c. Ban Xia Xie Xin Tang
    d. Gan Cao Xie Xin Tang

1454. Ban Xia Xie Xin Tang and Xiao Chai Hu Tang each contain which of the following ingredients?
    a. Ren Shen, Huang Qin, Ban Xia, Gan Jiang, and Gan Cao
    b. Ren Shen, Sheng Jiang, Ban Xia, Da Zao, and Gan Cao
    c. Ban Xia, Huang Qin, Ren Shen, Da Zao, and Gan Cao
    d. Ban Xia, Huang Qin, Gan Jiang, Da Zao, and Gan Cao

1455. Which formula would you select to treat a 30-year old female patient who has suffered from the following symptoms for four months: dull hypochondriac pain, dry mouth and throat, fatigue, reduced appetite, delayed menstrual period, distended breasts, pale red tongue, wiry-deficient pulse?
    a. Chai Hu Shu Gan San
    b. Xiao Yao San
    c. Si Wu Tang
    d. Hei Xiao Yao San

1456. How can Ban Xia Xin Xie Tang be modified to produce Sheng Jiang Xie Xin Tang?
    a. Add Sheng Jiang
    b. Remove Gan Jiang and add Sheng Jiang
    c. Reduce the dosage of Gan Jiang and add Sheng Jiang
    d. Remove Gan Cao and add Sheng Jiang

1457. Which formula would you select to treat this pattern: high fever, profuse sweating, severe thirst, red face, aversion to heat, flooding-forceful-rapid pulse?
    a. Bai Hu Tang
    b. Bai Hu Jia Ren Shen Tang
    c. Zhu Ye Shi Gao Tang
    d. Bai Hu Jia Gui Zhi Tang

1458. Which formula would you select to treat this pattern: Heat in the Heart meridian, sores around the mouth, warm sensation in the chest, thirst, red face, dark scanty rough and painful urination?
    a. Dao Chi San
    b. Xie Xin Tang
    c. Zhu Ye Shi Gao Tang
    d. Yi Yi Ren Tang

1459. Which formula would you select to treat this pattern: coughing caused by Heat in the Lungs, wheezing, skin that feels hot to the touch, fever which worsens in the late afternoon, red tongue with yellow fur, thin-rapid pulse?
    a. Ma Xing She Gan Tang
    b. Xie Bai San
    c. Wei Jing Tang
    d. Qing Qi Hua Hua Tan Wan

1460. Which formula would you select to treat this pattern: toothache and headache for more than a week that respond favorably to cold and worsen with heat, warm sensation in the face, bad breath, red tongue with yellow fur, slippery-rapid pulse?
    a. Zhu Ye Shi Gao Tang
    b. Xie Huang San
    c. Huang Lian Jie Du Tang
    d. Qing Wei San

1461. Which formula would you select to treat dysentery with bloody stool caused by Heat toxins?
    a. Bai Tou Weng Tang
    b. Huang Qin Tang
    c. Ge Gen Huang Lian Huang Qin Tang
    d. Shao Yao Tang

1462. Which formula would you select to treat this pattern: hectic fever caused by Deficient Yin, night sweats, emaciation, red lips and cheeks, coughing with bloody sputum, faint-rapid pulse?
    a. Qing Huo Bie Jie Tang
    b. Qin Jiao Bie Jie Tang
    c. Liu Wei Di Huang Wan
    d. Qing Gu San

1463. Which formula would you select to treat this pattern: mild Summer-Heat injuring the Lung meridian, slight fever and thirst, blurred vision with light-headedness, pink tongue with thin white fur?
    a. Liu Yi San
    b. Qing Luo Yin
    c. Huo Xiang Zheng Qi San
    d. Xiang Ru San

1464. Which formula would you select to treat a patient who comes to you during the summer with these symptoms: fever, headache, aversion to cold with no sweating, thirst, flushed face, tight sensation in the chest, greasy white tongue fur, floating-rapid pulse?
    a. Liu Yi San
    b. Huo Xiang Zheng Qi San
    c. Xin Jia Xiang Ru Yin
    d. Xiang Ru San

1465. Which formula would you select to treat this pattern: Exterior Cold and Interior Damp, heavy sensation in the head, headache, no sweating, stifling sensation in the chest, abdominal pain, vomiting, diarrhea, greasy white tongue fur, floating-rapid pulse?
    a. Xiang Ru San
    b. Xiang Su San
    c. Ma Huang Jia Zhu Tang
    d. Jiu Wei Qiang Huo Tang

1466. Liu Yi San is *not* indicated for which of the following?
    a. Fever
    b. Headache
    c. Diarrhea and urinary difficulty
    d. Thirst and irritability

1467. How can Xiao Chai Hu Tang be modified to produce Da Chai Hu Tang?
    a. Combine with Xiao Cheng Qi Tang; add Bai Shao; subtract Ren Shen, Gan Cao, and Huo Po
    b. Combine with Xiao Cheng Qi Tang
    c. Combine with Tiao Wei Cheng Qi Tang
    d. Combine with Tiao Wei Cheng Qi Tang; subtract Da Zao

1468. Da Chai Hu Tang is *not* indicated for which of the following?
    a. Alternating fever and chills, fullness in the chest and hypochondria
    b. Continuous vomiting, hard focal distention or fullness and pain in the epigastrium
    c. Yellow tongue fur and a wiry-forceful pulse
    d. Loose stool

1469. Which formula releases the Exterior, drains Heat, and unblocks the bowels?
    a. Ge Gen Qin Liang Tang
    b. Fang Feng Tong Sheng San
    c. Shi Gao Tang
    d. None of the above

1470. Which formula would you select to treat this pattern: fever, dysenteric diarrhea, sensation of irritability and heat in the chest, burning sensation around the anus, thirst, red tongue with yellow fur, rapid pulse?
    a. Ge Gen Huang Lian Huang Qin Tang
    b. Yin Qiao Bai Du San
    c. Shao Yao Tang
    d. Bei Tou Weng Tang

1471. Shi Gao Tang is *not* indicated for which of the following?
    a. Strong fever with no sweating
    b. Tinnitus and red eyes
    c. Dry nasal passages and thirst
    d. Irritability, insomnia or delirium

1472. What are the five accumulations in syndromes treated with Wu Ji San?
    a. Qi, Blood, Cold, Damp and Phlegm
    b. Qi, Blood, Fire, Phlegm and food
    c. Qi, Blood, parasites, Phlegm and food
    d. Qi, Blood, parasites, Phlegm and Cold

1473. What is the composition of Shi Goa Tang?
    a. Huang Lian Jie Du Tang with Shi Gao, Gui Zhi and Xiang Fu
    b. Huang Lian Jie Du Tang with Shi Gao, Gui Zhi and Bai Shao
    c. Huang Lian Jie Du Tang with Ma Huang, Shi Gao and Dan Dou Chi
    d. Huang Lian Jie Du Tang with Ma Huang, Shi Gao and Gui Zhi

1474. Which formula is used in particular to leach out Damp and stop diarrhea?
    a. Si Jun Zi Tang
    b. Liu Jun Zi Tang
    c. Bu Zhong Yi Qi Tang
    d. None of the above

1475. Which formula would you select to treat a male patient in his 30's who contracted Summer-Heat one month ago and suffers from fever (which responds to medicine) and sweating (which does not), and who also suffers from fatigue, shortness of breath, laconic speech, dry mouth, thirst, pale red tongue with dry fur, and a deficient-thin pulse?
    a. Zhu Ye Shi Gai Tang
    b. Qing Luo Yin
    c. Sheng Mai San
    d. Qing Shu Yi Qi Tang

1476. Which formula does *not* contain Dang Gui and Chuan Xiong?
    a. Si Wu Tang
    b. Sheng Hua Tang
    c. Gui Pi Tang
    d. Wen Jing Tang

1477. Which formula would you select to treat this pattern: irregular menstruation that is sparse, pale-colored, and late, withered yellowish complexion, dizziness, blurred vision, pale tongue, thin pulse?
    a. Si Wu Tang
    b. Tao Hong Si Wu Tang
    c. Xiao Yao San
    d. Bu Zhong Yi Qi Tang

1478. Which formula augments Heart Qi, nourishes Heart Blood, enriches Heart Yin, and restores the pulse?
   a. Zhi Gan Cao Tang
   b. Gui Pi Tang
   c. Ga Zhen Tang
   d. Sheng Mai San

1479. Which formula would you select to nourish the Blood, augment the Qi, and calm the fetus of a woman with this pattern: Deficient Qi and Blood, pale face, loss of appetite, fatigue, history of miscarriage?
   a. Jiao Ei Tang
   b. Tai Shan Pan Shi San
   c. Wen Jing Tang
   d. Bu Zhen Tang

1480. Which formula would you select to treat a man in his 70's with this pattern: lower back pain, weakness in the lower extremities, cold sensation in the lower half of the body, tension in the lower abdomen, excessive urination, pale swollen tongue, deep-faint pulse (especially at the proximal position)?
   a. Ji Sheng Shen Qi Wan
   b. Jin Gui Shen Qi Wan
   c. Liu Wei Di Huang Wan
   d. Zhen Wu Tang

1481. Which formula would you select to treat a female patient with this pattern: hysteria, disorientation, frequent attacks of melancholy and crying, inability to control herself, frequent bouts of yawning, red tongue with sparse fur, thin-rapid pulse?
   a. Xiao Yao San
   b. Wen Pi Tang
   c. Gan Mai Da Zao Tang
   d. Gui Pi Tang

1482. Which formula would you select to treat this pattern: spontaneous sweating (worse at night), easily startled, palpitations, shortness of breath, irritability, debility, lethargy, pale red tongue, thin-frail pulse?
   a. Yu Ping Feng San
   b. Qing Huo Bie Jia Tang
   c. Gui Zhi Tang
   d. Mu Li San

1483. Which formula warms the Liver and Kidneys, promotes the movement of Qi, and alleviates pain?
   a. Tian Tai Wu Yao San
   b. Wu Zhu Yu Tang
   c. Ju He Wan
   d. Nuan Gan Jian

1484. Which formula treats Deficient Blood during the postpartum period where there is retention of lochia with Cold and pain in the lower abdomen?
   a. Wen Jing Tang
   b. Tao Hong Si Wu Tang
   c. Sheng Hua Tang
   d. Shao Fu Zhu Yu Tang

1485. Which formula does *not* treat bleeding caused by Deficient Yang?
   a. Li Zhong Wan
   b. Gui Pi Tang
   c. Huang Tu Tang
   d. Shi Hui San

1486. Which formula augments the Qi, relieves Wind, strengthens the Spleen, and promotes urination?
    a. Fang Ji Huang Qi Tang
    b. Fang Ji Fu Ling Tang
    c. Ling Gui Zhu Gan Tang
    d. Wu Ling San

1487. Which formula does *not* contain Jie Geng and Gan Cao?
    a. Yin Qiao San
    b. Huang Long Tan
    c. Bai He Gu Jin Tang
    d. Bei Mu Gua Lou San

1488. Which formula clears Heat, transforms Phlegm, regulates Qi, and stops coughing?
    a. Qing Qi Hua Tan Wan
    b. Wen Dan Tang
    c. Xiao Xian Xiong Tang
    d. Bei Mu Gua Lou San

1489. Which formula would you select to treat this pattern: itchy throat, slight aversion to cold, fever, thin white tongue fur?
    a. Ling Gan Wu Wei Jiang Xin Tang
    b. Qing Zao Jiu Fei Tang
    c. Zhi Sou San
    d. Cong Chi Tang

1490. Which formula consists of Ma Huang, Gui Zhi, Gan Jiang, Xi Xin, Wu Wei Zi, Bai Shao, Ban Xia, and Zhi Gan Cao?
    a. Ma Huang Tang
    b. Da Qing Long Tang
    c. Xiao Qing Long Tang
    d. Ding Chuan Tang

1491. Sang Bai Pi is classified as the chief (monarch or *jun*) component in which formula?
    a. Xie Huang San
    b. Zhi Sou San
    c. Qing Qi Hua Tan Wan
    d. Xie Bai San

1492. Which formula consists of Gui Zhi Tang plus Dang Gui, Xi Xin, Mu Tong, with Sheng Jiang subtracted?
    a. Xiao Jian Zhong Tang
    b. Hui Yang Jiu Ji Tang
    c. Gui Zhi Jia Shao Yao Tang
    d. Dang Gui Si Ni Tang

1493. Which formula contains Jie Geng?
    a. Gui Pi Tang
    b. Zhi Gan Cao Tang
    c. Bu Zhong Yi Qi Tang
    d. Shen Ling Bai Zhu Tang

1494. Which formula would you select to treat this pattern: Deficient Liver and Kidneys leading to upward rising of Deficiency-Fire, coughing up of blood, steaming bone disorder, afternoon tidal fever, night sweats, rapid-forceful pulse at the rear (*chi*) position?
    a. Qing Gu San
    b. Qing Hao Bie Jia Tang
    c. Da Bu Yin Wan
    d. Liu Wei Di Huang Wan

1495. What is the pathogenesis of the symptoms that Huang Tu Tang treats?
    a. Deficient Spleen Yang
    b. Spleen and Stomach Deficient Qi
    c. Spleen and Deficient Kidney Yang
    d. Damp-Heat in the Large Intestine

1496. What causes the retention of lochia that Sheng Hua Tang treats?
    a. Blood Stasis, Deficient Blood, and Cold
    b. Blood Stasis and Deficient Qi
    c. Blood Stasis and deficiency-Fire
    d. None of the above

1497. Di Tan Tang is created by subtracting Wu Mei from Er Chen Tang and adding which of the following?
    a. Zhi Shi and Tian Nan Xing
    b. Zhi Shi, Zhu Ru, and Da Zao
    c. Zhi Shi, Zhu Ru, Ge Gen, and Da Zao
    d. Zhi Shi, Zhu Ru, Ren Shen, Da Zao, Shi Chang Pu, and Dan Nan Xing

1498. Which formula would you select to treat dizziness caused by Wind-Phlegm?
    a. Ling Gui Zhu Gan Tang
    b. Er Chen Tang
    c. Ban Xia Bai Zhu Tian Ma Tang
    d. None of the above

1499. Which formula would you select to treat night sweats and fever caused by Deficient Yin?
    a. Mu Li San
    b. Dang Gui Liu Huang Wan
    c. Yu Ping Feng San
    d. Tian Wang Bu Xin Dan

1500. Which formula consists of Fu Zi, Bai Zhu, Fu Ling, Sheng Jiang and Bai Shao?
    a. Fu Zi Tang
    b. Fu Zi Li Zhong Tang
    c. Yang He Tang
    d. Zhen Wu Tang

1501. Which of the following is considered part of the materia medica?
    a. Properties and flavors
    b. Lifting, lowering, floating, and sinking characteristics
    c. Meridian tropism
    d. All of the above

1502. Bitter-warm herbs treat which of the following?
    a. Deficient Yin
    b. Deficient body fluids
    c. Deficiency-Cold
    d. Damp-Cold

1503. Bitter-cold herbs treat which of the following?
    a. Deficient Blood
    b. Deficient Yin
    c. Deficiency-Heat
    d. Damp-Heat

1504. Sweet-cold herbs treat which of the following?
   a. Deficient Yang
   b. Deficient Qi
   c. Deficient Yin
   d. Damp-Heat

1505. Salty-cold herbs treat which of the following?
   a. Damp-Heat
   b. Damp-Cold
   c. Deficient Yin
   d. Blood Heat

1506. Herbs that tend to lift and float do *not* perform which of the following functions?
   a. Relieve Exterior syndromes
   b. Elevate Yang
   c. Remove Damp and improving digestion
   d. Dispel Exterior Wind and Cold

1507. What would be a contraindication for the use of two herbs together?
   a. Mutual restraint
   b. Mutual detoxification
   c. Mutual inhibition
   d. Mutual assistance

1508. Which of the following is considered a contraindication for the use of Chinese medicinal herbs?
   a. Use of prescription drugs
   b. Pregnancy
   c. Restricted diet
   d. All of the above

1509. Which of the following is *not* a way that Ma Huang treats edema?
   a. Diaphoresis
   b. Induces diuresis
   c. Reinforces Yang
   d. Promote the flow of Lung Qi

1510. Chai Hu performs which of the following functions?
   a. Clear Liver fire
   b. Nourish Liver Blood
   c. Nourish Liver Yin
   d. Spread Liver Qi

1511. Bai Zhi is *not* indicated for which of the following?
   a. Exterior Wind-Damp syndrome
   b. Leukorrhea caused by Damp-Cold
   c. Diarrhea caused by Damp-Heat
   d. Headache caused by stuffy nose and rhinorrhea with turbid purulent nasal discharge

1512. Which function do Fang Feng and Gao Ben *not* have in common?
   a. Relieve pain
   b. Relieve spasms
   c. Drain Damp
   d. Relieve Exterior syndromes by expelling Wind pathogens

1513. Sang Ye and Ju Hua each perform which of the following functions?
    a. Clear Liver Heat
    b. Detoxification
    c. Cool the Blood and stop bleeding
    d. Clear and drain Damp-Heat

1514. Which herb invigorates Spleen Yang to stop diarrhea?
    a. Chai Hu
    b. Ge Gen
    c. Sheng Ma
    d. Sang Ye

1515. Which herb does *not* function to release the Exterior and expel Wind?
    a. Dan Zhu Ye
    b. Fang Feng
    c. Cheng Jiang
    d. Jing Jie

1516. Which herb does *not* function to release the Exterior and vent measles?
    a. Man Jing Zi
    b. Niu Bang Zi
    c. Sheng Ma
    d. Ge Gen

1517. Which two herbs release the Exterior and allow constrained Liver Qi to flow freely?
    a. Sang Ye and Ju Hua
    b. Bo He and Chai Hu
    c. Chan Tui and Ge Gen
    d. Xia Ku Cao and Sheng Ma

1518. Which two herbs treat cough caused by Wind-Cold?
    a. Bo He and Sang Ye
    b. Zi Su Ye and Sheng Jiang
    c. Bai Zhi and Chai Hu
    d. Gui Zhi and Xin Yi Hua

1519. Which herb treats headache caused by Wind-Cold?
    a. Ju Hua
    b. Sang Ye
    c. Bo He
    d. Xi Xin

1520. Which herb treats headache caused by sinusitis?
    a. Xin Yin Hua
    b. Xi Xin
    c. Bai Ji Cang Er Zi
    d. All of the above

1521. Which herb treats both the Deficiency and Excess form of Wind-Cold Exterior syndrome?
    a. Ma Huang
    b. Gui Zhi
    c. Xi Xin
    d. Zi Su Ye

1522. Which herb cools the blood, stops bleeding, expels phlegm, and alleviates cough?
   a. Huai Hua Mi
   b. Qian Cao Gen
   c. Ce Bai Ye
   d. Ou Jie

1523. Which herbs must be used very cautiously (if at all) during pregnancy?
   a. Chen Pi and Wu Yao
   b. Zhi Shi and Wang Bu Liu Xing
   c. Fo Shou and Chen Xiang
   d. Gao Liang Jiang and Mu Xiang

1524. Which herbs promote Blood circulation and stop bleeding?
   a. Pu Huang and Jiang Xiang
   b. Qian Cao Gen and Bai Mao Gen
   c. Xian He Cao and Bai Ji
   d. Dan Shen and Chuan Xiong

1525. Which herbs treat jaundice caused by Damp-Heat?
   a. Fu Ling and Tu Fu Ling
   b. Chi Xiao Dou and Bai Xian Pi
   c. Jin Yin Hua and Zi Hua Di Ding
   d. Bai Tou Weng and Pu Gong Ying

1526. Which type of Phlegm is Ban Xia best known for treating?
   a. Heat-Phlegm
   b. Dry-Phlegm
   c. Damp-Phlegm
   d. Wind-Phlegm

1527. Zi Cao and Niu Bang Zi each perform which of the following functions?
   a. Disperse Wind-Heat
   b. Benefit the throat
   c. Detoxify poison and encourage rashes to the surface
   d. Cool and invigorate the Blood

1528. Which herb clears Heat from the Lungs, expels Phlegm, softens hardness, and dissipates Phlegm nodules?
   a. Kun Bu
   b. Hai Zao
   c. Tian Zhu Huang
   d. Fu Hai Shi

1529. Which herb is beneficial to the breasts?
   a. Zhu Ling
   b. Dong Kui Zhi
   c. Deng Xin Cao
   d. Dong Qua Ren

1530. Which herb treats Deficient Spleen with congestion of fluids and Phlegm, causing edema, heart palpitations, and insomnia?
   a. Fu Ling
   b. Yi Yi Ren
   c. Bai Zhu
   d. Lian Zi

1531. Which two formulas each contain Ma Huang and Shi Gao?
   a. Da Qing Long Tang and Ma Xing Shi Gan Tang
   b. Xiao Qing Long Tang and Yue Ju Wan
   c. Xie Huang San and Zhu Ye Shi Gao Tang
   d. Ding Chuan Tang and Qing Won Bai Du Yin

1532. Which two formulas each contain Sheng Jiang?
   a. Jiu Wei Qiang Huo Tang and Xiao Qing Long Tang
   b. Li Zhong Wan and Hui Yang Jiu Ji Tang
   c. Qui Zhi Tang and Da Qing Long Tang
   d. All of the above

1533. Which of the following is an indication for Xiao Qing Long Tang?
   a. Fever, chills, absence of sweating, poor appetite, and belching
   b. Fever, chills, absence of sweating, and a floating moderate pulse
   c. Fever, chills, absence of sweating, headache, and a stiff neck
   d. Fever, chills, absence of sweating, coughing, and wheezing

1534. Which herbs serve as the chief (monarch or *jun*) component in Zai Zao San?
   a. Gui Zhi and Fu Zi
   b. Ren Shen and Huang Qi
   c. Xi Xin and Qiang Huo
   d. Fang Feng and Chuan Xiong

1535. Which two formulas **both** treat wheezing caused by Exterior Cold with Interior Heat?
   a. Da Qing Long Tang and Ding Chuan Tang
   b. Xiao Qing Long Tang and Su Zi Jiang Qi Tang
   c. Qing Qi Hua Tan Wan and Bei Mu Qua Lou San
   d. Zhi Sou San and Di Tan Tang

1536. Which formula treats Exterior syndromes complicated by other types of syndromes?
   a. Xiang Su San
   b. Xiao Qing Long Tang
   c. Huo Xiang Zhen Qi San
   d. All of the above

1537. Bai Du San is *not* indicated for which of the following?
   a. Exogenous Wind-Cold-Damp complicated by Deficiency?
   b. Damp-Heat pathogens
   c. Pyesis in the primary stage that has been brought on by Deficient Normal Qi
   d. Attack of exogenous Wind-Cold-Damp on the body's surface

1538. Which formula contains Du Huo, Qing Huo, Chai Hu, and Qian Hu?
   a. Jiu Wei Qing Huo Tang
   b. Chai Ge Jie Ji Tang
   c. Bai Du San
   d. Chuan Xiong Cha Tiao San

1539. Which of the following herbs do Sang Ju Yin and Yin Qiao San *not* have in common?
   a. Lian Qiao
   b. Bo He
   c. Jie Geng and Gan Cao
   d. Xing Ren and Lu Gen

1540. Which of these treat attack of Wind-Cold on the body surface that involves headache and body ache?
   a. Jiu Wei Qing Huo Tang
   b. Qing Huo Sheng Shi Tang
   c. Gui Zhi Tang and Zai Zao San
   d. Zhu Ling Tang and Huo Xiang Zheng Qi San

1541. Which of the following herbs clear Heat, resolve Damp, and treat Damp-Heat jaundice?
   a. Zi Hua Di Ding
   b. Lu Gen
   c. Pu Gong Ying and Zhi Zi
   d. All of the above

1542. Zhi Zi does *not* perform which of the following functions?
   a. Eliminate irritability
   b. Cool the Blood
   c. Nourish fluids
   d. Promote diuresis

1543. Zhi Mu does *not* perform which of the following functions?
   a. Clear Lung Heat
   b. Clear Stomach Heat
   c. Clear Heart Heat and Liver Heat
   d. Clear Excess-Heat and Deficiency-Heat

1544. Huang Qin does *not* perform which of the following functions?
   a. Clear Heart Heat and eliminate irritability
   b. Clear Lung Heat and stop coughing
   c. Clear Deficiency-Heat
   d. Clear Heat and have a calming influence on the fetus

1545. Huang Qin helps to relieve coughing be performing which of the following functions?
   a. Release inhibited Lung Qi and resolve sputum
   b. Drain Damp-Heat and resolve sputum
   c. Disperse Wind-Heat
   d. Clear Lung Heat

1546. Zi Cao performs which of the following functions?
   a. Tonify the Blood
   b. Stop bleeding
   c. Cool the Blood and detoxify Fire Poison
   d. Clear Lung Heat and alleviate cough

1547. Hu Huang Lian performs which of the following functions?
   a. Clear Blood Heat
   b. Clear Lung Heat
   c. Clear Heart Heat and Bladder Heat
   d. Clear Damp-Heat and Deficiency-Heat

1548. Which formula clears Damp-Heat and toxicity and regulates the Qi and Blood?
   a. Bai Tou Weng Tang
   b. Shao Yao Tang
   c. Yu Nu Jian
   d. Huang Lian Jie Du Tang

1549. What is the pathogenesis of Xue Fu Zhu Yu Tang?
    a. Stagnation of Excess-Heat in the Interior
    b. Stagnation of Phlegm
    c. Deficient Qi and Deficient Blood
    d. Blood Stasis in the chest and Stagnation of Qi

1550. Niu Xin performs which of the following functions in the formula Yu Nu Jian?
    a. Helps Shi Gao clear away Stomach Heat
    b. Nourish Kidney Yin
    c. Guides pathogenic Heat downward to reduce Fire and conduct the Blood downward
    d. None of the above

1551. Which herb has the biggest dosage in Liang Ge San?
    a. Huang Qin
    b. Da Huang
    c. Liao Qiao
    d. Zhi Zi

1552. Which herb serves as the primary (ruling or *jun*) component in Qing Wei San?
    a. Huang Lian
    b. Sheng Ma
    c. Mu Dan Pi
    d. Sheng Di Huang

1553. Which directions are appropriate for Bai Hu Tang?
    a. Decoct all herbs in water, remove residue, drink the decoction while warm
    b. Decoct all of the herbs in a mixture that is half wine and half water
    c. Decoct all of the herbs in water, remove residue, let cool and then drink
    d. None of the above

1554. Which formula treats the early stages of Summer Heat accompanied by a superimposed contraction of Cold, a condition characterized by fever and chills, absence of sweating, headache, thirst, flushed face, a sensation of lightness in the chest, greasy white tongue fur, and a floating-rapid pulse?
    a. Xiang Ru San
    b. Xin Jia Xiang Ru Yin
    c. Gui Ling Gan Lu Yin
    d. Liu Yi San

1555. Which formula treats Heat in the Liver meridian that causes pain in the hypochondria?
    a. Long Dan Xie Gan Tang
    b. Zuo Jin Wan
    c. Jin Ling Zi San
    d. All of the above

1556. Liu Yi San does *not* contain which of the following formulas?
    a. Gui Ling Gan Lu Yin
    b. Ji Su San
    c. Qing Shu Yi Qi Tang
    d. Hao Qin Qing Dan Tang

1557. Using Da Huang to treat Heat diseases in the upper portion of the body (e.g., blood shot eyes, sore throat, swollen painful gums) is an example of which treatment approach?
    a. Treating diarrhea with cathartics
    b. Taking drastic measures to treat a disease
    c. Using medicines with a cold nature to treat pseudo-cold syndromes
    d. The corrigent method

1558. What makes Fu Ling a good treatment for diarrhea and edema?
    a. It warms the Middle Energizer
    b. It clears Heat
    c. It dries Damp and unblocks the bowels
    d. It promotes urination and strengthens the Spleen

1559. Zhu Ling is a good treatment for edema thanks to its ability to perform which of the following?
    a. Strengthen the Spleen
    b. Dry Damp
    c. Promote urination
    d. All of the above

1560. Yi Yi Ren is a good treatment for diarrhea thanks to its ability to perform which of the following?
    a. Promote urination
    b. Clear Heat
    c. Strengthen the Spleen and leach out Damp
    d. All of the above

1561. Which of the following functions do Fu Ling and Yi Yi Ren *not* have in common?
    a. Promote urination and leach out Damp
    b. Quiet the Heart and calm the Spirit
    c. Strengthen the Spleen
    d. Treats diarrhea

1562. Which of the following is an indication for Bei Xie Fen Qing Yin?
    a. Painful urinary dysfunction
    b. Stranguria complicated by hematuria
    c. Stranguria caused by Heat
    d. Cloudy or white and turbid urine

1563. Which herb does *not* dispel Wind-Damp?
    a. Wu Jia Pi
    b. Fang Feng
    c. She Tui
    d. Guang Feng Ji

1564. Which herb dispels Wind-Damp, relaxes the sinews, and clears Deficiency-Heat?
    a. Du Huo
    b. Qin Jiao
    c. Wei Ling Qian
    d. Mu Gua

1565. Du Huo, Mu Gua, and Wu Jia Pin each perform which of the following functions?
    a. Dispel Wind-Damp and release the Exterior
    b. Transform Damp and reduce swelling
    c. Reduce food stagnation
    d. None of the above

1566. What makes Cang Zhu a good treatment for diarrhea?
    a. It expels Wind-Damp
    b. It raises the Yang
    c. It dries Damp and strengthens the Spleen
    d. All of the above

1567. Which of the following herbs transform Damp and release the Exterior?
   a. Sha Ren
   b. Hou Po
   c. Huo Xiang and Xiang Ru
   d. Mu Gua and Can Sha

1568. Which herb does *not* transform Damp and stop vomiting?
   a. Sha Ren
   b. Bai Zhu
   c. Bai Dou Kou
   d. Luo Xiang

1569. Which herb dries Damp, strengthens the Spleen, and expels Wind-Damp?
   a. Hou Po
   b. Cang Zhu
   c. Cao Guo
   d. Cao Dou Kou

1570. Cao Guo and Cao Dou Kou each perform which of the following functions?
   a. Treat malarial disorders
   b. Activate Qi
   c. Dry Damp and warm the Middle Energizer
   d. All of the above

1571. Which herb does *not* treat malarial disorders?
   a. Cao Guo
   b. Cao Dou Kou
   c. Qing Hao
   d. Chang Shan

1572. Which herb releases the Exterior, disperses Cold, and promotes the movement of Qi?
   a. Pei Lan
   b. Huo Xiang
   c. Zi Su Ye
   d. Qing Hao

1573. Ping Wei San is *not* indicated for which of the following?
   a. Distention and fullness in the epigastrium and abdomen
   b. Nausea, vomiting, loose stool or diarrhea
   c. Eructation and acid regurgitation
   d. Thick, greasy, yellow tongue fur

1574. Which property makes Sang Bai Pi a good treatment for coughing?
   a. Warm the Lungs
   b. Clear the Lungs
   c. Strengthen the Lungs
   d. Inhibit the leakage of Lung Qi

1575. Which property makes Ma Dou Ling a good treatment for coughing?
   a. Strengthen the Lungs
   b. Moisten the Lungs
   c. Release Stagnant Lung Qi
   d. Clear the Lungs and transform Plhegm

1576. Which of the following herbs drain the Lungs, calm wheezing, promote urination, and reduce edema?
    a. Cheng Pi
    b. Bai Bu
    c. Sang Bai Pi and Ting Li Zi
    d. Ma Dou Ling and Jie Geng

1577. What channel does Bai Jie Zi enter?
    a. Spleen
    b. Stomach
    c. Lung
    d. Large Intestine

1578. What type of Phlegm does Qian Hu treat?
    a. Heat
    b. Cold
    c. Wind
    d. Damp

1579. What is the relationship between Ban Xia and Sheng Jiang?
    a. Mutual assistance
    b. Mutual restraint
    c. Mutual detoxification
    d. Mutual inhibition

1580. Which herb aids digestion, stops food retention, promotes blood circulation, and resolves Blood stasis?
    a. Mai Ya
    b. Shan Chu
    c. Shan Zha
    d. Ji Nei Jin

1581. What is the relationship between Lai Fu Zi and Ren Sheng?
    a. Mutual reinforcement
    b. Mutual inhibition
    c. Mutual restraint
    d. Incompatibility

1582. Which of the following are Xiang Fu and Wu Yao both able to treat?
    a. Pain in the hypochondrium
    b. Abdominal pain
    c. Dysmenorrhea
    d. Periumbilical colic caused by invasion of Cold

1583. Which herb does *not* regulate Qi and transform Phlegm?
    a. Chen Pi
    b. Qing Pi
    c. Chen Xiang
    d. Fo Shou

1584. Which of the following herbs break up Stagnant Qi?
    a. Chen Pi
    b. Mu Xiang
    c. Fo Shou and Chen Xiang
    d. Zhi Shi and Qing Pi

1585. Which herb does *not* spread and regulate Liver Qi?
    a. Chen Pi
    b. Xiang Fu
    c. Fo Shou
    d. Qing Pi

1586. Which of the following herbs treat distention and pain in the chest, hypochondrium, and abdomen caused by Stagnation of Liver Qi?
    a. Zhi Shi
    b. Chen Xiang
    c. Xiang Fu and Qing Pi
    d. Xiao Hui Xiang and Chen Pi

1587. Which herb does *not* enter into the Liver and Stomach?
    a. Li Zhi He
    b. Chuan Lian Zi
    c. Wu Yao
    d. Fo Shou

1588. Which herb treats irregular menstruation and dysmenorrhea caused by Stagnant Liver Qi?
    a. Mu Xiang
    b. Xiang Fu
    c. Tan Xiang
    d. Wu Yao

1589. Which herb would you select to treat epigastric or abdominal distention caused by Stagnant Qi of the Spleen and Stomach?
    a. Xiang Fu
    b. Qui Zhi
    c. Xi Xin
    d. None of the above

1590. Yue Ju Wan performs which of the following functions?
    a. Lower adverse flow of Qi and resolve Phlegm
    b. Promote the circulation of Qi to relieve Stagnation
    c. Invigorate Qi and regulate the function of the Stomach
    d. Promote the circulation of Qi to stop pain

1591. Da Ji performs which of the following functions?
    a. Warm the womb and stop bleeding
    b. Cool the Blood and stop bleeding
    c. Disperse Blood Stasis and stop bleeding
    d. Restrain leakage of Blood and stop bleeding

1592. Which two herbs each invigorate Blood circulation and promote the movement of Qi?
    a. Chuan Xiong and Yan Hu Sao
    b. Huai Hua Mi and Pu Huang
    c. Tao Ren and Mu Dan Pi
    d. Chi Shao and Qian Cao Gen

1593. Which herb cools the Blood, stops bleeding, and promotes urination?
    a. Lu Gen
    b. Dan Zhu Ye
    c. Bai Mao Gen
    d. Ze Xie

1594. Fried Wu Ling Zhi performs which of the following functions?
    a. Promote the movement of Qi
    b. Promote the movement of Blood and alleviate pain
    c. Disperse Blood Stasis and stop bleeding
    d. Nourish the Blood

1595. Which herb serves as the chief (monarch or *jun*) component in Bu Yang Huan Wu Tang?
    a. Chi Shao
    b. Tao Ren
    c. Huang Qi
    d. Chuan Xiong

1596. What organ is associated with the coughing and bleeding problem that Ke Xue Fang can treat?
    a. Heart
    b. Spleen
    c. Kidney
    d. Liver

1597. Which herb serves as the chief (monarch or *jun*) component in Da Jian Zhong Tang?
    a. Gan Jiang
    b. Chuan Jiao
    c. Ren Shen
    d. Yi Tang

1598. Tai Zi Shen performs which of the following functions?
    a. Augment Qi and stabilize the Exterior
    b. Augment Qi and calm the fetus
    c. Augment Qi and generate body fluids
    d. Augment Qi and stabilize Essence

1599. Which two herbs do *not* both moisten the Lungs and stop coughing?
    a. Mai Men Dong and Tian Men Dong
    b. Bai He and Bai Bu
    c. Sha Shen and Xi Yang Shen
    d. Tai Zi Shen and Dang Shen

1600. Which of the following herbs nourish the Blood and moisten the Intestines?
    a. Bai Shao
    b. Da Zao
    c. Dang Gui and He Shou Wu
    d. Suo Yang and Rou Cong Rong

1601. Which two herbs do *not* both moisten the Intestines and unblock the bowels?
    a. Dang Gui and Rou Cong Rong
    b. He Shou Wu and Hu Tao Ren
    c. Bai He and Ba Dou
    d. Tao Ren and Xing Ren

1602. Bai Shao does *not* perform which of the following functions?
    a. Calm the Liver
    b. Nourish the Liver
    c. Warm the Liver
    d. Curb the Liver

1603. Which formula treats cold limbs resulting from Deficient Yang Qi?
   a. Si Ni San
   b. Wu Mei Wan
   c. Si Ni Tang
   d. All of the above

1604. What caution is associated with Da Jian Zhong Tang?
   a. Contraindication for eating food that has cold and acrid properties
   b. Contraindication for washing the next 24 hours after taking
   c. Eat only dilute gruel during the first 24-hour period after beginning to take this medicine
   d. None of the above

1605. Which formula does *not* treat patients with extremely cold extremities?
   a. Da Cheng Qi Tang
   b. Xiao Chai Hu Tang
   c. Dang Gui Si Ni Tang
   d. Si Ni Tang and Si Ni San

1606. Ding Xiang performs which of the following functions?
   a. Direct rebellious Qi downward and stop coughing
   b. Direct rebellious Qi downward and stop bleeding
   c. Direct rebellious Qi downward and stop vomiting and hiccups
   d. Direct rebellious Qi downward and transform Phlegm

1607. Which of the following serves as the chief (monarch or *jun*) component in Fu Yuan Huo Xue Tang?
   a. Dang Gui
   b. Hong Hua
   c. Tao Ren and Chuan Shan Jia
   d. Da Huang and Chai Hu

1608. Which herb tonifies the Spleen and calms the fetus?
   a. Ban Xia
   b. Zi Su Ye
   c. Cang Zhu
   d. Bai Zhu

1609. Which herb does *not* tonify the Liver and Kidneys, strengthen the sinews and bones, and calm the fetus?
   a. Du Zhong
   b. Niu Xi
   c. Sang Ji Sheng
   d. Xu Duan

1610. Which of the following is *not* a pathogenesis of Huang Tu Tang?
   a. Deficient Spleen Yang
   b. Deficiency-Cold in the Middle Energizer
   c. Heat evil attacking the Blood
   d. Spleen fails to control Blood

1611. Which of the following herbs tonify the Blood and nourish Yin?
   a. Long Yau Rou
   b. Da Zao
   c. Shu Di Huang and He Shou Wu
   d. Dang Gui and Ji Xue Teng

1612. Which herb treats coughing and wheezing caused by Deficient Lungs and Kidneys?
    a. Ge Jie
    b. Dong Chong Xia Cao
    c. Zi He Che
    d. All of the above

1613. Which of the following herbs treat diarrhea caused by Deficient Spleen and Kidneys?
    a. Ba Ji Tian
    b. Rou Cong Rong
    c. Dang Shen and Bai Zhu
    d. Yi Zhi Ren and Bu Gu Zhi

1614. Which formula contains Ren Shen, Bai Zhu, Fu Ling, and Gan Cao?
    a. Shen Ling Bai Zhu San
    b. Xiang Sha Yang Wei Tang
    c. Yi Gong Shan and Gu Zhen Tang
    d. All of the above

1615. Which formula contains Ren Shen, Gan Cao, and Da Zao
    a. Ban Xia Xie Xin Tang
    b. Xuan Fu Dai Zhe Tang
    c. Zi Gan Cao Tang and Ju Pi Zhu Ru Tang
    d. All of the above

1616. Zhi Gan Cao Tang does *not* perform which of the following functions?
    a. Augment Heart Qi
    b. Tonify Heart Yang
    c. Nourish Heart Blood
    d. Enrich Heart Yin

1617. Which formula treats Deficient Qi and Deficient Blood?
    a. Sheng Mai San
    b. Shen Ling Bai Zhu San
    c. Ba Zhen Tang and Zhi Gan Cao Tang
    d. All of the above

1618. Which formula does *not* treat night sweats caused by Deficient Yin?
    a. Dang Gui Di Huang Yin
    b. Da Bu Yin Wan
    c. Di Huang Yin Zi
    d. Liu Wei Di Huang Wan

1619. Which of Ying Su Ke's functions make it a good treatment for diarrhea?
    a. Warm the Middle Energizer
    b. Bind up the Intestines
    c. Move Qi
    d. Stabilize the Kidneys

1620. Chi Shi Zhi performs which of the following functions?
    a. Stop sweating
    b. Stop spermatorrhea
    c. Stop leukorrhea and coughing
    d. Stop diarrhea and bleeding

1621. Sang Piao Xiao performs which of the following functions?
   a. Stop diarrhea
   b. Stop bleeding
   c. Stop excessive leukorrhea and spermatorrhea
   d. Stop sweating and coughing

1622. Hai Piao Xiao does *not* perform which of the following functions?
   a. Stop diarrhea
   b. Stop leukorrhea
   c. Stop bleeding
   d. Stop spermatorrhea

1623. Which herb does *not* bind up the Intestines and stop diarrhea?
   a. Wu Wei Zi
   b. Wu Bei Zi
   c. Wu Mei
   d. Shan Yu Rou

1624. Which of the following herbs generate fluids and stop thrist?
   a. Wu Bei Zi
   b. Wu Shao She
   c. Wu Yi and Wu Ju Pi
   d. Wu Wei Zi and Wu Mei

1625. The seed of which herb has medicinal value?
   a. Wu Mei
   b. Wu Bei Zi
   c. Wu Wei Zi
   d. Chi Xiao Dou

1626. Which of the following functions do Yu Ping Feng Shan and Mu Li San *not* have in common?
   a. Stabilize the Exterior to consolidate resistance
   b. Tonify Qi
   c. Stop excessive sweating
   d. Dispel pathogens

1627. Which formula treats dysentery or diarrhea caused by Damp-Heat?
   a. Si Shen Wan
   b. Tao Hua Tang
   c. Shao Yao Tang
   d. Zhen Ren Yang Zang Tang

1628. Which formula contains Ren Shen?
   a. Tao Hua Tang
   b. Si Shen Wan
   c. Gu Chong Tang
   d. Sang Piao Xiao San

1629. Which of the following is an indication for Suo Quan Wan?
   a. Frequent urination caused by Deficient Kidneys and Heart
   b. Frequent urination caused by Deficiency-Cold in the Lower Energizer
   c. Excessive sweating
   d. All of the above

1630. Which herb relieves constraint and calms the Spirit?
   a. Bai Shao
   b. Xian Fu
   c. He Huan Pi
   d. Chai Hu

1631. Which of the following herbs calm the Liver, anchor Floating Yang, and calm the Spirit?
   a. Zhu Sha
   b. Shi Jue Ming
   c. Long Gu and Ci Shi
   d. He Huan Pi and Yuan Zhi

1632. Which of the following functions do Mu Li and Long Gu *not* have in common?
   a. Calm the Liver and anchor Floating Yang
   b. Benefit Yin, soften hardness, and dissipate nodules
   c. Settle and calm the Spirit
   d. Prevent leakage of fluids

1633. Which of the following is *not* a caution or contraindication associated with Zhu Sha?
   a. Should not be used in large amounts
   b. Should not be prescribed for long term use
   c. Should not be calcined
   d. Should not be used to treat patients who are aged or frail

1634. Which of the following formulas is used to treat Deficient Heart and Deficient Kidneys?
   a. Qui Pi Tang
   b. Jin Suo Gu Jing Wan
   c. Tian Wang Bu Xin Dan and Sang Piao Xiao San
   d. Ci Zhu Wan and Qi Ju Di Huang Wan

1635. Which formula contains Zhu Sha and Suan Zao Ren
   a. Suan Zao Ren Tang
   b. Zhu Sha An Shen Wan
   c. Tian Wang Bu Xin Dan
   d. Ci Zhu Wan

1636. Which of the following herbs treats Phlegm that is veiling and blocking the sensory orifices?
   a. Zhu Ru
   b. Shi Chang Pi
   c. Yuan Zhi and Bing Pian
   d. Shi Jue Ming and Di Long

1637. Which caution is associated with formulas that open the orifices?
   a. Only for short-term use
   b. Should only be taken in pill or powder form or as an injection
   c. Do not decoct
   d. All of the above

1638. Gou Teng does *not* perform which of the following functions?
   a. Calm Liver Yang
   b. Nourish Liver Blood
   c. Clear Liver Fire
   d. Extinguish Liver Wind

1639. Tian Ma performs which of the following functions?
 a. Clear Liver Fire
 b. Transform Phlegm and stop coughing
 c. Warm and nourish the Blood
 d. Calm the Liver and extinguish Liver Wind

1640. Which statement is *not* true?
 a. Jue Ming Zi moistens the Intestines and the bowels
 b. Di Long clears Heat and calms wheezing
 c. Jiang Can expels Wind and stops itching
 d. Bai Ji Li clears Liver Heat and benefits the eyes

1641. Which herb dispels Wind and brightens the eyes?
 a. Xia Ku Cao
 b. Bai Ji Li
 c. Ju Hua
 d. Gou Qi Zi

1642. Which herb does *not* calm the Liver and improve vision?
 a. Mu Li
 b. Ling Yang Jiao
 c. Shi Jue Ming
 d. Jue Ming Zi

1643. Which herb does *not* calm the Liver?
 a. Shi Jue Ming
 b. Gou Teng
 c. Zhen Zhu Mu
 d. Jiang Can

1644. Which herb does *not* extinguish Wind and stop spasms?
 a. Quan Xie
 b. Wu Gong
 c. Can Sha
 d. Jiang Can

1645. What are the properties of Ling Yang Jiao and the meridians it enters?
 a. Salty, cold, and Heart, Liver
 b. Sweet, cold, and Heart, Liver
 c. Salty, cold, and Kidney, Liver
 d. Sweet, neutral, and Heart, Liver

1646. Which herb does *not* calm the Liver and extinguish Liver Wind?
 a. Tian Ma
 b. Ling Yang Jiao
 c. Shi Jue Ming
 d. Gou Teng

1647. Which herb clears Heat, calms the Liver, extinguishes Wind, stops spasms, and releases the Exterior?
 a. Tian Ma
 b. Gou Teng
 c. Bai Shao
 d. Sang Ye

1648. Which of the following functions do Shi Jue Ming and Zhen Zhu Mu *not* have in common?
    a. Clear Liver Fire
    b. Improve vision
    c. Calm the Liver and anchor the Yang
    d. Soften hardness and dissipate nodules

1649. Which of the following is an indication for Qian Zheng San?
    a. Hemiplegia and deviation of the eyes and mouth
    b. Liver Wind stirring inside and deviation of the mouth
    c. Wind-Cold Phlegm obstructing the meridians and collaterals on the head and face, deviation of the eyes and mouth
    d. Wind-Heat Phlegm obstructing the meridians and collaterals on the head and face, deviation of the eyes and mouth

1650. Which formula would you use to treat infantile convulsions caused by Heat in the Liver meridian stirring up internal movement of Wind?
    a. Zhen Gan Xi Feng Tang
    b. Ling Jiao Gou Teng Tang
    c. Di Huang Yin Zi
    d. Do Ding Feng Zhu

1651. Which herb serves as the chief (monarch or *jun*) component in Zhen Gan Xi Feng Tang?
    a. Dai Zhe Shi
    b. Mu Li
    c. Huai Niu Xi
    d. Long Gu

1652. Tian Ma Gou Teng Yin does *not* perform which of the following functions?
    a. Calm the Liver, extinguish Wind
    b. Transform Phlegm, relieve spasms
    c. Clear Heat, invigorate the Blood
    d. Tonify the Liver and Kidneys

1653. Which of the following formulas treat internal movement of Wind arising from Deficient Blood and Yin, causing muscle spasms and twitching of the extremities?
    a. Di Huang Yin Zi
    b. Tian Ma Gou Teng Yin
    c. E Jiao Ji Zi Huang Tang and Da Ding Feng Zhu
    d. San Jia Fu Mai Tang and Zhan Gan Xi Feng Tang

1654. Da Ding Feng Zhu and E Jiao Zi Huang Tang each contain which of the following ingredients?
    a. E Jiao and Bai Shao
    b. Mu Li and Zhi Gan Cao
    c. Gou Teng and Ren Shen
    d. Di Huang and Ji Zi Huang

1655. When taking a decocted formula to expel parasites, how should it be taken?
    a. In several small doses
    b. While also drinking a draft lager
    c. On an empty stomach
    d. While feeling the pain caused by the parasites

1656. Wu Mei Wan performs which of the following functions?
   a. Reduce accumulation
   b. Clear Heat
   c. Warm the Intestines and calm round worms
   d. Strengthen the Spleen and Stomach

1657. Which properties of the herbs in Wu Mei Wan treat colic associated with ascariasis?
   a. Cool the upper body, warm the lower body
   b. Cool the Exterior, warm the Interior
   c. Cool the Stomach, warm the Interior
   d. Cool the Intestines, warm the Stomach

1658. Liu Huang and Xiong Huang each are applied topically to perform which of the following functions?
   a. Stop pain
   b. Stop bleeding
   c. Kill parasites
   d. Reduce swelling

1659. Which of the following herbs generate flesh?
   a. Xiong Huang
   b. Qing Fen
   c. Lu Gan Shi and Qian Dan
   d. She Chuang Zi and Ming Fan

1660. Which of the following is *not* an alternate name for Qian Dan?
   a. Huang Dan
   b. Guang Dan
   c. San Xian Dan
   d. Dong Dan

1661. Which of the following mineral medicines should *not* be heated in preparation for use?
   a. Ci Shi
   b. Qian Dan
   c. Xiong Huang and Zhu Sha
   d. Shi Gao and Long Gu

1662. Which herb contains arsenic?
   a. Mi Yuo Seng
   b. Qian Dan
   c. Lu Gan Shi
   d. Xiong Huang

1663. Which herb is an emetic?
   a. Chang Shan
   b. Li Lu
   c. Gua Di
   d. All of the above

1664. Which of the following herbs contain mercury?
   a. Xiong Huang
   b. Ming Fan
   c. Mi Tuo Seng and Qian Dan
   d. Qing Fen and Zhu Sha

1665. Which of the following herbs contain lead?
- a. Lu Gan Shi
- b. Liu Huang
- c. Mi Tuo Seng and Qian Dan
- d. Xiong Huang and Pong Sha

1666. Xian Fang Huo Ming Yin is *not* indicated for which of the following?
- a. Swelling and pain in the affected area
- b. Feverishness with slight aversion to cold
- c. Thin-whitish or slightly yellow tongue fur
- d. Deep-weak pulse

1667. Which formula treats Lung abscesses caused by Heat and Blood Stasis?
- a. Wei Jing Tang
- b. Yi Yi Ren Tang
- c. Tou Nong San
- d. Da Huang Mu Dan Tang

1668. Which formula treats periappendicular abscesses caused by obstruction of Damp-Heat and Phlegm?
- a. Yi Yi Fu Zi Bai Jiang San
- b. Da Huang Mu Dan Tang
- c. Wei Jing Tang
- d. Xie Huang San

1669. Yang He Tang does *not* contain which of the following?
- a. E Jiao
- b. Shu Di Huang
- c. Ma Huang
- d. Gui Zhi

1670. Which of the following is *not* a caution associated with Yang He Tang?
- a. Avoid using when Yang carbuncles are present
- b. Avoid using when Deficient Yin carbuncles are present
- c. Avoid using when pregnant
- d. All of the above *(Changed from "None of the preceding" in Dr. Wu's manuscript)*

1671. Wei Jing Tang and Da Huang Mu Dan Tang each contain which of the following ingredients?
- a. Mu Dan Pi
- b. Yi Yi Ren
- c. Tao Ren and Dong Gua Ren
- d. Wei Jing and Da Huang

1672. How can you treat unremitting vomiting associated with Gua Di San?
- a. Administer Gan Cao
- b. Administer Sheng Jiang
- c. Administer 0.3 - 0.6 grams of Ding Xiang or 0.03 - 0.06 grams of She Xiang
- d. All of the above

1673. Which of the following is *not* a caution associated with the use of emetics?
- a. Avoid using with weak patients
- b. Avoid using if the Phlegm is not lodged in the chest
- c. Avoid using when stagnant food has already passed into the intestines
- d. Avoid using if covering the patient with warm blankets causes him or her to sweat

1674. Di Gu Pi does *not* perform which of the following functions?
    a. Clear away Heat in the Lungs
    b. Invigorate Blood circulation to remove Blood Stasis
    c. Remove Heat from the Blood, bringing down hectic fever
    d. Drain Floating Fire from the Kidneys

1675. Chai Hu performs which of the following functions?
    a. Anchor the Floating Yang
    b. Fortify the Yang
    c. Raise the Yang
    d. Tonify the Yang

1676. Gou Qi Zi and Sha Yuan Ji Li each improve sharpness of vision by performing which of the following functions?
    a. Calm the Liver
    b. Clear Liver Heat
    c. Nourish the Liver
    d. None of the above

1677. Su Zi treats coughing and wheezing by performing which of the following functions?
    a. Clear Lung Heat
    b. Moisten the Lungs
    c. Tonify the Lungs
    d. Lower the adverse flow of Qi and dissolve Phlegm

1678. Dong Chong Xia Cao treats coughing and wheezing by performing which of the following functions?
    a. Tonify Kidney Yang
    b. Moisten Lung Yin
    c. Stop bleeding and dissolve Phlegm
    d. All of the above

1679. Rou Dou Kou treats diarrhea by performing which of the following functions?
    a. Bind the Intestines and warm the Middle Energizer
    b. Tonify the Kidneys and Liver
    c. Reinforce the Spleen and Stomach
    d. All of the above

1680. Which of the following functions is *not* a reason why Yu Jin is used to treat abdominal pain?
    a. Warm the Middle Energizer
    b. Promote Blood circulation
    c. Invigorate the flow of Qi
    d. Normalize the Gallbladder

1681. Which of the following functions is *not* a reason why Wu Zhu Yu is used to treat abdominal pain?
    a. Relieve constraint in the Liver meridian
    b. Warm the Middle Energizer
    c. Invigorate Blood circulation to remove Blood Stasis
    d. Disperse Cold

1682. Sang Ye, Ju Hua, and Mu Zei each improve sharpness of vision by performing which of the following functions?
    a. Nourish the Liver and Kidneys
    b. Transform Damp and induce diuresis
    c. Expel pathogenic Wind and clear Liver Heat
    d. Normalize the Gallbladder

1683. Huang Bai does *not* perform which of the following functions?
    a. Clear away Heat and remove Damp
    b. Purge Fire and detoxify
    c. Clear away Deficiency-Heat
    d. Clear Stomach-Heat to stop vomiting

1684. Shan Yao does *not* perform which of the following functions?
    a. Reinforce the Spleen and Stomach
    b. Strengthen the Kidneys
    c. Nourish the Lungs
    d. Induce diuresis

1685. Fu Ling does *not* perform which of the following functions?
    a. Strengthen the Spleen
    b. Induce diuresis
    c. Strengthen the Kidneys
    d. Quiet the Heart

1686. Shu Di Huang and E Jiao each perform which of the following functions?
    a. Tonify the Blood and stop bleeding
    b. Moisten the Lungs and stop coughing
    c. Nourish the Blood and moisten the Yin
    d. Nourish the Blood and moisten the Intestines

1687. Which of the following functions do Rou Cong Rong and Suo Yang *not* have in common?
    a. Tonify the Kidneys
    b. Fortify the Yang
    c. Strengthen the sinews and bones
    d. Moisten the Intestines and unblock the bowels

1688. Which of the following functions do Tu Si Zi and Sha Yuan Zi Li *not* have in common?
    a. Secure the Essence
    b. Reserve urine
    c. Improve vision
    d. Stop diarrhea

1689. Yan Hu Suo is *not* indicated for which of the following?
    a. Abdominal pain and hernial pain
    b. Pain in the chest caused by Obstruction of Qi
    c. Traumatic injuries
    d. Wind-Damp-Cold painful obstruction

1690. Bai Shao is *not* indicated for which of the following?
    a. Irregular menstruation, dysmenorrhea, metrorrhagia, and metrostaxis caused by Deficient Blood
    b. Pain in the hypochondrium, stomach, and abdomen caused by a disorder of Liver Qi
    c. Poisonous snake bites
    d. Hyperactive Liver Yang marked by headaches and vertigo

1691. Which of the following is an indication for Ge Gen?
    a. Diarrhea caused by Deficient Kidneys
    b. Dysentery caused by Fire toxins
    c. Dysentery caused by Damp-Cold
    d. Diarrhea caused by pathogenic Damp-Heat or Deficient Spleen

1692. Which of the following is an indication for Bai Zhi in particular?
    a. Taiyang headache
    b. Shaiyang headache
    c. Jueyin headache and headache caused by Excess Liver Yang
    d. Yangming headache and headache caused by sinusitis

1693. Qiang Huo is *not* indicated for which of the following?
    a. Taiyang headache
    b. Yangming headache
    c. Headache caused by exopathogenic Wind-Cold
    d. Headache caused by Wind-Damp painful obstruction

1694. Which of the following is an indication for Ju Hua?
    a. Taiyang headache
    b. Yangming headache
    c. Headache associated with Wind-Cold patterns
    d. Headache caused by pathogenic Wind-Heat or Excess Liver Yang

1695. Which of the following is an indication for Tian Ma
    a. Yangming headache
    b. Taiyang headache
    c. Headache associated with Wind-Cold or Wind-heat patterns
    d. Headache caused by Wind-Phlegm or Excess Liver Yang

1696. Huang Lian does *not* perform which of the following functions?
    a. Clear Heart Heat
    b. Clear Stomach Heat
    c. Clear Deficiency-Heat
    d. Clear Damp-Heat

1697. Which herb does *not* astringe the Lungs and stop coughing?
    a. Wu Wei Zi
    b. He Zi
    c. Lian Zi
    d. Wu Bei Zi

1698. Long Dan Cao is *not* used to treat which of the following?
    a. Jaundice caused by Damp-Heat
    b. Excess-Fire in the Liver and Gallbladder
    c. Wind syndrome induced by excessive Heat in the Liver
    d. Excess Liver Yang

1699. Which of the following herbs drain Fire and guide out accumulation?
    a. Tong Cao
    b. Pu Gong Ying
    c. Lu Hui and Fax Xie Ye
    d. Zhi Zi and Zi Hua Di Ding

1700. Which of the following herbs clear Heat and dry Damp in order to stop dysentery?
    a. Ge Gen
    b. Mu Xiang
    c. Huang Lian and Ku Shou
    d. Huang Qi and Long Dan Cao

1701. Which herb does *not* warm the Stomach and stop vomiting?
   a. Gan Jiang
   b. Sheng Jiang
   c. Gao Laing Jiang
   d. Dou Chi Jiang

1702. Which herb does *not* purge Heart Fire and relieve dysphoria?
   a. Lu Gen
   b. Zhi Zi
   c. Huang Lian
   d. Lian Xin

1703. Which herb clears Liver Heat?
   a. Shi Jue Ming
   b. Ling Yang Jia
   c. Gou Teng
   d. All of the above

1704. Which herb does *not* release the Exterior through diaphoresis and reduce edema by inducing diuresis?
   a. Ma Huang
   b. Fang Feng
   c. Fu Ping
   d. Xiang Ru

1705. Which herb does *not* sedate the Heart and calm the Spirit?
   a. Zhu Sha
   b. Mu Li
   c. Zhen Zhu
   d. Long Gu

1706. Which of the following herbs does *not* help to prevent miscarriage?
   a. Sang Ji Sheng
   b. Bai Zhu
   c. Xu Duan and Sha Ren
   d. All of the above

1707. Which herb does *not* stop excessive loss of body fluids due to incessant sweating and seminal emission?
   a. Wu Wei Zi
   b. Shan Zhu Yu
   c. Jin Yin Zi
   d. Wu Bei Zi

1708. Which herb does *not* remove Blood Stasis and promote Blood circulation and the flow of Qi?
   a. Jiang Huang
   b. Chuan Xiong
   c. San Leng
   d. Ze Lan

1709. Which of the following herbs invigorate the meridians and unblock lactation?
   a. Wu Ling Zhi
   b. Niu Xi
   c. Wang Bu Liu Xing and Chuan Shan Jia
   d. Shan Yao and Bai Shao

1710. Which herb does *not* treat abdominal pain caused by round worms?
    a. Da Suan
    b. Wu Mei
    c. Shi Jun Zi
    d. Lei Wan

1711. Sheng Jiang and Da Zao each perform which of the following functions in formulas for relieving Exterior syndromes?
    a. Ameliorates the side effects associated with formulas that provide relief from Exterior syndrome
    b. Regulate the Ying-fen and Wei-fen
    c. Increase the patient's ability to absorb the medicine in the formula
    d. None of the above

1712. Which of the following herbs treat vomiting caused by accumulation of Damp in the Middle Energizer and Stagnant Qi?
    a. Zhu Ru
    b. Xuan Fu Hua
    c. Sha Ren and Bai Dou Kou
    d. Fu Ling and Bai Bian Dou

1713. Which herb does *not* treat dysentery caused by Damp-Heat?
    a. Ku Shen
    b. Qin Pi
    c. Hu Huang Lian
    d. Yin Chai Hu

1714. Which herb does *not* treat edema caused by Deficient Spleen?
    a. Fu Ling
    b. Bai Zhu
    c. Qian Niu Zi
    d. Yi Yi Ren

1715. Which of the following herbs treat lumbago caused by Deficient Liver and Kidneys?
    a. Bu Gu Zi
    b. Gang Fang Ji
    c. He Shou Wu and Ji Xue Teng
    d. Xu Duan and Du Zhong

1716. Which herb is *not* appropriate for treating vomiting during pregnancy?
    a. Zhu Ru
    b. Huo Xiang
    c. Huo Po
    d. Sha Ren

1717. Which herb does *not* treat amenorrhea and abdominal masses caused by Blood Stasis?
    a. Ji Nei Jin
    b. Tu Bie Chong
    c. Chuan Shan Jia
    d. Shui Zhi

1718. Which of the following functions do Wu Gong and Quan Xie *not* have in common?
    a. Extinguish Wind and stop tremors and convulsions
    b. Promote Blood circulation and remove Blood Stasis
    c. Attack toxins and dissipate nodules
    d. Unblock the collaterals and stop pain

1719. Which herb does *not* promote the discharge of pus?
   a. Bai Zi
   b. Tian Hua Fen
   c. Zao Jiao Ci
   d. Fu Hai Shi

1720. Which herb tonifies the Kidneys, moistens the Intestines, and unblocks the bowels?
   a. Bu Gu Zhi
   b. Hu Tao Ren
   c. Yu Li Ren
   d. Tu Si Zi

1721. Which herb would *not* be used to treat Retention of Cold-Phlegm in the Lungs, which is manifested as coughing, dyspnea, a chilly sensation in the back, and profuse clear sputum?
   a. Qian Hu
   b. Gan Jiang
   c. Ban Xia
   d. Xi Xin

1722. Which herb would *not* be used to treat an attack on the Exterior of exopathogenic Wind-Cold complicated by pathogenic Damp?
   a. Du Huo
   b. Qiang Huo
   c. Xi Xian Cao
   d. Cang Zhu

1723. Which of the following herbs tonify the Kidneys, strengthen Yang, dispel Wind, and eliminate Damp?
   a. Xu Duan
   b. Gu Sui Bu
   c. Rou Cong Rong and Suo Yang
   d. Yin Yang Huo and Ba Ji Tian

1724. Which herb does *not* tonify the Yin nor enter the Stomach and Lung meridians?
   a. Sha Shen
   b. Mai Men Dong
   c. Tian Men Dong
   d. Yu Zhu (Wei Rui)

1725. Which herb does *not* nourish the Yin and tonify the Qi?
   a. Shan Yao
   b. Xi Yang Shen
   c. Sha Shen
   d. Huang Jing

1726. Which of the following herbs assist the Kidney Yang and help the Kidneys to grasp Qi?
   a. Ba Ji Tian
   b. Rou Cong Rong
   c. Xian Mao and Yin Yang Huo
   d. Bu Gu Zhi and Ge Jie

1727. Shu Di Huang and E Jiao each perform which of the following functions?
   a. Tonify the Blood and stop bleeding
   b. Tonify the Blood and Tonify the Yin
   c. Tonify the Blood and tonify the Qi
   d. Tonify the Lungs and stop coughing

1728. Dang Gui and Ji Xue Tang each perform which of the following functions?
    a. Promote Blood circulation and regulate the menses
    b. Tonify the Yin and moisten the Intestines
    c. Tonify the Yang and relieve pain
    d. Cool the Blood and stop bleeding

1729. Which herb would you select to treat a patient suffering from prodomal manifestation of prostration syndrome caused by Deficient Qi, where the limbs are cold and the pulse is almost imperceptibly weak?
    a. Lu Rong
    b. Suo Yang
    c. Ren Shen and Fu Zi
    d. Huang Qi and Wu Zhu Yu

1730. Which of the following herbs would treat a patient suffering from Yang Depletion syndrome with intolerance for cold and profuse sweating?
    a. Dang Shen
    b. Huang Qi
    c. Ren Shen and Fu Zi
    d. Rou Gui and Fu Zi

1731. Wu Wei Zi could be used with which of the following herbs to treat a patient whose Qi and Yin are impaired as a result of Heat, causing palpitations, feeble pulse, thirst, and profuse sweating?
    a. Yu Zhu
    b. Shi Hu
    c. Ren Shen and Mai Men Dong
    d. Huang Qi and Sha Shen

1732. Niu Bang Zi and Ge Gen each perform which of the following functions?
    a. Disperse Wind-Heat and vent measles
    b. Nourish the fluids and alleviate thirst
    c. Relieve toxicity and benefit the throat
    d. Moisten the Intestines

1733. Sheng Jiang alleviates vomiting by performing which of the following functions?
    a. Dry Damp
    b. Warm the Middle Energizer
    c. Direct the Qi downward
    d. Regulate Stomach Qi

1734. Which of the following is an indication for Chi Shao?
    a. Epidemic febrile disease with Heat in the Blood, manifested as macules or skin eruptions
    b. Hematemesis and epistaxis caused by invasion of the Blood by Heat
    c. Amenorrhea and metrorrhagia caused by Blood Stasis
    d. All of the above

1735. Which herb is *not* used for treating diabetes caused by Deficient Yin?
    a. Yu Zhu (Wei Rui)
    b. Zhi Zi
    c. Zhi Mu
    d. Tian Hua Fen

1736. Which herb does *not* treat dizziness and blurred vision caused by Deficient Yin of the Kidneys and Liver?
    a. Sha Shen
    b. He Shou Wu
    c. Gu Gi Zi
    d. Nu Zhen Zi

1737. Which of the following herbs cool the Blood and relieve toxicity?
   a. Mu Dan Pi
   b. Sheng Di Huang
   c. Zi Cao and Xuan Shen
   d. Yin Chai Hu and Di Gu Pi

1738. Purgatives should be used cautiously with patients suffering from which of the following?
   a. Deficient Qi after chronic illness
   b. Women who are pregnant
   c. Women who are in the postpartum phase or who are menstruating
   d. All of the above

1739. How would you treat vomiting caused by Deficiency-Cold of the Spleen and Stomach?
   a. Warm the Middle Energizer
   b. Direct Qi downward
   c. Strengthen the Spleen and regulate the Stomach
   d. All of the above

1740. Which formula treats disorders of the Exterior as well as the Interior?
   a. Bei Xie Fen Qing Yin
   b. Xuan Bi Tang
   c. Huo Xiang Zheng Qi San
   d. Gan Lu Xiao Du Dan

1741. Which of the following formulas contain Ren Shen, Ban Xia, Sheng Jiang, Da Zao, and Gan Cao?
   a. Wu Zhu Yu Tang
   b. Da Chai Hu Tang
   c. Xiao Chai Hu Tang and Xuan Fu Dai Zhe Tang
   d. Ban Xia Xie Xin Tang and Sheng Jiang Xie Xia Tang

1742. Which of the following formulas treat conditions marked by cold limbs?
   a. Si Ni Tang
   b. Da Huang Fu Zi Tang
   c. Shen Fu Tang and Wu Mei Wan
   d. All of the above

1743. Xiao Yao San is *not* indicated for which of the following?
   a. Pain in the hypochondria
   b. Headache and dizziness
   c. Abdominal pain and diarrhea
   d. Irregular menstruation and distension in the chest

1744. Which of the following formulas moderate spasms and relieve pain through the ingredient Bai Shao?
   a. Xiao Jian Zhong Tang
   b. Da Ding Feng Zhu
   c. Shao Yao Tang and Bai Zhu Shao Yao Tang
   d. All of the above

1745. Which formula does *not* contain Chuan Li Zi?
   a. Zhe Gan Xi Fing Tang
   b. Nuan Gan Jian
   c. Ju He Wan
   d. Yi Guan Juan

1746. Pu Ji Xiao Du Yin and Bu Zhong Yi Qi Tang each contain which of the following ingredients?
   a. Chen Pi
   b. Gan Cao
   c. Chai Hu and Sheng Ma
   d. All of the above

1747. What is the pathogenesis of Bu Yang Huan Wu Tang?
   a. Deficient Blood
   b. Deficient Yin
   c. Deficient Yang and Stagnant Qi
   d. Deficient Qi and Blood Stasis

1748. Huang Qi performs which of the following functions in Bu Yang Huan Wu Tang?
   a. Invigorate Primordial Qi to promote Blood circulation
   b. Invigorate Primordial Qi to generate Blood
   c. Benefit the Qi to astringe sweating
   d. Benefit the Qi to lift up the Yang

1749. What is the pathogenesis of Mu Li San?
   a. Deficient Blood
   b. Deficient Yang Qi
   c. Deficient Qi and Yin
   d. Excess-Heat and Qi Stagnation

1750. In which of the following formulas does Huang Qi serve as the chief (monarch or *jun*) component?
   a. Bu Zhong Yi Qi Tang
   b. Bu Yang Huan Wu tang
   c. Fang Ji Huang Qi Tang and Yu Ping Feng San
   d. All of the above

1751. Which of the following is true of Huang Tu Tang?
   a. Herbs of a cold and hot nature are used in combination
   b. Herbs of a bitter and sweet nature are used in combination
   c. The herbs relieve the primary and secondary symptoms at the same time
   d. All of the above

1752. Which of the following functions do Mu Li San and Yu Ping Feng San *not* have in common?
   a. Benefit Qi
   b. Stop sweating
   c. Alleviate depression
   d. Consolidate the resistance of the Exterior

1753. Which of the following is an indication for Si Shen Wan?
   a. Chronic diarrhea or dysentery caused by Deficient and Cold Spleen and Kidneys, incontinence of the feces caused by lingering diarrhea or prolapse of the anus
   b. Diarrhea that occurs before dawn which is caused by Deficient Yang of the Spleen and Kidneys, accompanied by anorexia, abdominal pain, lumbago, cold limbs, and listlessness
   c. Chronic dysenteric disorders with dark blood or pus in the stool
   d. None of the above

1754. Which of the following formulas treat chronic diarrhea or dysentery?
   a. Zhen Ren Yang Zang Tang
   b. Bu Zhong Yi Qi Tang
   c. Tao Hua Tang
   d. All of the above

1755. What is the pathogenesis of Jin Suo Gu Jing Wan when used to treat impotence and spermatorrhea?
    a. Heart and Liver Heat
    b. Deficient Heart and Kidneys
    c. Unconsolidation of the Essence Gate caused by Deficeint Kidneys
    d. Damp-Heat evil attacking the Lower Energizer

1756. Zhi Bao Dan is *not* indicated for which of the following?
    a. Coma and delirium, abundant expectoration, harsh breathing
    b. Feverish body, irritability
    c. Dark brown urine, constipation
    d. Red tongue coated with thick, greasy, yellow fur, slippery-rapid pulse

1757. Which formula contains Suan Zao Ren and Zhu Sha?
    a. Suan Zao Ren Tang
    b. Tian Wang Bu Xin Dan
    c. Zhu Shu An Shen Wan
    d. Ci Zhu Wan

1758. Wen Jing Tang is *not* indicated for which of the following?
    a. Cold in the lower abdomen, long-term failure to conceive
    b. Fever at nightfall, a feverish sensation in the palms
    c. Irregular menstruation or persistent menstrual duration
    d. Hemiplegia after apoplexy

1759. Tian Ma Gou Teng Yin does *not* perform which of the following functions?
    a. Remove Phlegm and Blood Stasis
    b. Calm the Liver to stop endogenous Wind
    c. Clear pathogenic Heat to promote Blood circulation
    d. Nourish the Liver and Kidneys

1760. Xing Su San and Er Chen Tang both do *not* contain which of the following?
    a. Fu Ling
    b. Chen Pi and Ban Xia
    c. Sheng Jiang and Gan Cao
    d. Qian Hu and Zhi Ke

1761. Which of the following herbs serve as the chief (monarch or *jun*) component in Bai He Gu Jin Tang?
    a. Xuan Shen
    b. Bai Shao
    c. Bei Mu and Bai He
    d. Sheng Di Huang and Shu Di Huang

1762. Which of the following is *not* the pathogenesis of Xing Su San?
    a. Dry-Cool exopathic factors
    b. Injured Stomach Yin
    c. Sluggish Lung Qi
    d. Accumulation of Phlegm-Damp in the body

1763. Which of the following formulas treat edema caused by Deficient Yang of the Spleen and Kidneys?
    a. Wu Ling San
    b. Wu Pi San
    c. Shi Pi Yin and Zhen Wu Tang
    d. Wu Lin San and Shao Yao Tang

1764. Which of the following formulas warm and invigorate the Spleen?
    a. Jian Pi Wan
    b. Gui Pi Tang
    c. Wu Pi San and Wu Pi Yin
    d. Wen Pi Tang and Shi Pi Yin

1765. Bai Shao performs which of the following functions in Zhen Wu Tang?
    a. Nourish the Blood
    b. Regulate the menses
    c. Calm and curb Liver Yang
    d. Preserve Yin and alleviate pain

1766. Wu Wei Zi performs which of the following functions in Ling Gan Wu Wei Jiang Xin Tang?
    a. Inhibit sweating and generate fluids
    b. Tonify the Kidneys and bind up Essence
    c. Quiet the Spirit and calm the Heart
    d. Astringe Lung Qi to arrest cough and prevent over-expelling so as not to damage Lung Qi

1767. Jie Geng performs which of the following functions in Shen Ling Bai Shu San?
    a. Ventilate the Lungs and resolve Phlegm
    b. Benefit the throat
    c. Guide the other drugs upward to replenish the Lungs
    d. All of the above

1768. What method does Tou Nong San use to treat carbuncles?
    a. Eliminating
    b. Clearing Heat
    c. Warming
    d. Promoting pus drainage

1769. Which of the following is *not* the pathogenesis of Sheng Hua Tang?
    a. Obstruction of the uterus by childbirth
    b. Deficient Blood after childbirth
    c. Deficient Qi caused by Cold evil
    d. Cold evil invading the Interior

1770. Xian Fang Huo Ming Yin does *not* perform which of the following functions?
    a. Activate Qi and remove Blood Stasis
    b. Clear away Heat and toxic materials
    c. Subdue swelling and resolve masses
    d. Activate Blood flow and alleviate pain

1771. What is the pathogenesis of Qing Qi Hua Tan Wan?
    a. Externally contracted Wind-Cold
    b. Fire evil consuming Yin
    c. Dry-Warm exopathic factors
    d. Stagnation of Phlegm or Heat in the Lungs or accumulation of Phlegm-Damp in the body

1772. Zhen Wu Tang performs which of the following functions?
    a. Warm the Yang to induce diuresis
    b. Warm the Yang to excrete Damp
    c. Expel Cold evil by warming the meridians
    d. Warm the Stomach and strengthen the Middle Energizer

1773. Which herb do Zhu Ling Tang and Wu Ling San *not* have in common?
   a. Zhu Ling
   b. Fu Ling
   c. Ze Xie
   d. Hua Shi

1774. Which herb does *not* clear Lung Heat?
   a. Di Gu Pi
   b. Huang Qin
   c. Huang Lian
   d. Lu Gen

1775. Which herb does *not* clear Heat, dry Damp, and stop dysentery?
   a. Ma Chi Xian
   b. Huang Lian
   c. Huang Bai
   d. Ku Shen

1776. Which herb does *not* clear Stomach Heat and stop vomiting?
   a. Lu Ge
   b. Huang Lian
   c. Zhi Zi
   d. Zhu Ru

1777. Which of the following herbs treat Deficient Yin accompanied by fever and Steaming Bone Disorder?
   a. Zhi Mu and Bie Jia
   b. Di Gu Pi
   c. Mu Dan Pi
   d. All of the above

1778. Which herb clears Stomach Heat?
   a. Mu Dan Pi
   b. Di Gu Pi
   c. Huang Lian
   d. None of the above

1779. Which of the following herbs disperse Wind and benefit the eyes?
   a. Ye Ming Sha
   b. Mi Meng Hua
   c. Ju Hua and Man Jing Zi
   d. Niu Bang Zi and Fu Ping

1780. Which of the following herbs do *not* clear the Liver and benefit the eyes?
   a. Jue Ming Zi
   b. Qing Xiang Zi
   c. Mu Zei and Xia Ku Cao
   d. Lu Gen and Dan Zhu Ye

1781. Which of the following would you *not* use to treat intestinal abscesses?
   a. Pu Gong Ying
   b. Zi Hua Di Ding
   c. Bai Jiang Cao
   d. Yi Yi Ren

1782. Which of the following functions do Bai Tou Weng and Ma Chi Xian *not* have in common?
    a. Cool the Blood
    b. Stop dysenteric disorders
    c. Clear Heat and relieve toxicity
    d. Reduce swelling and promote discharge of pus

1783. Sheng Di Huang, Xuan Shen, and Mai Men Dong are contained in which of the following formulas?
    a. Qing Ying Tang
    b. Qing Wen Bai Du Yin
    c. Bai He Gu Jin Tang
    d. All of the above

1784. Which of the following indicates use of a formula that treats invasion of the Blood by pathogenic Heat?
    a. Fever, bleeding, dark purple rashes, deep red tongue with prickled fur
    b. Parched throat, thirst but no desire to swallow water once it is in the mouth
    c. Abdominal distension and fullness with delirium
    d. All of the above

1785. Qing Ying Tang is *not* indicated for which of the following?
    a. Feverishness which is worse at night
    b. Occasional delirium
    c. Insomnia resulting from vexation or faint skin rashes
    d. Deep red tongue with slippery white fur

1786. Which herb is *not* one of the three Huangs in Shao Yao Tang?
    a. Huang Lian
    b. Da Huang
    c. Huang Bai
    d. Huang Qin

1787. Which statement is incorrect regarding the components that make up Qing Wen Bai Du Yin?
    a. Bai Hu Tang clears Heat and promotes the production of body fluids
    b. Huang Lian Jie Du Tang purges pathogenic Fire and Heat from the Triple Energizer
    c. Jie Geng Tang promotes the discharge of pus
    d. Xi Jiao Di Huang Tang clears Heat and toxicity and removes Blood Stasis

1788. Which of the following formulas would you select to treat diarrhea with a cathartic treatment method?
    a. Huang Qin Tang
    b. Bai Tou Weng Tang
    c. Shao Yao Tang and Da Cheng Zi Tang
    d. All of the above

1789. Which type of Heat is Shi Gao well suited to clear?
    a. Heart Heat
    b. Liver and Gallbladder Heat
    c. Lung and Stomach Heat
    d. Large Intestine and Small Intestine Heat

1790. Which of the following cautions are associated with formulas that relieve Exterior syndromes?
    a. Do not decoct for a long time
    b. Drink the decoction while it is warm
    c. After drinking the decoction lie in a warm bed to induce perspiration and prevent Wind
    d. All of the above

1791. Green tea performs which of the following functions in Chuan Xiong Cha Tiao San?
   a. Clear Heat from the eyes
   b. Moderate undesirable effects of the elevating and lowering ingredients
   c. Moderate undesirable effects of the warming and drying ingredients
   d. All of the above

1792. Which herb does Sheng Ma Ge Gen Tang and Chai Ge Jie Ji Tang *not* have in common?
   a. Sheng Ma
   b. Ge Gen
   c. Gan Cao
   d. Shao Yao

1793. Gui Zhi Tang is *not* associated with which of the following cautions or contraindications?
   a. Avoid using in cases of Exterior-Deficiency syndrome caused by pathogenic Wind and Cold
   b. Avoid using in cases of Exterior-Excess syndrome caused by pathogenic Wind and Cold
   c. Avoid using in cases of Exterior Wind-Heat syndrome
   d. Avoid using in cases of Exterior Cold and Interior Heat

1794. Qiang Huo is *not* indicated for which of the following?
   a. Exterior Wind-Damp syndrome
   b. Exterior Wind-Cold syndrome
   c. Exterior Wind-Heat syndrome
   d. Arthralgia caused by Wind-Cold-Damp

1795. Which herb serves as the chief (monarch or *jun*) component in Ji Chuan Jian?
   a. Dang Gui
   b. Niu Xi
   c. Rou Cong Rong
   d. Sheng Ma

1796. Which formula is *not* used to treat Cold-Heat combinations?
   a. San Wu Bei Ji Wan
   b. Wen Pi Tang
   c. Dan Huang Mu Dan Tang
   d. Ban Xia Xie Xin Tang

1797. Which formula does *not* contain all of the herbs from Tiao Wei Cheng Qi Tang?
   a. Tao Ren Cheng Qi Tang
   b. Liang Ge San
   c. Zeng Ye Cheng Qi Tang
   d. Huang Long Tang

1798. Which of the following is an indication for Bei Xie?
   a. Cloudy urine
   b. Painful urinary dysfunction that involves stones
   c. Stranguria complicated with hematuria
   d. Heat stranguria

1799. Which of the following herbs are especially effective for treating Lung abscesses?
   a. Yi Yi Ren
   b. Dong Gua Ren
   c. Yu Xing Cao
   d. All of the above

1800. Yin Chen Hao Tang is *not* indicated for which of the following?
   a. Bright yellow coloration of the skin and eyes
   b. A sensation of fullness in the abdomen
   c. Greasy yellow tongue fur and a slippery-rapid pulse
   d. Loose stool or diarrhea

B. In the next section (questions 1801–2500), questions comes in sets of two to five. To the right of each set of questions, you will find five possible answers. Use these to answer all of the questions in that set. *Each question has only one correct answer.* More than one question may share the same correct answer, however.

1801. What is a function associated with sweet substances?

1802. What is a function associated with salty substances?

a. Release the Exterior
b. Astringe
c. Drain
d. Soften
e. Harmonize

1803. Which answer best describes the relationship between Shi Gao and Zhi Mu?

1804. Which answer best describes the relationship between Da Huang and Huang Qin?

a. Mutual promotion
b. Mutual incompatibility
c. One increases the effect of the other
d. One counteracts the other's toxicity
e. Mutual antagonism

1805. Which herb has antagonism with Li Lu?

1806. Which herb is incompatible with Wu Tou?

a. Hai Zao
b. Bei Mu
c. Ren Shen
d. Mang Xiao
e. Wu Ling Zhi

1807. Which type of herbs tend to drain and dry Damp?

1808. Which type of herbs tend to release the Exterior and move Qi?

1809. Which type of herbs tend to astringe, stabilize, and bind?

a. Acrid
b. Sweet
c. Bitter
d. Sour
e. Salty

1810. Ma Huang and Xiang Ru each Release the Exterior, disperse Cold, and perform which of the functions at right?

1811. Fang Feng and Qiang Huo each Release the Exterior, disperse Cold, and perform which of the functions at right?

a. Promote urination
b. Expel Wind-Damp
c. Transform Phlegm
d. Unblock the Qi of the nasal orifices
e. Warm the Middle Energizer and stop vomiting

1812. Chan Tui vents rashes/measles and performs which of the functions at right?

1813. Sheng Ma vents rashes/measles and performs which of the functions at right?

a. Raise the Yang and stop diarrhea
b. Clear Heat and relieve toxicity
c. Stop spasms and extinguish Wind
d. Cool the Blood and stop bleeding
e. Relieve toxicity and benefit the throat

1814. Ge Gen performs which of the functions at right?

1815. Chan Tui performs which of the functions at right?

a. Clear and benefit the head and eyes
b. Benefit the throat and reduce swelling
c. Vent measles and release the muscles
d. Clear the eyes and remove superficial visual obstruction
e. Resolve lesser Yang disorders and reduce fever

1816. Xiang Ru releases the Exterior and performs which of the functions at right?

1817. Jiang Jie releases the Exterior and performs which of the functions at right?

a. Regulate Qi
b. Transform Damp
c. Stop bleeding
d. Expel pus
e. Unblock nasal passages

1818. Xiang Ru releases the Exterior and performs which of the functions at right?

1819. Cong Bai releases the Exterior and performs which of the functions at right?

a. Promote movement of Qi and expand the chest
b. Warm the Middle Energizer and alleviate pain
c. Promote urination and reduce swelling
d. Unblock the Yang
e. Stop bleeding

1820. Bo, He disperses Wind-Heat and performs which of the functions at right?

1821. Sang Ye disperses Wind-Heat and performs which of the functions at right?

1822. Sheng Ma disperses Wind-Heat and performs which of the functions at right?

a. Disperse Wind-Heat, relieve toxicity and vent measles
b. Disperse Wind-Heat, stop spasms and extinguish Wind
c. Expel Wind, clear Heat from the Lungs, cool the Blood, and stop bleeding
d. Disperse Wind-Heat, clear the head and eyes, and vent rashes
e. Disperse Wind-Heat and moisten the Intestines

1823. Sheng Jiang performs which of the functions at right?

1824. Bai Zhi performs which of the functions at right?

1825. Xin Yi Hua performs which of the functions at right?

a. Expel Wind, release the Exterior, and stop bleeding,
b. Warm the Lungs and transform Phlegm
c. Expel Wind, release the Exterior, and unblock the Yang
d. Expel Wind-Cold and unblock the nasal passages
e. Expel Wind-Cold, stop coughing, and reduce the toxicity of other herbs

1826. Which two herbs each release the Exterior and dispel Wind-Damp?

1827. Which two herbs each Expel Wind-Cold and unblock the nasal passages?

a. Ma Huang and Gui Zhi
b. Sheng Jiang and Zi Su
c. Qiang Huo and Du Huo
d. Fang Feng and Jing Jie
e. Xin Yi Hua and Cang Er Zi

1828. Which two herbs each disperse Wind-Heat and relieve toxicity?

1829. Which two herbs each isperse Wind-Heat and clear the Liver and eyes?

a. Bo He and Niu Bang Zi
b. Sang Ye and Ju Hua
c. Chai Hu and Ju Hua
d. Sheng Ma and Niu Bang Zi
e. Chan Tui and Ge Gen

1830. Which herb serves to expel Wind and relax muscular spasms?

1831. Which herb serves to expel pus and reduce swelling?

a. Fang Feng
b. Jing Jie
c. Qiang Huo
d. Bai Zhi
e. Gao Ben

1832. Which of the herbs at right would you combine with Bo He to treat patterns of Wind-Heat or seasonal febrile disease that begin with fever and a slight aversion to cold?

1833. Which of the herbs at right would you combine with Bo He to treat externally contracted Wind-Heat patterns that involve a swollen and painful throat?

a. Su Ye and Jing Jie
b. Lian Qiao and Jin Yin Hua
c. Jie Geng and Niu Bang Zi
d. Chan Tui and Gu Jing Cao
e. Chai Hu and Bai Shao

1834. Which herb would you combine with Gui Zhi to treat patterns of Deficient Heart Yang that involve palpitations and a pulse that is slow-uneven-intermittent or feeble-rapid?

1835. Which herb would you combine with Gui Zhi to treat patterns of Deficient Yang that involve painful obstruction, chills, and pain in the extremities?

a. Bai Shao
b. Bai Zhu
c. Zhi Gan Cao
d. Fu Zi
e. Dang Gui

1836. Which herb treats Exterior patterns of Wind-Cold that involve Qi Stagnation and a stifling sensation in the chest?

1837. Which herb treats Exterior patterns of Wind-Cold that involve headache and pain in the upper limbs and back?

a. Ma Huang
b. Zi Su
c. Gui Zhi
d. Sheng Jiang
e. Qiang Huo

1838. Which herb treat patterns of dizziness, blurry vision, and headache caused by Excess Liver Yang?

1839. Which herb treats Yangming headaches?

a. Bai Zhi
b. Qing Huo
c. Gao Ben
d. Man Jing Zi
e. Ju Hua

1840. Which condition would you treat with Xiao Qing Long Tang?

1841. Which condition would you treat with Da Qing Long Tang?

1842. Which condition would you treat with Xiang Su San?

a. Exterior Wind-Cold complicated by Qi Constrained in the Interior
b. Externally contracted Wind-Cold-Damp complicated by Internal accumulation of Heat
c. Exterior Wind-Cold complicated by Congealed fluids in the Interior
d. Exterior Wind-Cold complicated by Interior Heat
e. Externally contracted Wind-Cold leading to an Interior Cold-Deficiency condition

---

1843. She Gan Ma Huang Tang contains Ma Huang, Xi Xin, Ban Xia, Wu Wei Zi, and which of the herbs at right?

1844. Xiao Qing Long Tang contains Ma Huang, Xi Xin, Ban Xia, Wu Wei Zi, and which of the herbs at right?

a. Sheng Jiang
b. Gan Jiang
c. Sang Bai Pi
d. Shi Gao
e. Zi Su Ye

1845. Which formula releases Exterior Damp and clears Interior Heat?

1846. Which formula releases pathogenic influence from the muscle layer and regulates the Nutritive (Ying) and Protective (Wei) Qi?

a. Xiao Qing Long Tang
b. Ma Huang Tang
c. Gui Zhi Tang
d. Cong Chi Tang
e. Jiu Wei Qiang Huo Tang

1847. Chuan Xiong Cha Tiao San performs which of the functions at right?

1848. Sang Ju Yin performs which of the functions at right?

a. Release Exterior Wind-Heat, open inhibited Lung energy, and stop coughing
b. Disperse Wind-Heat, clear Heat, and relieve toxicity
c. Release the muscle layer and vent rashes
d. Release pathogenic influences from the muscle layer and clear Interior Heat
e. Disperse Wind and alleviate pain

1849. Which formula would you select to treat this pattern: increasing fever and decreasing chills accompanied by headache, stiff extremities, orbital and eye pain, dry nasal passages, irritability, insomnia, thin yellow tongue fur, and a floating and slightly flooding pulse?

1850. Which formula would you select to treat this pattern: slight fever, cough, slight thirst, thin white tongue fur, and a floating-rapid pulse?

a. Yin Qiao San
b. Sang Ju Yin
c. Chai Ge Jie Ji Tang
d. Jia Jian Wei Rui Tang
e. Jing Fang Bai Du San

1851. Xiao Yao San can be created by altering Si Ni San in which way?

1852. Chai Hu Shu Gan San can be created by altering Si Ni San in hich way?

a. Add Chuan Xiong, Mu Xiang, Chen Pi
b. Add Chuan Xiong, Xiang Fu, Chen Pi
c. Add Bai Zhu, Fu Ling, Dang Gui, Sheng Jiang, and Bo He
d. Subtract Zhi Shi and add Bai Zhu, Fu Ling, Dang Gui, Sheng Jiang, Bo He
e. Subtract Zhi Shi and add Zhi Ke, Chuan Xiong, Xiang Fu, Chen Pi

---

1853. Bo He performs what function in Yang Yin Qing Fei Tang?

1854. Bo He performs what function in Xiao Yao San?

1855. Bo He performs what function in Xuan Du Fa Biao Tang?

1856. Bo He performs what function in Yin Qiao San?

a. Relieve Liver Constraint
b. Release Exterior Heat
c. Vent rashes/measles
d. Disperse pathogenic influences and benefit the throat
e. None of the above

1857. Chuan Xin Lian clears Heat, relieves toxicity, and performs which of the functions at right?

1858. Bai Jiang Cao clears Heat, relieves toxicity, and performs which of the functions at right?

1859. Da Qing Ye clears Heat, relieves toxicity, and performs which of the functions at right?

a. Cool the Blood, reduce blotches
b. Dispel Blood Stasis, stop pain
c. Dry Damp
d. Reduce abscesses, promote urination
e. Clear away Liver Fire to treat diseases of the eye

1860. Huang Qin performs which of the functions at right?

1861. Ku Shen performs which of the functions at right?

1862. Qin Pi performs which of the functions at right?

a. Disperse Wind, kill parasites
b. Drain Liver Fire, benefit the eyes
c. Drain Kidney Fire
d. Clear Heart Fire, stop bleeding
e. Calm the fetus, stop bleeding

1863. Tian Hua Fen performs which of the functions at right?

1864. Lu Gen performs which of the functions at right?

1865. Xuan Shen performs which of the functions at right?

a. Generate fluids, stop vomiting, relieve irritability
b. Nourish Yin, Soften hardness, dissipate nodules
c. Drain Fire, cool the Blood, stop bleeding
d. Drain Fire, enrich Yin, moisten Dry
e. Generate fluids, expel pus

1866. Shan Dou Gen clears Heat, relieves toxicity, and performs which of the functions at right?

1867. Bai Tou Weng clears Heat, relieves toxicity, and performs which of the functions at right?

1868. Pu Gong Ying clears Heat, relieves toxicity, and performs which of the functions at right?

a. Benefit the throat, relieve swelling
b. Benefit the throat, transform Phlegm
c. Benefit the throat, stop bleeding
d. Expel Damp, stop dysentery
e. Promote lactation, reduce abscesses

1869. Huang Bai performs which of the functions at right?

1870. Huang Lian performs which of the functions at right?

1871. Long Dan Cao performs which of the functions at right?

a. Drain and pacify excessive Liver Fire
b. Relieve toxicity, drain Deficiency-Fire
c. Calm the fetus, stop bleeding
d. Expel Wind, kill parasites
e. Stop bleeding and diarrhea

1872. Jue Ming performs which of the functions at right?

1873. Qing Xiang Zi performs which of the functions at right?

1874. Gu Jing Cao performs which of the functions at right?

a. Clear the Liver, benefit the eyes, and calm the Liver to stop Wind
b. Clear the Liver, benefit the eyes, invigorate the Blood, and reduce swelling
c. Clear the Liver, benefit the eyes, moisten the Intestines, and unblock the bowels
d. Disperse Wind-Heat, eliminate superficial visual obstruction, and brightens the eyes
e. Treats hypertension associated with Ascendant Liver yang

1875. What type of Fire is Huang Bai particularly known for clearing?

1876. What type of Fire is Huang Qin particularly known for clearing?

1877. What type of Fire is Long Dan Cao particularly known for clearing?

a. Heart Fire
b. Lung Fire
c. Bladder Fire
d. Stomach Fire
e. Liver Fire

1878. Which two herbs each clear Heat and generate fluids?

1879. Which two herbs each clear Heart Heat and eliminate irritability?

a. Shi Gao and Zhi Mu
b. Lu Gen and Tian Hua Fu
c. Huang Lian and Zhi Zi
d. Huang Bai and Long Dan Cao
e. Huang Qin and Zhi Zi

1880. Which two herbs each cool and invigorate the Blood?

1881. Which two herbs each cool the Blood and nourish the Yin?

a. Xi Jiao and Mu Dan Pi
b. Xuan Shen and Zi Cao
c. Chi Shao and Mu Dan Pi
d. Sheng Di Huang and Xi Jiao
e. Xuan Shen and Sheng Di Huang

1882. Which two herbs each clear Heat, relieve toxicity, and benefit the throat?

1883. Which two herbs each clear Heat, relieve toxicity, and reduce abscesses?

1884. Which two herbs each clear Heat, relieve toxicity, and expel externally contracted Wind-Heat?

a. She Gan and Shan Dou Gen
b. Pu Gong Ying and Zi Hua Di Ding
c. Jin Yin Hua and Lian Qiao
d. Da Qing Ye and Qing Dai
e. Ye Ju Hua and Bai Jiang Cao

1885. Which herb would you use with Shi Gao to clear Lung Heat?

1886. Which herb would you use with Shi Gao to clear the Blood and clear the Qifen?

1887. Which herb would you use with Shi Gao to clear Qi-level Heat and generate fluids?

a. Ma Huang
b. Xi Jiao
c. Mai Men Dong
d. Zhi Mu
e. Niu Xi

1888. Which herbs would you use with Ge Gen to release the muscles and release the Exterior?

1889. Which herbs would you use with Ge Gen to nourish the fluids and alleviate thirst?

a. Gui Zhi and Ma Huang
b. Chai Hu and Shi Gao
c. Sheng Ma and Gan Cao
d. Huang Qin and Huang Lian
e. Tian Hua Fen and Mai Men Dong

1890. Which herb treats syphilis?

1891. Which herb treats lung abscesses involving a cough that produces sputum containing bloody pus?

a. Yu Xing Cao
b. Bai Jiang Cao
c. Tu Fu Ling
d. Bai Xian Pi
e. Zi Hua Di Ding

1892. Which herb treats coughing caused by Lung Heat?

1893. Which herb treats vomiting caused by Stomach Heat?

1894. Which herb treats irritability caused by Heart Fire?

a. Huang Lian
b. Huang Bai
c. Huang Qin
d. Ku Shen
e. Long Dan Cao

1895. Ma Bo is especially effective at treating which of these ailments?

1896. Hong Teng is especially effective at treating which of these ailments?

1897. Lou Lu is especially effective at treating which of these ailments?

a. Lung abscesses
b. Intestinal abscesses
c. Breast abscesses
d. Cancer
e. Bleeding in the oral cavity or lips

1898. Bai Hua She She Cao is especially effective at treating which of these ailments?

1899. Tu Fu Liang is especially effective at treating which of these ailments?

a. Breast abscesses
b. Stomach abscesses
c. Lung abscesses
d. Skin lesions caused by Damp-Heat
e. Snake bites

1900. Ban Zhi Lian clears Heat, relieves toxicity, and performs which of the functions at right?

1901. Hong Teng clears Heat, relieves toxicity, and performs which of the functions at right?

1902. Pu Gong Ying clears Heat, relieves toxicity, and performs which of the functions at right?

1903. Da Qing Ye clears Heat, relieves toxicity, and performs which of the functions at right?

a. Resolve Damp
b. Cool the Blood, reduce blotches
c. Dispel Blood Stasis and stop pain
d. Treat dysentery and stop diarrhea
e. Treat cancer and chronic hepatitis

1904. Xie Xin Tang performs which of the functions at right?

1905. Bing Wan Bai Du Yin performs which of the functions at right?

1906. Pu Ji Xiao Du Yin performs which of the functions at right?

a. Drain Fire, relieve toxicity, and cool the Blood
b. Drain Fire, relieve toxicity, and disperse Wind-Heat
c. Drain Fire, relieve toxicity, dry Damp, and relieve swelling
d. Drain Fire, relieve toxicity, invigorate the Blood, and alleviate pain
e. None of the above

1907. Which formula would you select to treat the latter stages of a Warm-Febrile disease with these symptoms: Yin and body fluids depleted by Heat, night fevers are followed by morning coolness, fine-rapid pulse?

1908. Which formula would you select to treat the latter stages of warm-febrile disease where the Yin and body fluids have been depleted by Heat, the Qi and body fluids have been injured by Heat, the chest has a lingering stifling sensation, and there is a deficient-rapid pulse?

a. Bai Hu Jia Ren Shen Tang
b. Zhu Ye Shi Gao Tang
c. Bai Hu Tang
d. Sheng Mai San
e. Qing Hao Bie Jia San

1909. Which formula would you select to treat this pattern: delirium caused by accumulation of Stagnant Blood, abdominal distention and fullness, thirst with an inability to swallow, black and tarry stool?

1910. Which formula would you select to treat this pattern: high fever, irritability, dry mouth and throat, incoherent speech, insomnia, nosebleeds, vomiting of blood, red tongue with yellow fur, rapid-forceful pulse?

a. Huang Lian Jie Du Tang
b. Qing Wen Bai Du Yin
c. Xi Xiao Di Huang Tang
d. Pu Ji Xiao Du Yin
e. Tao Ren Cheng Qi Tang

1911. Which formula would you select to treat this pattern: coughing, wheezing, fever that worsens in the afternoon, red tongue, thin-rapid pulse?

1912. Which formula would you select to treat this pattern: cough that produces foul-smelling sputum, slight fever and chest pain, dry or scaly skin, red tongue with greasy yellow fur, slippery-rapid pulse?

a. Wei Jing Tang
b. Xie Bai San
c. Zuo Jin Wan
d. Sang Ju Yin
e. Sang Xing Tang

1913. Which formula would you select to treat Stomach Heat and Deficient Yin with these symptoms: irritability, fever, thirst with a desire to drink cold beverages, and toothache or bleeding from the teeth?

1914. Which formula would you select to treat Excess-Stomach Heat resulting in bleeding gums, toothache, and swollen cheeks?

a. Bai Hu Tang
b. Yu Nu Jian
c. Qing Wei San
d. Xie Huang Tang
e. Xie Xin Dao Chi Tang

1915. Xie Huang Tang performs which of the functions at right?

1916. Qing Wei San performs which of the functions at right?

a. Drain Heat from the Stomach and nourish the Yin
b. Drain smoldering Fire from the Spleen and Stomach
c. Drain Stomach Fire, cool the Blood
d. Clear Heat, regulate Stomach Qi, generate body fluids, nourish the Yin
e. None of the above

1917. Shao Yao Tang performs which of the functions at right?

1918. Bai Tou Weng performs which of the functions at right?

a. Relieve toxicity, cool the Blood, alleviate dysenteric disorders
b. Transform Damp, promote movement of Qi, alleviate dysenteric disorders
c. Relieve toxicity, nourish the Blood, enrich the Yin
d. Relieve toxicity, regulate Qi, invigorate the Blood
e. Resolve Damp, alleviate dysenteric disorders

1919. Sheng Jiang Xie Xin Tang can be created by altering Ban Xia Xie Xin Tang in which way?

1920. Gan Cao Xie Xin Tang can be created by altering Ban Xia Xie Xin Tang in which way?

a. Add Sheng Jiang and subtract Gan Jiang
b. Add Gan Cao
c. Add Gan Cao and Sheng Jiang
d. Subtract Gan Cao and Sheng Jiang
e. Add Gan Cao and subtract Gan Jiang

1921. Which formula would you select to treat a Stomach Qi disorder with these symptoms: localized firm epigastric distention, dry heaves that emit a foul odor, watery sound in the hypochondria, very loud borborygmus and diarrhea?

1922. Which formula would you select to treat this pattern: undigested food in the stool, very loud borborygmus and diarrhea, focal epigastric hardness and distention, dry heaves that emit a foul odor, irritability?

a. Sheng Jiang Xie Xin Tang
b. Can Cao Xie Xin Tang
c. Xie Xin Tang
d. Bai Zhu Shao Yao Tang
e. None of the above

1923. Gan Sui performs which of the functions at right?

1924. Lu Hui performs which of the functions at right?

1925. Mang Xiao performs which of the functions at right?

a. Clear Heat, purge accumulation, soften hardness
b. Drain Heat, purge accumulation, reduce toxicity, dispel Blood Stasis
c. Purge accumulation, kill parasites, clear the Liver
d. Drain water downward, purge accumulation, drive out congested fluids, kill parasites
e. Drain water downward, drive out congested fluids, reduce swelling and nodules

---

1926. Gua Lou Ren treats constipation caused by which of the factors at right?

1927. Ba Dou treats constipation caused by which of the factors at right?

a. Cold accumulation
b. Food accumulation
c. Heat accumulation
d. Deficiency-Cold
e. Dry Intestines

1928. Da Huang invigorates the Blood, dispels Blood Stasis, and performs which of the functions at right?

1929. Mu Dan Pi invigorates the Blood, dispels Blood Stasis, and performs which of the functions at right?

1930. Dan Shen invigorates the Blood, dispels Blood Stasis, and performs which of the functions at right?

a. Cool the Blood, clear the liver
b. Reduce abscesses, stop pain
c. Clear Heat toxins, reduce abscesses
d. Clear Heat, calm the Spirit
e. Clear Heat, reduce Fire toxins

1931. Which formula would you select to treat accumulation of Blood Stasis and Heat, with Blood building up in the Lower Energizer?

1932. Which formula would you select to treat mild organ stage disorder in the Yang Brightness meridian that causes distention, hardness, and fullness?

a. Da Cheng Qi Tang
b. Tiao Wei Cheng Qi Tang
c. Xiao Cheng Qi Tang
d. Fu Fang Da Cheng Qi Tang
e. Tao Ren Cheng Qi Tang

1933. Which formula would you select to treat an organ stage disorder in the Yang Brightness meridian with these symptoms: constipation, abdominal distention, fullness and pain, tidal fever, delirious speech, prickly and dry yellow tongue fur, submerged-excessive pulse?

1934. Which formula would you select to treat accumulation of Heat evil with these symptoms: constipation with occasional watery discharge, watery diarrhea, abdominal pain that increases when pressure is applied, dry mouth and tongue, slippery-excessive pulse?

1935. Which formula would you select to treat accumulation of Heat evil with these symptoms: constipation with occasional watery discharge caused by, watery green diarrhea, abdominal pain that increases when pressure is applied, thirst, dry tongue and mouth, shortness of breath, lethargy, yellow-black tongue fur, deficient pulse?

a. Da Cheng Qi Tang
b. Tiao Wei Cheng Qi Tang
c. Zeng Ye Cheng Qi Tang
d. Liang Ge San
e. Huang Long Tang

1936. Da Huang Fu Zi Tang treats constipation caused by which of the factors at right?

1937. Ma Zi Ren Wan treats constipation caused by which of the factors at right?

1938. Ji Chuan Jian treats constipation caused by which of the factors at right?

a. Cold accumulation in the Interior
b. Heat-induced Dry of the Stomach and Intestines
c. Deficient Yang and Qi of the Kidneys
d. Deficient Qi and Blood
e. Desiccated Intestines

1939. San Wu Bei Ji Wan performs which of the functions at right?

1940. Run Chang Wan performs which of the functions at right?

1941. Huang Long Tang performs which of the functions at right?

a. Harshly purge Cold accumulation
b. Moisten the Intestines, unblock the bowels
c. Support healthy energy and purgation
d. Warm and moisten to unblock bowels
e. Warm the Interior to unblock the bowels

1942. Which formula would you select to treat this pattern: constipation, abdominal pain, cold extremities, deep-wiry pulse, may involve chronic red or white dysenteric disorders?

1943. Which formula would you select to treat this pattern: constipation, abdominal pain, chills, low-grade fever, cold hands and feet, tight-wiry pulse, may involve slight pain in the hypochondria,?

1944. Which formula would you select to treat this pattern: epigastric and abdominal pain and distention, the pain so intense that the patient's mouth remains tightly clenched and consciousness is sometimes lost?

a. Da Huang Fu Zi Tang
b. Wen Pi Tang
c. San Wu Bei Ji Wan
d. Huang Long Tang
e. Ma Zi Ren Wan

1945. Di Fu Zi performs which of the functions at right?

1946. Shi Wei performs which of the functions at right?

1947. Bei Xie performs which of the functions at right?

a. Clear Damp-Heat, unblock painful urinary dysfunction, stop coughs
b. Separate the pure from the turbid, expel Wind-Damp
c. Clear Heat, promote urination, disperse Blood Stasis
d. Clear Damp-Heat, promote urination, stop itching
e. Clear Damp-Heat, relieve jaundice

1948. Hua Shi promotes urination and performs which of the functions at right?

1949. Che Qian Zi promotes urination and performs which of the functions at right?

1950. Fang Ji promotes urination and performs which of the functions at right?

a. Expel Wind-Damp
b. Unblock the bowels
c. Improve eyesight
d. Promote lactation
e. Release Summer Heat

1951. Which two herbs each promote urination, unblock urinary difficulty, leach out Damp, and stop diarrhea?

1952. Which two herbs each promote urination unblock painful urinary dysfunction, and promote lactation?

1953. Which two herbs each clear Damp-Heat from the Liver and Gallbladder and relieve jaundice?

a. Di Fu Zi and Hua Shi
b. Mu Tong and Tong Cao
c. Yi Yi Ren and Fu Ling
d. Yin Chen Hao and Jin Qian Cao
e. Shi Wei and Hai Jin Sha

1954. Which herb is combined with Fu Ling to strengthen the Spleen and promote urination?

1955. Which herb is combined with Fu Ling to warm the Yang and promote urination?

1956. Which herb is combined with Fu Ling to stop vomiting and nausea and to move the Qi?

a. Bai Zhu
b. Ze Xie
c. Zhu Ling
d. Chen Pi
e. Fu Zi

1957. Which meridians are entered by Fu Ling?

1958. Which meridians are entered by Hua Shi?

1959. Which meridians are entered by Chi Xiao Dou?

a. Kidney, Liver, Lung
b. Bladder, Large Intestine, Small Intestine
c. Heart, Small Intestine
d. Heart, Spleen, Lung
e. Stomach, Bladder

1960. Bu Huan Jin Zheng Qi San can be created by adding which herbs to Ping Wei San?

1961. Chai Ping Tang can be created by adding which herbs to Ping Wei San?

a. Ban Xia and Huo Xiang
b. Ban Xia and Pei Lan
c. Ban Xia and Chai Hu
d. Ban Xia, Hu Xiang, Ren Shen, and Huang Qin
e. Ban Xia, Chai Hu, Ren Shen, and Huang Qin

1962. Which type of jaundice is an indication for Yin Chen Hao Tang?

1963. Which type of jaundice is an indication for Yin Chen Zhu Fu Tang?

a. Jaundice caused by heavy Heat and heavy Damp
b. Jaundice caused by heavy Heat and slight Damp
c. Jaundice caused by slight Heat and heavy Damp
d. Yin-type jaundice (Damp-Cold) with Deficient Kidney Yang
e. Yin-type jaundice with Deficient Spleen Yang

1964. Ba Zheng San and Zong Man Fen Xiao Wan each perform which of the functions at right?

1965. Yin Chen Hao Tang and San Ren Tang each perform which of the functions at right?

1966. Gan Lu Xiao Du Dan and Xuan Bi Tang each perform which of the functions at right?

1967. Ji Ming San and Shi Pi Yin each perform which of the functions at right?

a. Clear Heat, expel Damp
b. Release the Exterior, transform Damp
c. Warm and transform water and Damp
d. Dispel Wind, overcome Damp
e. Promote urination, drain Damp

1968. Da Qing Long Tang contains which of the herbs at right?

1969. Ma Huang Jia Zhu Tang contains which of the herbs at right?

1970. Wu Ling San contains which of the herbs at right?

1971. Jin Gui Shen Qi Wan contains which of the herbs at right?

a. Gui Zhi and Fu Ling
b. Gui Zhi and Bai Shao
c. Gui Zhi and Ma Huang
d. Gui Zhi and Tao Ren
e. Gui Zhi and Da Huang

1972. Which of the functions at right does Sheng Jiang perform in Ji Ming San?

1973. Which of the functions at right does Sheng Jiang perform in Zhen Wu Tang?

1974. Which of the functions at right does Sheng Jiang perform in Wu Zhu Yu Tang?

a. Warm and dispel pathogenic water
b. Warm the Stomach, stop vomiting
c. Warm the Lungs, stop coughing
d. Warm and disperse Cold-Damp, assist treatment of leg Qi
e. None of the above

1975. Which formula would you select to treat a Damp Warm-Febrile disease in its early stages with these symptoms: headache, chills, a heavy sensation in the body, pain, pale yellow complexion, stifling sensation in the chest, lost appetite, afternoon fever, absence of thirst, white tongue fur, thin-wiry-soggy pulse?

1976. Which formula would you select to treat the clumping of Damp-Heat in the Lower Energizer with these symptoms: difficult and painful urination that produces scanty and turbid dark urine (may sometimes involve urinary retention), abdominal distension and pain, dry mouth and throat, greasy yellow tongue fur, slippery-rapid pulse?

1977. Which formula would you select to treat Damp-Cold stagnation in the Spleen and Stomach with these symptoms: distention and fullness in the epigastrium and abdomen, loss of taste and appetite, nausea and vomiting, belching, acid regurgitation, is easily fatigued, sleeps longer, thick greasy white tongue fur?

a. Ping Wei San
b. San Ren Tang
c. Gan Lu Xiao Du Dan
d. Huo Xiang Zheng Qi San
e. Ba Zheng San

1978. Which choice at right is an indication for Xiao Ji Yin Zi?

1979. Which choice at right is an indication for Bei Xie Fen Qing Yin?

1980. Which choice at right is an indication for Ba Zhong San?

a. Stranguria caused by urinary stones
b. Stranguria complicated by hematuria
c. Stranguria caused by a vital energy disorder
d. Stranguria caused by Damp-Heat
e. Cloudy painful urinary dysfunction caused by Deficiency-Cold

---

1981. Which of the ailments at right would you treat with Qiang Huo?

1982. Which of the ailments at right would you treat with Bai Hua She?

1983. Which of the ailments at right you treat with Fang Ji?

a. Chronic arthralgia
b. Wind arthralgia
c. Damp-Heat arthralgia
d. Arthralgia chiefly caused by Damp evil
e. Numbness caused by Deficient Blood

1984. Luo Shi Ten dispels Wind-Damp and performs which of the functions at right?

1985. Qin Jiao dispels Wind-Damp and performs which of the functions at right?

1986. Du Huo dispels Wind-Damp and performs which of the functions at right?

a. Release the Exterior
b. Reduce jaundice
c. Reduce food stagnation
d. Cool the Blood, reduce swelling
e. Open the nasal passages

1987. Wei Ling Xian dispels Wind-Damp and performs which of the functions at right?

1988. Can Sha dispels Wind-Damp and performs which of the functions at right?

1989. Qian Nian Jian dispels Wind-Damp and performs which of the functions at right?

a. Unblock the channels, alleviate pain
b. Strengthen the sinews and bones
c. Nourish the Blood, unblock the channels
d. Clear Heat caused by Deficiency
e. Harmonize the Stomach, transform turbid Damp

1990. Which herb would you select to treat arthralgia throughout the body?

1991. Which her would you select to treat arthralgia in the upper lumbar region?

1992. Which herb would you select to treat arthralgia in the lower lumbar region?

a. Qiang Huo
b. Du Huo
c. Wei Ling Xian
d. Shan Zhu Yu
e. Wu Zhu Yu

1993. Which two herbs each dispel Wind-Damp and promote urination?

1994. Which two herbs each dispel Wind-Damp and strengthen the sinews and bones?

1995. Which two herbs each dispel Wind-Damp and treat hypertension?

a. Luo Shi Teng and Bai Hua She
b. Wu Jia Pi and Sang Ji Sheng
c. Fang Ji and Wu Jia Pi
d. Wei Ling Xian and Hai Tong Pi
e. Xi Xian Cao and Chou Wu Tong

1996. Sha Ren performs which of the functions at right?

1997. Cao Guo performs which of the functions at right?

1998. Cang Zhu performs which of the functions at right?

a. Dry Damp, strengthen the Spleen
b. Dry Damp, warm the Middle Energizer
c. Aromatically transform Damp, release Summer Heat
d. Treat malaria
e. Calm the fetus

1999. Huo Xiang and Xiang Ru each perform which of the functions at right?

2000. Bai Dou Kou and Sha Ren each perform which of the functions at right?

2001. Cang Zhu and Pei Lan each perform which of the functions at right?

a. Transform Damp, promote movement of Qi, transform Stagnation
b. Release Summer Heat, transform Damp, harmonize the Middle Energizer
c. Warm the Middle Energizer, strengthen the Spleen
d. Induce sweating, improve vision
e. None of the above

2002. Cao Guo performs which of the functions at right?

2003. Bai Dou Kou performs which of the functions at right?

2004. Huo Xiang performs which of the functions at right?

a. Harmonize the Middle Energizer, release the Exterior
b. Harmonize the Middle Energizer, promote the movement of Qi
c. Harmonize the Middle Energizer, check malarial disorders
d. Stop vomiting, promote the movement of Qi
e. None of the above

2005. Bai Bu moistens the Lungs and performs which of the functions at right?

2006. Tian Hua Fen moistens the Lungs and performs which of the functions at right?

2007. Gua Lou Ren moistens the Lungs and performs which of the functions at right?

a. Expel parasites
b. Clear the voice
c. Expel pus
d. Moisten the Intestines
e. Transform Damp

2008. Bai Guo and Wu Wei Zi each perform which of the functions at right?

2009. Zhe Bei Mu and Ban Xia each perform which of the functions at right?

2010. Zhu Ru and Gua Lou each perform which of the functions at right?

a. Transform Phlegm, dissipate nodules
b. Dry Damp, transform Phlegm
c. Clear and transform Phlegm-Heat
d. Moisten the Lungs, stop coughing
e. Stop coughing and wheezing with styptic pectorals

2011. Gua Lou Pi clears Heat, transforms Phlegm, and performs which of the functions at right?

2012. Zhu Ru clears Heat, transforms Phlegm, and performs which of the functions at right?

2013. Bei Mu clears Heat, transforms Phlegm, and performs which of the functions at right?

a. Stop coughing, dissipate nodules
b. Expand the chest, benefit Qi
c. Stop vomiting and bleeding
d. Promote urination, reduce edema
e. Calm the Liver to stop Wind

2014. Kuan Dong Hua performs which of the functions at right?

2015. Xing Ren performs which of the functions at right?

2016. Ting Li Zi performs which of the functions at right?

a. Clear the Lungs, transform Phlegm, stop coughing and wheezing
b. Moisten the Lungs, redirect Qi downward, stop coughing, transform Phlegm
c. Transform Phlegm, stop coughing, harmonize the Stomach, cause rebellious Qi to descend
d. Stop coughing and wheezing, moisten the Intestines, unblock the bowels
e. Stop coughing and wheezing, move water, reduce edema

2017. Which herb redirects Qi downward and moistens the Intestines?
2018. Which herb clears the Lungs and calms wheezing?
2019. Which herb treats acute, chronic cough, especially one that results from Deficiency?

a. Kuan Dong Hua
b. Zi Wan
c. Su Zi
d. Bai Bu
e. Ting Li Zi

2020. Which herb treats coughing caused by Lung Dry syndrome?
2021. Which herb treats coughing caused by Damp-Phlegm?
2022. Which herb treats spasm caused by Wind?

a. Qian Hu
b. Bai Qian
c. Gua Lou
d. Ban Xia
e. Tian Nan Xing

2023. Jie Geng performs which of the functions at right?
2024. Sang Ye performs which of the functions at right?
2025. Ma Dou Ling performs which of the functions at right?
2026. Gua Di performs which of the functions at right?

a. Open up and disseminate Lung Qi
b. Warm and moisten the Lungs
c. Clear the Lungs, moisten Dry
d. Clear the Lungs, reduce blood pressure
e. Clear Damp-Heat, relieve jaundice

2027. Tian Zhu Huang performs which of the functions at right?
2028. Hai Zao performs which of the functions at right?
2029. Bai Qian performs which of the functions at right?
2030. Tian Nan Xing performs which of the functions at right?

a. Expel Phlegm, stop coughing, redirect Qi downward
b. Dry Damp, expel Phlegm, disperse Wind, stop spasms
c. Dry Damp, expel Phlegm, disperse Wind, dissipate nodules
d. Reduce Phlegm, promote urination, dissipate nodules
e. Clear Phlegm-Heat, clear the Heart, arrest convulsions

2031. Which herbs are part of the formula Gun Tan Wan?
2032. Which herbs are part of the formula Xiao Xian Xiong Tang?
2033. Which herbs are part of the formula Xiao Luo Wan?

a. Gua Lou, Huang Lian, Jiang Ban Xia
b. Xuan Shen, Mu Li, Bei Mu
c. Bai Jie Zi, Su Zi, Lai Fu Zi
d. Gua Di, Chi Xiao Dou
e. Da Huang, Huang Qin, Duan Meng Shi, Chen Xiang

2034. Which formula treats externally contracted Wind that moves upward to the head and causes headaches?
2035. Which formula treats excessive Heat and chronic Phlegm leading to dizziness or vertigo?
2036. Which formula treats Wind-Phlegm leading to headaches and dizziness or vertigo?

a. Dao Tan Tang
b. Gun Tan Wan
c. Ban Xia Bai Zhu Tian Ma Tang
d. Er Chen Tang
e. Chuan Xiong Cha Tiao San

2037. Which formula would you select to treat this pattern: coughing and wheezing, copious sputum, focal distention in the chest, loss of appetite, digestive difficulty, greasy white tongue fur, slippery pulse?

2038. Which formula would you select to treat this pattern: dizziness or vertigo, fullness in the chest and hypochondria, shortness of breath, palpitations, slippery white tongue fur, wiry-slippery pulse?

2039. Which formula would you select to treat this pattern: dizziness or vertigo, headache, a stifling sensation in the chest, nausea or vomiting, copious sputum, greasy white tongue fur, slippery pulse?

a. San Zi Yang Qin Tang
b. Ling Gan Wu Wei Jiang Xin Tang
c. Er Chen Tang
d. Ban Xia Bai Zhu Tian Ma Tang
e. Ling Gui Zhu Gan Tang

2040. Which formula dries Damp, transforms Phlegm, regulates the Qi, and harmonizes the Middle Energizer?

2041. Which formula dries Damp, transforms Phlegm, promotes the movement of Qi, and opens up areas of constraint?

2042. Which formula regulates the Qi, transforms Phlegm, clears the Gallbladder, and harmonizes the Middle Energizer?

a. Er Chen Tang
b. Dao Tan Tang
c. Gun Tan Wan
d. Wen Dan Tang
e. Ji Shui Liu Jun Jian

2043. Which pattern indicates the use of Gun Tan Wan?

2044. Which pattern indicates the use of Qing Qi Hua Tan Wan

2045. Which pattern indicates the use of Zhi Sou San?

a. Focal distention and a feeling of fullness in the chest and diaphragm, coughing that produces viscous yellow sputum with great difficulty, greasy yellow tongue fur, slippery-rapid pulse
b. Focal distention and a stifling sensation in the chest and epigastrium, coughing and wheezing that produces thick viscous sputum, constipation, thick greasy yellow tongue fur, rapid-forceful pulse
c. Focal distention and a stifling sensation in the chest and diaphragm, coughing that easily produces copious white sputum, nausea or vomiting, thick white greasy tongue fur, slippery pulse
d. Focal distention in the chest and epigastrium that is painful when pressed, coughing up of viscous yellow sputum, constipation, greasy yellow tongue fur, slippery-rapid pulse
e. None of the above

2046. Which herb reduces food stagnation, transforms accumulation, and reduces Phlegm?

2047. Which herb reduces food stagnation, harmonizes the Middle Energizer, and inhibits lactation?

2048. Which herb reduces food stagnation, harmonizes the Stomach, and aids the digestion and absorption of mineral herbs?

a. Shan Zha
b. Shen Qu
c. Lai Fu Zi
d. Mai Ya
e. Ji Nei Jin

2049. Which herb reduces food stagnation, secures the Essence, and dissolves stones?

2050. Which herb reduces food stagnation and harmonizes the Stomach?

2051. Which herb reduces and guides out food stagnation, transforms Blood Stasis, and dissipates clumps?

a. Shan Zha
b. Gu Ya
c. Ji Nei Jin
d. Shen Qu
e. Bai Bian Dou

2052. Which formula would you select to treat this pattern: focal distention and fullness in the chest and epigastrium, aversion to food, abdominal distention with occasional pain, rotten-smelling belching, acid regurgitation, nausea and vomiting, loose stool, slippery pulse?

2053. Which formula would you select to treat this pattern: focal distention of the epigastrium and abdomen, reduced appetite with digestive difficulty, loose watery diarrhea, slightly yellow tongue fur, deficient-frail pulse?

2054. Which formula would you select to treat this pattern: focal distention in the epigastrium and abdomen, loss of appetite, white tongue fur, deficient pulse?

a. Zhi Zhu Wan
b. Zhi Shi Xiao Pi Wan
c. Jian Pi Wan
d. Bao He Wan
e. De An Wan

2055. Which pattern is an indication for Bao He Wan?

2056. Which pattern is an indication for Jian Pi Wan?

2057. Which pattern is an indication for Zhi Zhu Wan?

a. Overeating that injures the Spleen and Stomach, accumulation of undigested food
b. Deficient Spleen and Stomach, reduced appetite with digestive difficulty, stagnation and accumulation of undigested food
c. Deficient Spleen and Stomach, loss of appetite, tendency for food to stagnate in the digestive system, focal distention in the epigastrium
d. Food stagnation that transforms into Damp-Heat
e. None of the above

2058. What are the relative dispersing and strengthening powers of Jian Pi Wan?

2059. What are the relative dispersing and strengthening powers of Zhi Zhu Wan?

2060. What are the relative dispersing and strengthening powers of Bao He Wan?

a. Disperses, but does not strengthen
b. Strengthens, but does not disperse
c. Primarily disperses, but also strengthens
d. Primarily strengthens, but also disperse
e. Disperses and strengthens equally

2061. Jian Pi Wan contains which of the herbs at right?

2062. Bao He Wan contains which of the herbs at right?

2063. Zhi Shi Dao Zhi Wan contains which of the herbs at right?

2064. Mu Xiang Bing Lang Wan contains which of the herbs at right?

a. Shen Qu, Fu Ling, Chen Pi
b. Shen Qu, Fu Ling, Bai Zhu
c. Shen Qu, Fu Ling, Bai Zhu, Shan Zha
d. All of the above
e. None of the above

2065. Mu Xiang Bing Lang Wan treats focal and generalized distention caused by what?

2066. Zhi Shi Xiao Pi Wan treats focal distention and fullness in the upper epigastrium that is caused by what?

2067. Jian Pi Wan treats focal distention of the epigastrium and abdomen that is caused by what?

a. Deficient Spleen and Stomach, Cold-Heat complex Qi obstruction
b. Deficient Spleen and Stomach, food stagnation
c. Deficient Spleen causing food stagnation, which transforms to Heat
d. Food stagnation that has become complicated by Damp-Heat
e. None of the above

2068. Fo Shou performs which of the functions at right?

2069. Tan Xiang performs which of the functions at right?

2070. Xie Bai performs which of the functions at right?

a. Spread and regulate Liver Qi, regulate menstruation, alleviate pain
b. Spread and regulate Liver Qi, harmonize the Stomach, transform Phlegm
c. Promote movement of Qi, expel Cold, alleviate pain, treat diseases of the coronary arteries
d. Promote the movement of Qi and Blood, direct the Qi downward, reduce stagnation
e. None of the above

2071. Chuan Lian Zi promotes movement of Qi, alleviates pain, and performs which of the functions at right?

2072. Wu Yao promotes movement of Qi, alleviates pain, and performs which of the functions at right?

2073. Mu Xiang promotes movement of Qi, alleviates pain, and performs which of the functions at right?

a. Kill parasites, treat tinea
b. Warm the Kidneys, expel Cold
c. Strengthen the Spleen, prevent stagnation
d. Harmonize the Blood, disperse stasis
e. Disperse Cold, disperse stagnation

2074. Which two herbs each promote the movement of Qi and alleviate pain?

2075. Which two herbs each dry Damp and transform Phlegm?

2076. Which two herbs each spread and regulate Liver Qi?

a. Chen Pi and Ju Hong
b. Zhi Shi and Qing Pi
c. Chen Xiang and Ding XIang
d. Wu Yao and Mu XIang
e. Fo Shou and Xiang Fu

2077. Which herb is especially useful for treating breast abscesses caused by Phlegm-Damp?

2078. Which herb treats coughing caused by Damp-Phlegm and also treats Stagnant Qi of the Spleen or Stomach?

2079. Which herb treats dysenteric diarrhea with tenesmus?

a. Chen Pi
b. Ju Hong
c. Zhi Shi
d. Zhi Ke
e. Qing Pi

2080. Which herb treats constrained Liver Qi and irregular menstruation?

2081. Which herb treats constrained Liver Qi, hernial pain, and pain in the chest or hypochondriac regions?

2082. Which herb treats accumulation and Stagnant Qi, abdominal pain, constipation, and fullness in the chest and epigastrium?

a. Chen Pi
b. Qing Pi
c. Xiang Fu
d. Zhi Shi
e. Hou Po

2083. Which herb treats hiccups caused by Stomach dysfunction?

2084. Which herb treats asthma and wheezing caused by inability of the Kidneys to grasp Qi?

2085. Which herb treats nausea and vomiting caused by Phlegm-Damp in the Stomach rebelling upward?

a. Shi Di
b. Wu Yao
c. Chen Xiang
d. Mu Xiang
e. None of the above

2086. Qing Pi performs which of the functions at right?

2087. Chai Hu performs which of the functions at right?

2088. Fo Shou performs which of the functions at right?

a. Spread Liver Qi, break up stagnant Qi, dissipate clumps, reduce stagnation
b. Spread and regulate Liver Qi, harmonize the Stomach, and transforms Phlegm
c. Spread Liver Qi, relieve constraint, resolve Lesser Yang disorders, reduce fever
d. Spread Liver Qi, promote the movement of Qi, regulate menstruation, alleviate pain
e. None of the above

2089. Which formula spreads Liver Qi, drains Heat, regulates the Qi, and alleviates pain?

2090. Which formula promotes the movement of Qi, spreads Liver Qi, scatters Cold, and alleviates pain?

2091. Which formula warms the Middle Energizer, dispels Cold, prmotes the movement of Qi, and alleviates pain?

a. Jin Ling Zi San
b. Tian Tai Wu Yao San
c. Ban Xia Hou Po Tang
d. Ju He Wan
e. Liang Fu Wan

2092. Ban Xia Hou Po Tang performs which of the functions at right?

2093. Hou Po Wen Zhong Tang performs which of the functions at right?

2094. Ju He Wan performs which of the functions at right?

a. Dissipate clumps, direct rebellious Qi downward, transform Phlegm
b. Expel Phlegm, unblock the Yang
c. Warm the Middle Energizer, dry Damp, eliminate fullness
d. Spread Liver Qi, scatter Cold, alleviate pain
e. None of the above

2095. Zhi Shi Gua Gui Zhi Tang can be created by altering Gua Lou Xie Bai Bai Jiu Tang in which way?

2096. Gua Lou Xie Bai Ban Xia Tang can be created by altering Gua Lou Xie Bai Bai Jiu Tang in which way?

2097. Gua Lou Zhi Shi Tang can be created by altering Gua Lou Xie Bai Bai Jiu Tang in which way?

a. Add Ban Xia
b. Add Ban Xia, subtract Bai Jiu
c. Add Ban Xia, subtract Bai Jiu
d. Add Zhi Shi, Gui Zhi, Hou Po, subtract Bai Jiu
e. None of the above

2098. Nuan Gan Jian treats lower abdominal pain caused by what?

2099. Tian Tai Wu Yan San treats lower abdominal pain caused by what?

2100. Ju He Wan treats lower abdominal pain caused by what?

a. Deficiency-Cold in the Liver and Kidneys, stagnant Qi
b. Damp-Cold in the Spleen and Stomach, stagnant Qi
c. Cold stagnation in the Liver meridian, stagnant Qi
d. Damp-Cold invading the Liver meridian, stagnant Qi, Blood Stasis
e. Exogenous Cold evil attacking the Stomach, stagnant Qi

2101. Which formula treats wheezing caused by Excess above and Deficiency below, with Excess being the primary factor?

2102. Which formula treats wheezing caused by Excess above and Deficiency below, with Deficiency being the primary factor?

a. Ding Chuan Tang
b. Su Zi Jiang Qi Tang
c. Xiao Qing Long Tang
d. Da Qing Long Tang
e. Hei Xi Dan

2103. Which formula would you select to treat this pattern: coughing and wheezing that produces copious thick yellow sputum, labored breathing, greasy yellow tongue fur, slippery-rapid pulse, may involve simultaneous fever and chills?

2104. Which formula would you select to treat this pattern: coughing and wheezing that produces copious watery sputum, a stifling sensation in the chest and diaphragm, shortness of breath, slippery-greasy white tongue fur,?

2105. Which formula would you select to treat this pattern: coughing and wheezing that produces copious sputum, focal distention in the chest, loss of appetite, digestive difficulties, greasy white tongue fur, slippery pulse?

a. Ding Chuan Tang
b. Su Zi Jiang Qi Tang
c. San Zi Yang Qin Tang
d. Shen Mi Tang
e. Bei Mu Gua Lou San

2106. Liang Fu Wan warms the Middle Energizer, alleviates pain, and performs which of the functions at right?

2107. Hou Po Wen Zhong Tang warms the Middle Energizer, alleviates pain, and performs which of the functions at right?

a. Treats the Spleen and Stomach, expel Cold, dry Damp
b. Strengthen the Liver and Kidneys
c. Treats the Stomach, spread Liver Qi
d. Expel Damp-Cold evil with herbs of a warm nature
e. Strengthen the Spleen, dispel Damp

2108. Ju Pi Zhu Ru Tang performs which of the functions at right?

2109. Xuan Fu Dai Zhe Tang performs which of the functions at right?

2110. Ding Xiang Shi Di Tang performs which of the functions at right?

a. Augment the Qi, warm the Middle Energizer, direct rebellious Qi downward, stop hiccups
b. Augment the Qi, harmonize the Stomach, direct rebellious Qi downward, transform Phlegm
c. Augment the Qi, clear Heat, direct rebellious Qi downward, stop vomiting
d. Warm and tonify the Middle Energizer, direct rebellious Qi downward, stop vomiting
e. None of the above

2111. In a case of focal distention, Xuan Fu Dai Zhe Tang is indicated for which of the causes at right?

2112. In a case of focal distention, Bao He Wan is indicated for which of the causes at right?

2113. In a case of focal distention, Ban Xia Xie Xin Tang is indicated for which of the causes at right?

a. Cold-Heat complex
b. Deficient Stomach, Phlegm obstruction, and abnormal rising of Qi
c. Food-Heat complex
d. Dry-Heat in the Stomach and Intestines
e. Damp turbidity obstruction

2114. Ai Ye stops bleeding through what influence?

2115. Huai Hua Mi stops bleeding through what influence?

2116. Lian Fang stops bleeding through what influence?

a. It restrains leakage of Blood
b. It cools the Blood
c. It warms the womb
d. It disperses Blood Stasis
e. It tonifies Deficiency

2117. Bai Mao Gen cools the Blood, stops bleeding, and performs which of the functions at right?

2118. Qian Cao Gen cools the Blood, stops bleeding, and performs which of the functions at right?

2119. Da Ji (Cirsium) cools the Blood, stops bleeding, and performs which of the functions at right?

a. Promote healing of burns
b. Invigorate the Blood, dispel Blood Stasis
c. Cool the Liver
d. Reduce swelling, regenerate the flesh of sores
e. Clear Heat, promote urination

2120. Yi Mu Cao performs which of the functions at right?

2121. Yu Jin performs which of the functions at right?

2122. San Leng performs which of the functions at right?

a. Invigorate the Blood, alleviate pain, promote the movement of Qi, spread Liver Qi, cool the Blood, benefit the Gallbladder
b. Invigorate the Blood, alleviate pain, promote the movement of Qi, unblock menstruation, expel Wind, promote the Blood
c. Invigorate the Blood, regulate menses, promote urination, reduce swelling,
d. Promote the movement of Qi, alleviate pain, break up Blood Stasis, unblock menses, dissolve accumulation
e. None of the above

2123. Which two herbs can each be applied topically to treat burns?

2124. Which two herbs each invigorate the Blood, dispel Blood Stasis, and stop bleeding?

2125. Which two herbs each cool the Blood and stop bleeding?

a. San Qi and Bai Ji
b. Pu Huang and Qian Cao Gen
c. Han Lian Cao and Ce Bai Ye
d. Da Huang and Di Yu
e. Da Ji and Xian He Cao

2126. Which herb treats red, painful, swollen eyes that have been caused by Liver Heat?

2127. Which herb treats headaches caused by Blood Stasis and Qi Stagnation?

2128. Which herb treats swelling in the neck and scrofula?

a. Chuan Xiong
b. Dang Gui
c. Dan Shen
d. Chong Wei Zi
e. Yue Ji Hua

2129. Tao Ren invigorates Blood circulation and performs which of the functions at right?

2130. Niu Xi invigorates Blood circulation and performs which of the functions at right?

2131. Ru Xiang invigorates Blood circulation and performs which of the functions at right?

2132. Hu Zhang invigorates Blood circulation and performs which of the functions at right?

2133. Dan Shen invigorates Blood circulation and performs which of the functions at right?

a. Drain Heat downward, transform Phlegm, stop coughing
b. Dispel Blood Stasis, Clear Heat, sooth irritability
c. Dispel Blood Stasis, moisten the Intestines, unblock the bowels
d. Alleviate pain, reduce swelling, regenerate flesh
e. Dispel Blood Stasis, supplement and restore the Liver and Kidneys

---

2134. Qi Li San contains which of the herbs at right?

2135. Huo Luo Xiao Ling Dan contains which of the herbs at right?

2136. Fu Yuan Huo Xue Tang contains which of the herbs at right?

a. Ru Xiang and Mo Yao
b. Wu Ling Zhi and Pu Huang
c. Hong Hua and Tao Ren
d. Hong Hua and Chi Shao
e. Hong Hua and Pu Huang

2137. Which of the herbs at right treat a variety of skin problems caused by Wind?

2138. Which of the herbs at right treat childhood nutritional impairment involving focal distention?

2139. Which of the herbs at right treat postpartum abdominal pain involving lochioschesis in cases resulting from Blood Stasis?

2140. Which of the herbs at right stop bleeding?

2141. Which of the herbs at right treat hot Phlegm that is obstructing the Heart orifices?

a. Chuan Xiong
b. Yi Mu Cao and Shan Zha
c. Wu Ling Zhi
d. Xue Jie and Su Mu
e. Yu Jin and Ming Fan

2142. Which formula would you select to treat a case where Stagnant Blood has accumulated in the Lower Energizer causing acute lower abdominal pain, urinary incontinence, night fevers, delirious speech, thirst, and a deep-full-choppy pulse?

2143. Which formula would you select to treat a case where Stagnant Blood has accumulated in the Lower Energizer causing manic behavior, firmness and distention of the lower abdomen, forgetfulness, black stool that is easily expelled, deep-slow-irregular pulse?

a. Tao He Cheng Qi Tang
b. Di Dang Tang
c. Xue Fu Zhu Yu Tang
d. Xi Jiao Di Huang Tang
e. Dan Shen Yin

2144. Dan Shen Yin contains Dan Shen, Tan Xiang, and which of the herbs at right?

2145. Huo Luo Xiao Ling Dan contains Dan Shen, Ru Xiang, Mo Yao, and which of the herbs at right?

a. Chuan Xiong
b. Chi Shao
c. Dang Gui
d. Sha Ren
e. Xiang Fu

2146. Which formula would you select to treat a case of Deficient Spleen where there is blood in the stool and vomiting of blood?

2147. Which formula would you select to treat a patient who has bleeding hemorrhoids, typically bleeds bright red blood from the rectum before passing stool that is bloody as well, and has a red tongue and wiry-rapid pulse?

a. Huang Tu Tang
b. Huai Hua Tang
c. Shi Hui San
d. Si Sheng Wan
e. Jiao Ai Tang

2148. Fu Zi and Gan Jiang each perform which of the functions at right?

2149. Hua Jiao and Gao Liang Jiang each perform which of the functions at right?

a. Recuperate depleted Yang and rescue the patient from danger
b. Warm the Lungs, transform Phlegm
c. Warm the Middle Energizer, alleviate pain
d. Warm the Liver, alleviate pain
e. Warm the Fire, assist the Yang

2150. Gan Jiang performs which of the functions at right?

2151. Wu Zhu Yu performs which of the functions at right?

a. Warm the Middle Energizer, expel Cold, warm the Lungs, transform Phlegm
b. Disperse Cold, alleviate pain, dry Damp
c. Disperse Cold, alleviate pain, warm the Kidneys, assist the Yang
d. Disperse Cold, alleviate pain, regulate Qi, harmonize the Stomach
e. Disperse Cold, alleviate pain, disperse the Depressed Liver Qi, redirect rebellious Qi downward

2152. Ding Xiang performs which of the functions at right?

2153. Sheng Jiang performs which of the functions at right?

2154. Hua Jiao performs which of the functions at right?

a. Warm the Middle Energizer, alleviate pain, kill parasites
b. Warm the Middle Energizer, alleviate pain, warm the Lungs, transform Phlegm
c. Expel Cold, alleviate pain, disperse depressed Liver Qi, redirect rebellious Qi downward
d. Warm the Middle Energizer, redirect rebellious Qi downward, warm the Kidneys, assist the Yang
e. Warm the Middle Energizer, expel Cold, expel Wind, alleviate vomiting

---

2155. Which herb at right releases the Exterior and disperses Cold?

2156. Which herb at right recuperates depleted Yang and rescues the patient from danger?

2157. Which herb at right stops bleeding?

a. Sheng Jiang
b. Gan Jiang
c. Pao Jiang
d. Sheng Jiang Pi
e. None of the above

2158. What are the properties of Fu Zi?

2159. What are the properties of Xi Xin?

a. Acrid, hot, toxic, enters the Heart, Kidney, and Spleen meridians
b. Acrid, hot, enters the Heart, Stomach, Lung, and Spleen meridians
c. Acrid, bitter, hot, slightly toxic, enters the Liver, Spleen, and Stomach meridians
d. Acrid, warm, enters the Lung and Kidney meridians
e. Acrid, hot, slightly toxic, enters the Spleen, Stomach, and Kidney meridians

---

2160. Which two herbs each supplement the Fire and assist the Yang?

2161. Which two herbs each warm the Lungs and transform Phlegm?

a. Fu Zi and Gan Jiang
b. Fu Zi and Rou Gui
c. Xi Xin and Wu Zhu Yu
d. Xi Xin and Gan Jiang
e. Gao Liang and Jiang Gan Jiang

2162. Which of the herbs at right would you combine with Fu Zi to treat this pattern: cold extremities, sweating, weak breathing, dizziness, an extremely pale complexion?

2163. Which of the herbs at right would you combine with Fu Zi to treat Deficient Yang of the Spleen and Kidneys where there is retention of pathogenic water and urinary difficulty?

2164. Which of the herbs at right would you combine with Fu Zi to treat a case of collapsed Yang of the Spleen and Kidneys involving chills, cold extremities, and diarrhea containing undigested food?

2165. Which of the herbs at right would you combine with Fu Zi to treat this pattern: strong sensation of cold in the epigastrium, vomiting to the point of being unable to eat, excruciating epigastric and abdominal pain, will not tolerate being touched in those areas, slippery white tongue fur, thin-light or slow-wiry pulse?

a. Ren Shen
b. Bai Zhu and Fu Ling
c. Ren Shen and Gan Jiang
d. Gui Zhi and Bai Zhu
e. Gan Jiang and Gan Cao

2166. Which formula would you select to treat a case of Deficiency-Cold of the Spleen and Stomach where there is diarrhea with watery stool, no particular thirst, vomiting and pain in the abdomen, and loss of appetite?

2167. Which formula would you select to treat this pattern: intermittent spasmodic abdominal pain that responds favorably to local application of warmth and pressure, occasional fever?

a. Li Zhong Wan
b. Xiao Jian Zhong Tang
c. Da Jian Zhong Tang
d. Huang Qi Jian Zhong Tang
e. None of the above

2168. Xiao Jian Zhong Tang performs which of the functions at right?

2169. Wu Zhu Yu Tang performs which of the functions at right?

2170. Li Zhong Wan performs which of the functions at right?

a. Warm the Middle Energizer, strengthen the Spleen and Stomach
b. Warm the meridians, disperse Cold, nourish the Blood, unblock the blood vessels
c. Warm and tonify the Liver and Stomach, direct rebellious Qi downward, stop vomiting
d. Rescue devastated Yang, warm the Middle Energizer, stop diarrhea
e. Warm and tonify the Middle Energizer, moderate spasmodic abdominal pain

---

2171. Xiao Jian Zhong Tang warms the Middle Energizer, tonifies Deficiency, and performs which of the functions at right?

2172. Da Jian Zhong Tang warms the Middle Energizer, tonifies Deficiency, and performs which of the functions at right?

a. Expel Cold, strengthen the Spleen and Stomach
b. Moderate spasmodic abdominal pain
c. Direct rebellious Qi downward, alleviate pain
d. Direct rebellious Qi downward, stop vomiting
e. Alleviate diarrhea with astringents

2173. Which pattern indicates the use of Si Ni Tang?

2174. Which pattern indicates the use of Dang Gui Si Ni Tang?

2175. Which pattern indicates the use of Tong Mai Si Ni Tang?

a. Extremely cold extremities, sweating, weak breathing, faint pulse
b. Extremely cold extremities, lack of thirst, sore extremities, pale tongue, deep-thin pulse
c. Extremely cold extremities, diarrhea containing undigested food, intolerance to cold, flushed face, imperceptible pulse
d. Extremely cold extremities, intolerance to cold, sleeping with the knees drawn up, diarrhea containing undigested food, lack of thirst, lethargy with a constant desire to sleep, thin-deep-faint pulse
e. Incessant diarrhea, patient feels extremely cold, dry heaves, irritability, faint pulse

---

2176. Yang He Tang performs which of the functions at right?

2177. Wen Jing Tang performs which of the functions at right?

2178. Bu Yang Huan Wu Tang performs which of the functions at right?

2179. Sheng Hua Tang performs which of the functions at right?

a. Warm the meridians, disperse Cold, nourish the Blood, unblock the blood vessels
b. Warm the meridians, disperse Cold, nourish the Blood, dispel Blood Stasis
c. Tonify the Qi, invigorate the Blood, unblock the meridians
d. Invigorate the Blood, transform and dispel Blood Stasis, warm the menses, alleviate pain
e. Warm the Yang, tonify the Blood, disperse Cold, unblock areas of stagnation

---

2180. Which of the functions at right does Rou Cong Rong perform?

2181. Which of the functions at right does He Shou Wu perform?

a. Relieve cough, expel phlegm, moisten the Intestines, unblock the bowels
b. Tonify Kidneys, strengthen the Yang, moisten the Intestines, facilitate passage of stool
c. Tonify the Liver and Kidneys, moisten the Intestines, unblock the bowels
d. Promote the movement of Blood, moisten the Intestines, unblock the bowels
e. Promote urination, reduce swelling, moisten the Intestines, unblock the bowels

---

2182. Zi He Che and Long Yau Rou each perform which of the functions at right?

2183. Sang Ji Sheng and Xu Duan each perform which of the functions at right?

a. Tonify the Kidneys, strengthen the Yang
b. Tonify the Liver and Kidneys
c. Tonify the Lungs and Kidneys
d. Tonify the Spleen and Kidneys
e. Augment the Qi, nourish the Blood

2184. Which of the functions at right can be achieved by combining Dang Gui with Huang Qi?

2185. Which of the functions at right can be achieved by combining Ren Shen with Mai Men Dong?

2186. Which of the functions at right can be achieved by combining Fu Zi with Shu Di?

a. Strengthen the Qi, fortify the Yang
b. Strongly tonify the Yuan Qi, nourish the Yin
c. Strengthen the Qi, generate Blood
d. Strengthen the Yin and the Yang
e. Nourish the Yin and the Blood

2187. Shan Yao performs which of the functions at right?

2188. Bai Zhu performs which of the functions at right?

a. Tonify the Spleen, augment the Qi, nourish the Blood, calm the Spirit
b. Tonify and augment both the Spleen and the Qi, stop sweating, calm the fetus
c. Tonify the Qi, nourish the Yin, tonify the Spleen, Lungs, and Kidneys
d. Tonify the Spleen, augment the Qi, promote urination, reduce edema, nourish the Blood
e. Strengthen the Spleen, augment the Qi, generate fluids

2189. Mai Men Dong and Bai He each perform which of the functions at right?

2190. Tian Men Dong and Huang Jing each perform which of the functions at right?

a. Nourish the Liver and Kidneys
b. Nourish the Lungs and Heart
c. Nourish the Liver, Kidneys, and Lungs
d. Nourish the Lungs and Kidneys
e. Nourish the Lungs and Stomach

2191. Mai Men Dong performs which of the functions at right?

2192. Tian Men Dong performs which of the functions at right?

2193. Huang Jing performs which of the functions at right?

a. Nourish the Yin, clear Heat, moisten the Intestines, calm the Spirit
b. Nourish the Yin, moisten the Lungs, tonify Spleen Qi
c. Nourish the Yin, clear Heat, moisten the Lungs, nourish the Kidneys
d. Nourish the Yin, augment the Stomach, moisten the Lungs, clear the Heart
e. Nourish the Stomach, generate body fluids, sterngthen Kidney Qi, stop asthma

---

2194. Which herb tonifies and augments the Liver and Kidneys, retains Essence, and retains excessive urination?

2195. Which herb tonifies and augments the Spleen and Stomach and tonifies the Lungs and Kidneys?

a. Shan Yao
b. Shan Zha
c. Shan Dou Gen
d. Shan Zhu Yu
e. Shan Zhi Zi

2196. Which herb strengthens the Spleen, dries Damp, and stabilizes the Exterior?

2197. Which herb tonifies the Spleen, augments the Qi, eliminates Phlegm, and stops coughing?

a. Huang Qi
b. Bai Zhu
c. Gan Cao
d. Shan Yao
e. Xi Yang Shen

2198. Which herb benefits the Spleen, stops diarrhea, nourishes the Liver, and improves vision?

2199. Which herb warms the Spleen, stops diarrhea, tonifies the Kidneys, and fortifies the Yang?

a. Bu Gu Zhi
b. Xu Duan
c. Gu Sui Bu
d. Tu Si Zi
e. Gou Ji

2200. Which herb calms and curbs Liver Yang and alleviates pain?

2201. Which herb moistens the Lungs and stops bleeding?

a. Shu Di Huang
b. E Jiao
c. He Shou Wu
d. Bai Shao
e. Dang Gui

2202. Which herbs at right benefit the Kidneys and tonify the Lungs?

2203. Which herbs at right tonify the Kidneys and secure the Essence?

a. Ba Ji Tian and Rou Cong Rong
b. Xian Mao and Yin Yang Huo
c. Tu Si Zi and Sha Yuan Zi
d. Ge Jie and Dong Chong Xia Cao
e. Gou Ji and Du Zhong

2204. Which herb augments the Qi and promotes urination?

2205. Which herb tonifies the Qi and nourishes the Yin?

2206. Which herb augments the Qi and stabilizes the Exterior?

a. Huang Qi
b. Hai Er Shen
c. Dang Shen
d. Xi Yang Shen
e. Dan Shen

2207. What is another name for Yin Yang Huo?

2208. What is another name for Bu Gu Zhi?

a. Huai Shan
b. Bei Qi
c. Hai Er Shen
d. Xian Ling Pi
e. Po Gu Zhi

2209. Liu Jun Zi Tang can be created by adding which of the following to Si Jun Zi Tang?

2210. Xiang Sha Liu Jun Ji Tang can be created by adding which of the following to Si Jun Zi Tang?

a. Chen Pi, Ban Xia
b. Mu Xiang, Sha Ren
c. Ban Xia, Sheng Jiang
d. Ban Xia, Chen Pi, Mu Xiang, and Sha Ren
e. Chen Pi

2211. Which formula would you select to treat intermittent fever caused by Deficient Qi?

2212. Which formula would you select to treat a fever that occurs after a severe loss of Blood?

a. Si Jun Zi Tang
b. Bu Zhong Yi Qi Tang
c. Dang Gui Bu Xue Tang
d. Sheng Mai San
e. Shen Ling Bai Zhu San

2213. Which of the dosages at right are correct for Dang Gui Bu Xue Tang?

2214. Which of the dosages at right are correct for Bu Yang Huan Wu Tang?

a. 30 g. of Huang Qi; 6 g. of Dang Gui
b. 120 g. of Huang Qi; 6 g. of Dang Gui
c. 30 g. of Huang Qi; 3 g. of Dang Gui
d. 6 g. of Huang Qi; 15 g. of Dang Gui
e. 20 g. of Huang Qi; 10 g. of Dang Gui

2215. Which choice at right is used in Da Bu Yin Wan?

2216. Which choice at right is used in Zhi Gan Cao Tang?

2217. Which choice at right is used in Qi Bao Mei Ran Dan?

2218. Which choice at right is used in He Ren Yin?

a. Shu Di Huang
b. Sheng Di Huang
c. Shu Di Huang steamed in rice wine
d. Prepared He Shou Wu
e. Unprepared He Shou Wu

2219. Which two herbs each stabilize the Essence and stop diarrhea?

2220. Which two herbs each contain leakage of the Lungs and bind up the Intestines?

a. Shan Yu Rou and Wu Zei Gu
b. He Zi and Ying Su Ke
c. Lian Zi and Qian Shi
d. Sang Piao Xiao and Fu Pen Zi
e. Shi Liu Pi and Chun Pi

2221. Which herb is known especially for containing leakage of the Lungs?

2222. Which herb is known especially for generating fluids?

a. Fu Xiao Mai
b. Wu Wei Zi
c. Ma Huang Gen
d. Long Gu
e. Mu Li

2223. Rou Dan Kou performs which of the functions at right?

2224. Wu Wei Zi performs which of the functions at right?

2225. Wu Mei performs which of the functions at right?

2226. Chi Shi Zhi performs which of the functions at right?

2227. Hai Piao Xiao performs which of the functions at right?

a. Expel roundworms and alleviate pain
b. Treat chronic intractable diarrhea and daybreak diarrhea caused by Deficiency-Cold
c. Control acidity and alleviate pain
d. Quiet the Spirit and calm the Heart
e. Promote healing of wounds

2228. Which formula would you select to treat this pattern: spontaneous sweating, aversion to drafts, pale shiny complexion, pale tongue with white fur, floating-deficient-soft pulse?

2229. Which formula would you select to treat this pattern: spontaneous sweating that worsens at night, palpitations, shortness of breath, general debility, lethargy, pale red tongue, thin-frail pulse?

a. Mu Li San
b. Yu Ping Feng San
c. Dang Gui Liu Huang Tang
d. Sheng Mai San
e. Gui Zhi Tang

2230. Qing Dai Tang is indicated for which pattern?

2231. Yi Huang Tang is indicated for which pattern?

2232. Wan Dai Tang is indicated for which pattern?

2233. Bu Zhong Yi Qi Tang is indicated for which pattern?

a. Continuous, thin, clear (or red) vaginal discharge, sore and weak lower back, pale tongue with white fur, submerged-thin pulse
b. Long-term, unremitting, viscous, yellowish-white vaginal discharge that is fishy-smelling, dizziness, a heavy sensation in the head, pale tongue with white fur, soft-slippery or submerged pulse
c. Profuse, thin, white (or pale yellow) vaginal discharge that is not too foul smelling, lethargy, pale shiny complexion, loose stool, pale tongue with white fur, soggy-frail or moderate pulse
d. Yellow vaginal discharge, urine that is yellowish or reddish and passed with a sensation of heat, red tongue with greasy yellow fur, wiry-slippery pulse
e. White vaginal discharge, shortness of breath, laconic speech, poor appetite, weak limbs, pale tongue with white fur, deficient-rootless pulse

---

2234. Mu Li performs which of the functions at right?

2235. Zhen Zhu performs which of the functions at right?

2236. Zi Shi Ying performs which of the functions at right?

2237. Dai Zhe Zhi performs which of the functions at right?

a. Calm the Spirit, soften hardness, and dissipate nodules
b. Calm the Spirit, promote healing, and generate flesh
c. Calm the Liver, anchor the floating Yang, cool the Blood, and stop bleeding
d. Sedate the Heart, settle tremors and palpitations, warm the Lungs, and direct the Qi downwards
e. Absorb acidity, alleviate pain, calm the Liver, and prevent leakage of fluids

---

2238. Yuan Zi performs which of the functions at right?

2239. Suan Zao Ren performs which of the functions at right?

2240. Ye Jiao Teng performs which of the functions at right?

2241. He Huan Pi performs which of the functions at right?

a. Nourish the Heart, calm the Spirit, and moisten the Intestines
b. Nourish the Heart, calm the Spirit, and astringe sweating
c. Nourish the Heart, calm the Spirit, unblock the meridians, alleviate itching
d. Quiet the Heart, calm the Spirit, expel phlegm, and clean the orifices
e. Relieve constraint, calm the Spirit, invigorate the Blood, and dissipate swelling

2242. Zhu Sha performs which of the functions at right?

2243. Ci Shi performs which of the functions at right?

2244. Mu Li performs which of the functions at right?

2245. Hu Po performs which of the functions at right?

a. Calm the Spirit, clear Heat, and relieve toxicity
b. Calm the Spirit and prevent leakage of fluids
c. Calm the Spirit, aid in grasping the Qi, and alleviate asthma
d. Calm the Spirit and tonify the Qi and Blood
e. Calm the Spirit, promote urination, and reduce swelling

2246. Bai Zi Yang Xin Wan performs which of the functions at right?

2247. Suan Zao Ren Tang performs which of the functions at right?

2248. Gan Mai Da Zao Tang performs which of the functions at right?

2249. Zhu Sha An Shen Wan performs which of the functions at right?

a. Nourish the Heart, calm the Spirit, and harmonize the Middle Energizer
b. Nourish the Heart, calm the Spirit, and tonify Kidney Yin
c. Sedate the Heart, calm the Spirit, clear Heat, and nourish the Yin
d. Nourish the Blood, clam the Spirit, clear Heat, and eliminate irritability
e. Enrich the Yin, calm the Spirit, nourish the Blood, and tonify the Heart

---

2250. Which formula at right would you select to treat insomnia caused by Deficient Liver Blood?

2251. Which formula at right would you select to treat insomnia caused by Deficient Heart and Kidneys?

2252. Which formula at right would you select to treat insomnia caused by Deficient Heart and Spleen?

2253. Which formula at right would you select to treat insomnia caused by an imbalance between the Heart Yang and Kidney Yin?

a. Suan Zao Ren Tang
b. Tian Wang Bu Xin Du
c. Gui Pi Tang
d. Ci Zhu Wang
e. Gan Mai Da Zao Tang

2254. Ci Zhu Wan performs which of the functions at right?

2255. Zhen Zhu Mu performs which of the functions at right?

2256. Zhu Sha An Shen Wan performs which of the functions at right?

2257. Sheng Tie Luo Yin performs which of the functions at right?

a. Sedate the Heart, calm the Spirit, enrich the Yin, and nourish Blood
b. Sedate the Heart, calm the Spirit, and eliminate Phlegm
c. Sedate the Heart, calm the Spirit, drain Fire, and nourish the Yin
d. Heavily sedate and calm the Spirit, weigh down the Yang, and improve vision and hearing
e. Sedate and calm the Spirit and unblock the three Yang stages

2258. Niu Huange performs which of the functions at right?

2259. Bing Pian performs which of the functions at right?

2260. Shi Chang Pu performs which of the functions at right?

a. Open the orifices and invigorate the Blood
b. Open the orifices and transform Damp
c. Open the orifices and alleviate pain
d. Open the orifices and extinguish Wind
e. Open the orifices and dissipate clumps

2261. Which herb vaporizes Phlegm and opens the orifices?

2262. Which herb clears the Liver and eliminates superficial visual obstructions?

2263. Which herb opens the orifices and clears away filth?

a. Su He Xiang
b. Niu Huang
c. She Xiang
d. Zhen Zhu
e. Gou Teng

2264. Zi Xue Dan performs which of the functions at right?

2265. Hui Chun Dan performs which of the functions at right?

2266. An Gong Niu Huang Wan performs which of the functions at right?

a. Clear heat, relieve toxicity, dislodge Phlegm, and open the orifices
b. Clear Heat, relieve toxicity, control spasms and convulsions,
c. Clear Heat, relieve toxicity, transform turbidity, and open the orifices
d. Clear Heat, transform Phlegm, arrest convulsions, and open the orifices
e. Clear Heat, relieve toxicity, cool the Blood, and open the orifices

---

2267. Which formula at right would you select to treat this pattern: high fever, irritability, restlessness, delirious speech, stiffness of the tongue, frigid-feeling extremities, rapid-sthenic pulse?

2268. Which formula at right would you select to treat this pattern: high fever, irritability, restlessness, delirious speech, impaired consciousness, muscle twitches, spasms and convulsions, thirst, parched lips, deep red tongue, rapid-sthenic pulse?

2269. Which formula at right would you select to treat this pattern: fever, irritability, restlessness, delirious speech, copious sputum, labored raspy breathing, spasms and convulsions, deep red tongue with foul greasy yellow fur, rapid-slippery pulse?

a. An Gong Niu Huang Wan
b. Zi Xue Dan
c. Hui Chun Dan
d. Su He Xiang Wan
e. Zhi Bao Dan

2270. Di Long and Jiang Can each perform which of the functions at right?

2271. Pi Pa Ye and Fu Long Gan each perform which of the functions at right?

a. Stop vomiting
b. Stop diarrhea
c. Stop coughing
d. Stop convulsions
e. Stop pain

2272. Dai Zhe Shi performs which of the functions at right?

2273. Shi Jue Ming performs which of the functions at right?

2274. Bai Shao performs which of the functions at right?

2275. Bai Ji Li performs which of the functions at right?

2276. Long Gu performs which of the functions at right?

a. Calm the Liver, anchor the Yang, clear the Liver, and improve vision
b. Calm the Liver, anchor the Yang, direct rebellious Qi downward, and stop bleeding
c. Calm and curb Liver Yang, nourish the Blood, and preserve the Yin
d. Calm the Liver, anchor the Yang, and settle and calm the Spirit
e. Calm the Liver, anchor the Yang, dispel Wind, and stop itching

---

2277. Jiang Can performs which of the functions at right?

2278. Wu Gong performs which of the functions at right?

2279. Di Long performs which of the functions at right?

2280. Tian Ma performs which of the functions at right?

2281. Gou Teng performs which of the functions at right?

a. Extinguish Wind, stop convulsions, attack toxins, and dissipate nodules
b. Extinguish Wind, stop convulsions, drain Liver Heat, and release the Exterior
c. Extinguish Wind, stop convulsions, unblock the collaterals, and calm wheezing
d. Extinguish Wind, stop convulsions, calm the Liver, and alleviate pain
e. Extinguish Wind, stop convulsions, transform Phlegm, and stop itching

---

2282. Which herb calms and curbs the Liver and stops pain?

2283. Which herb calms the Liver, softens hardness, and dissipates nodules?

2284. Which herb calms the Liver, anchors the Yang, and prevents leakage of fluids?

a. Shi Jue Ming
b. Zhen Zhu Mu
c. Mu Li
d. Bai Shao
e. Ling Yang Jiao

2285. Which herb would you select to treat Wind syndrome resulting from the domination of Heat evil?

2286. Which herb would you select to treat sudden onset or recurrence of convulsive seizures?

2287. Which herb would you select to treat tremors, seizures, or stroke caused by Phlegm-Heat?

a. Shi Jue Ming
b. Ling Yang Jiao
c. Tian Ma
d. Long Gu
e. Dan Nan Xing

2288. What function does Bo He serve in Chuan Xiong Cha Tiao San?

2289. What function does Bo He serve in Di Huang Yin Zi?

a. Soften the Liver Qi
b. Disperse Wind-Heat
c. Clear the head and eyes
d. Benefit the throat
e. Vent rashes

2290. Which formula is indicated for headaches caused by Exterior Wind evil?

2291. Which formula is indicated for headaches caused by Exterior Wind-Damp?

a. Qiang Huo Sheng Shi Tang
b. Chuan Xiong Cha Tiao San
c. Ma Huang Tang
d. Jiu Wei Qian Huo Tang
e. Xiang Su San

2292. Which cause of dizziness and vertigo is an indication for Ma Gou Teng Yin?

2293. Which cause of dizziness and vertigo is an indication for Zhen Gan Xi Feng Tang?

a. Deficient Qi and Blood
b. Ascendant Liver Yang
c. Deficient Essence
d. Spleen Damp that becomes Phlegm
e. Excessive Liver-Fire

2294. Zhen Gan Xi Feng Tang performs which of the functions at right?

2295. Ling Jiao Gou Teng Tang performs which of the functions at right?

a. Sedate the Liver and extinguish Wind
b. Cool the Blood and extinguish Wind
c. Soften the Liver and extinguish Wind
d. Calm the Liver, extinguish and clear Heat, and calm the Spirit
e. Clear Heat, cool the Liver, extinguish Wind, and stop spasms

---

2296. Which formula at right cools the Liver and extinguishes Wind?

2297. Which formula at right nourishes the Yin and extinguishes Wind?

a. Ling Jiao Gou Teng Tang
b. Tian Ma Gou Teng Yin
c. Da Ding Feng Zhu
d. E Jiao Ji Zi Huang Tang
e. Di Huang Yin Zi

2298. Which formula at right treats Excess-Heat in the Liver meridian that stirs up internal movement of Wind?

2299. Which formula at right treats internal movement of Wind caused by Deficient True Yin?

2300. Which formula at right treats internal movement of Wind arising from Deficient Blood and Yin caused by Heat injuring the True Yin?

2301. Which formula at right treats Deficient Yin of the Liver and Kidneys accompanied by ascendant Liver Yang, which in severe cases leads to internal movement of Liver Wind?

a. Ling Jiao Gou Teng Tang
b. E Jiao Ji Zi Huang Tang
c. Zhen Gan Xi Feng Tang
d. Da Ding Feng Zhu
e. Tian Ma Gou Teng Yin

2302. Bai Bu performs which of the functions at right?

2303. Ku Lian Gen Pi performs which of the functions at right?

2304. Shi Jun Zi performs which of the functions at right?

a. Kill parasites and reduce stagnation
b. Kill parasites and treat tinea infection
c. Kill parasites, clear Heat, relieve toxicity, and stop bleeding
d. Kill pinworms and lice, moisten the Lungs, and stop coughing
e. Kill parasites, reduce stagnation, drain downward, and drive out water

---

2305. Which herb kills parasites, cools the Blood, and stops bleeding?

2306. Which herb kills parasites, reduces accumulation, and promotes the movement of Qi?

2307. Which herb kills parasites and treats tinea infection?

a. Shi Jun Zi
b. Lei Wan
c. Wu Yi
d. Guan Zhong
e. Bing Lang

2308. What function does Tian Hua Fen perform in Xian Fang Huo Ming Yin?

2309. What function does Tian Hua Fen perform in Fu Yuan Huo Xue Tang?

a. Clear Heat and transform Phlegm
b. Clear Heat and dry Damp
c. Relieve toxicity and expel pus
d. Promote the growth of new tissue and reduce swelling
e. Promote urination and dispel Blood Stasis

2310. What function does Wu Mei Wan perform in order to expel roundworms?

2311. What function does Bu Dai Wan perform in order to expel roundworms?

2312. What function does Fei Er Wan perform in order to expel roundworms?

a. Warm the Lower Energizer and clear Upper Energizer Heat
b. Strengthen Spleen Qi, alleviate accumulations, and clear Heat
c. Warm the Middle Energizer and support the Middle Energizer Yang
d. Relieve food stagnation, dry Damp and clear the Liver
e. Tonify the Spleen and Stomach using methods for eliminating evil factors and restoring healthy Qi

---

2313. Chuan Niu Xi performs which of the functions at right?

2314. Huai Niu Xi performs which of the functions at right?

2315. Du Zhong performs which of the functions at right?

a. Tonify the Liver and Kidneys and strengthen the sinews and bones
b. Tonify the Yin
c. Invigorate the Blood to clear away obstruction in the meridians
d. Tonify the Qi
e. None of the above

2316. Wu Wei Xiao Du Yin is useful for treating which of the patterns at right?

2317. Xian Fang Huo Ming Yin is useful for treating which of the patterns at right?

2318. Huang Lian Jie Du Tang is useful for treating which of the patterns at right?

2319. Niu Huang Shang Qing Wan is useful for treating which of the patterns at right?

a. Boils and carbuncles with erythema and extremely painful swelling, fever accompanied by restlessness and thirst, red tongue, rapid pulse
b. Early stage sores and carbuncles with hot, painful, red swollen skin lesions, fever, slight aversion to cold, thin or slightly yellow fur, rapid-forceful pulse
c. Boils and carbuncles with localized erythema and hot painful swelling that appears like millet but is hard and with a deep root like a nail, red tongue, rapid pulse
d. Redness, swelling, and burning pain of the head and facedysfunction of the throat, dryness, thirst, red tongue, floating-rapid-forceful pulse
e. Headache, red eyes, pain and swelling in the throat and gums, ulcerations of the mouth and tongue

---

2320. Which condition would you treat with Ji Zue Teng?

2321. Which symptom would you treat with Mu Tong?

2322. Which symptom would you treat with Cao Wu?

a. Migratory arthralgia
b. Arthralgia chiefly caused by Damp evil
c. Arthralgia chiefly caused by Cold evil
d. Arthralgia chiefly caused by Heat evil
e. Numbness in the limbs caused by Deficient Blood

2323. Xu Duan performs which of the functions at right?

2324. Gou Ji performs which of the functions at right?

2325. Sang Ji Sheng performs which of the functions at right?

a. Tonify the Liver and Kidneys, strengthen the sinews and bones, and expel Cold-Damp
b. Tonify the Liver and Kidneys, strengthen the sinews and bones, and stabilize the Kidneys
c. Tonify the Liver and Kidneys, strengthen the sinews and bones, and promote the movement of Blood
d. Tonify the Liver and Kidneys, strengthen the sinews and bones, and calm the womb
e. Expel Wind, strengthen the sinews and bones, and promote urination

---

2326. Xi Xin performs which of the functions at right?

2327. Rou Dou Kou performs which of the functions at right?

2328. Pao Jiang performs which of the functions at right?

a. Stop bleeding
b. Stop vomiting
c. Stop itching
d. Stop diarrhea
e. Alleviate pain

2329. In addition to absorbing acidity and alleviating pain, Hai Piao Xiao performs which of the functions at right?

2330. In addition to absorbing acidity and alleviating pain, Wa Leng Zi performs which of the functions at right?

2331. In addition to absorbing acidity and alleviating pain, Mu Li performs which of the functions at right?

a. Calm the Liver and treat through astringency
b. Dissolve phlegm and dissipate nodules
c. Stop bleeding and vaginal discharge
d. Invigorate the Blood and unblock the collateral meridians
e. Promote urination and reduce swelling

2332. Which herb clears Damp-Heat, promotes urination, and stops itching?

2333. Which herb warms the Kidneys, fortifies the Yang, dries Damp, and kills parasites?

2334. Which herb reduces swelling, disperses clumps, unblocks the channels, and alleviates pain?

a. Ma Qian Zi
b. Di Fu Zi
c. Tu Si Zi
d. Fu Pen Zi
e. She Chuang Zi

2335. Which herb clears Heat-Phlegm, controls acidity, and alleviates pain?

2336. Which herb retains Essence, stops vaginal discharge, controls acidity, and alleviates pain?

2337. Which herb clears Heat, promotes urination, and dispels stones?

a. Hai Ge Ke
b. Hai Jin Sha
c. Hai Fu She
d. Hai Piao Xiao
e. Hai Zao

2338. Which herb dries Damp, transforms Phlegm, expels Wind, and stops spasms?

2339. Which herb expels Wind, releases the Exterior, eliminates Damp, and stops leukorrhagia?

2340. Which herb restrains leakage of Blood, stops bleeding, reduces swelling, and generates flesh?

a. Bai Zhu
b. Bai Fu Zi
c. Bai Ji
d. Bai Jie Zi
e. Bai Zhi

2341. Which herb clears Heat and dispels Wind-Damp?

2342. Which herb invigorates the Blood, dispels Blood Stasis, promotes urination, and reduces swelling?

2343. Which herb dispels Blood Stasis, stops pain, clears Heat, and expels pus?

a. Bai Jiang Cao
b. Xi Xian Cao
c. Yi Mu Cao
d. Xian He Cao
e. Xia Ku Cao

2344. Which herb promotes urination, reduces edema, and reduces hypertension?

2345. Which herb dispels Wind-Damp, promotes urination, and reduces swelling?

2346. Which herb calms the Spirit, relieves constraint, invigorates the Blood, and dissipates swelling?

a. Da Fu Pi
b. He Huan Pi
c. Wu Jia Pi
d. Di Gu Pi
e. Sang Bai Pi

2347. Which herb expels Cold, alleviates pain, regulates the Qi, and harmonizes the Stomach?

2348. Which herb aromatically transforms Damp and releases Summer Heat?

2349. Which herb coordinates the functions of the Spleen and Stomach, promotes the movement of Qi, and alleviates pain?

a. Su He Xiang
b. Mu Xiang
c. Qing Mu Xiang
d. Xiao Hui Xiang
e. Huo Xiang

2350. Which herb unblocks the bowels, drives out water, expels parasites, and reduces stagnation?

2351. Which herb tonifies the Liver and Kidneys, invigorates the Blood, and expels Blood Stasis?

2352. Which herb disperses Wind-Heat, vents rashes, and benefits the throat?

a. Niu Bang Zi
b. Niu Huang
c. Niu Xi
d. Tu Niu Xi
e. Qian Niu Zi

2353. Which herb drains Damp-Heat and Deficiency-Heat?

2354. Which herb releases Wind from the Exterior, expels Phlegm, and redirects the Qi downward?

2355. Which herb clears Deficiency-Heat and reduces childhood nutritional impairment?

a. Yan Hu Suo
b. Qian Hu
c. Chai Hu
d. Yin Chai Hu
e. Hu Huang Lian

2356. Which herb warms the Middle Energizer, moves the Qi, binds up the Intestines, and stops diarrhea?

2357. Which herb dries Damp and checks malarial disorders?

2358. Which herb aromatically transforms Damp, redirects rebellious Qi downward, and transforms stagnation?

a. Bai Dou Kou
b. Cao Dou Kou
c. Rou Dou Kou
d. Cao Gou
e. Sha Ren

2359. Which herb attacks toxins, wears away sores, and disperses clumps?

2360. Which herb extinguishes Wind, alleviates pain, and stops itching?

2361. Which herb extinguishes Wind stroke, calms wheezing, and promotes urination?

a. Quan Xie
b. Di Long
c. Wu Gong
d. Jiang Can
e. Ban Mao

2362. Which herb directs rebellious Qi downward, anchors the Floating Yang, and stops bleeding?

2363. Which herb clears Heat-Phlegm, promotes urination, and dissipates Phlegm?

2364. Which herb anchors and calms the Spirit, aids the Kidneys to grasp the Qi, and improves hearing and vision?

a. Hua Shi
b. Ci Shi
c. Dai Zhe Shi
d. Fu Hai Shi
e. Yang Qi Shi

2365. Which herb sedates the Heart, calms the Spirit, expels Phlegm, and prevents putrefaction?

2366. Which herb calms the Spirit, invigorates the Blood, and promotes urination?

2367. Which herb calms the spirt, induces astringency, and promotes regeneration of tissue and healing of wounds?

a. Ci Shi
b. Yuan Zhi
c. Zhu Sha
d. Hu Po
e. Long Gu

2368. Which herb clears the Heart, calms the Spirit, moistens the Lungs, and stops coughing?

2369. Which herb moistens the Lungs, augments the Stomach, and clears the Heart?

2370. Which herb moistens the Lungs, nourishes the Kidneys, and generates fluids?

a. Yu Zhu
b. Tian Men Dong
c. Mai Men Dong
d. Sha Shen
e. Bai He

2371. Which herb tonifies the Kidneys, stabilizes the Essence, and calms the Spirit?

2372. Which herb augments the Spleen, tonifies Lung Qi, and tonifies the Kidneys?

2373. Which herb clears Heat, expels pus, and strengthens the Spleen?

a. Bai Zhu
b. Shan Yao
c. Lian Zi
d. Yi Yi Ren
e. Bai Bian Dou

2374. Which herb binds up the Intestines, stops bleeding, stops vaginal discharge, and kills parasites?

2375. Which herb binds up the Intestines, and contains the leakage of Lung Qi?

2376. Which herb retains the Essence and inhibits excessive salivation?

a. He Zi
b. Qian Shi
c. Jin Ying
d. Yi Zhi Ren
e. Chun Pi

2377. Which herb releases the Exterior and calms a restless fetus?

2378. Which herb releases the Exterior and promotes urination?

2379. Which herb releases the Exterior, transforms turbidity, and stops vomiting?

a. Pei Lan
b. Huo Xiang
c. Xiang Ru
d. Zi Su
e. Jing Jie

2380. Lou Lu performs which of the functions at right?

2381. Mu Tong performs which of the functions at right?

2382. Chuan Shan Jia performs which of the functions at right?

a. Promote urination, drain Heat, and promote lactation
b. Reduce swelling, expel pus, unblock menstruation, and promote lactation
c. Warm the Middle Energizer, expel Cold, and promote lactation
d. Invigorate the meridians, reduce swelling, and promote lactation
e. Clear Heat, relieve toxicity, and promote lactation

2383. Hu Lu Ba performs which of the functions at right?

2384. Chi Xiao Dou performs which of the functions at right?

2385. Yin Yang Huo performs which of the functions at right?

a. Expel Wind-Damp-Cold
b. Disperse Damp-Cold
c. Expel Damp-Heat
d. Expel Wind-Heat
e. Expel Wind-Cold

2386. Tai Zi Shen performs which of the functions at right?

2387. Sha Shen performs which of the functions at right?

2388. Huang Jing performs which of the functions at right?

a. Augment the Yin, moisten the Lungs, tonify the Spleen, and augment Qi
b. Strengthen the Spleen, augment the Qi, and generate fluids
c. Augment the Stomach Yin, moisten the Lungs, and clear the Heart
d. Augment the Yin, clear Heat, moisten the Lungs, and nourish the Kidneys
e. None of the above

2389. Which herb clears Summer Heat and raises Spleen Yang?

2390. Which herb disperses Blood Stasis, stops bleeding, and calms the fetus?

2391. Which herb stabilizes the Kidneys, binds up the Essence, clears the Heart, and stops bleeding?

a. Lian Xin
b. Lian Zi
c. Lian Fang
d. Lian Xu
e. He Ye

2392. Tao Ren performs which of the functions at right?

2393. Bing Lang performs which of the functions at right?

2394. Yuan Hua performs which of the functions at right?

a. Relax the bowels with demulcents
b. Relax the bowels with drugs of a lubricating nature
c. Relax the bowels with drugs of a warm nature
d. Purgation
e. Induce diarrhea with potent purgatives

2395. Bai Ji Li performs which of the functions at right?
2396. Tian Ma performs which of the functions at right?
2397. Ju Hua performs which of the functions at right?

a. Calm the Liver and facilitate the smooth flow of Liver Qi
b. Calm the Liver, dispel Wind, and unblock the meridians
c. Calm the liver, clear Heat, and relieve toxicity
d. Calm the Liver, clear the Liver, and clear the eyes
e. Calm the Liver and stop bleeding

2398. Herbs of which nature astringe and bind?
2399. Herbs of which nature disperse and move Qi?
2400. Herbs of which nature drain and dry Damp?

a. Acrid
b. Sweet
c. Bitter
d. Salty
e. Sour

2401. Yuan Zhi performs which of the functions at right?
2402. Bai Zi Ren performs which of the functions at right?
2403. Hu Po performs which of the functions at right?

a. Calm the Spirit, promote urination, and reduce swelling
b. Calm the Spirit, moisten the Intestines, and unblock stool
c. Calm the Spirit, expel Phlegm, and stop coughing
d. Calm the Spirit, promote healing, and generate flesh
e. Calm the Spirit and calm the Liver

2404. Shi Jue Ming performs which of the functions at right?
2405. Di Long performs which of the functions at right?
2406. Wu Gong performs which of the functions at right?

a. Extinguish Wind, stop spasms, attack toxins, and dissipate nodules
b. Extinguish Wind, stop spasms, unblock the meridians, and stop wheezing
c. Extinguish Wind, stop spasms, transform Phlegm, and stop itching
d. Extinguish Wind, stop spasms, clear the Liver, and improve vision
e. Extinguish Wind, stop spasms, drain Liver Heat, and release the Exterior

---

2407. Which symptom is an indication for Rou Dou Kou?
2408. Which symptom is an indication for Bai Zhu?
2409. Which symptom is an indication for Wei Ling Xian?

a. Night blindness or diminished vision
b. Swollen, painful, red eyes
c. Fish bone lodged in the throat
d. Inhibited lactation
e. Chronic intractable diarrhea

2410. Shi Gao and Zhi Mu are each used to treat which type of coughing?

2411. Lai Fu Zi and She Gan are each used to treat which type of coughing?

2412. Dong Chong Xia Cao and Hu Tao Ren are each used to treat which type of coughing?

a. Coughing and wheezing due to Lung Heat
b. Coughing and wheezing due to Cold-Phlegm
c. Coughing and wheezing due to copious sputum
d. Chronic coughing due to Deficient Lungs
e. Coughing due to Dry-Phlegm

2413. Bai Zhi and Xi Xin each are used to treat which of the ailments at right?

2414. Jie Geng and Xuan Shen each are used to treat which of the ailments at right?

a. Red, painful, swollen eyes
b. Red, painful, swollen throat
c. Sinus congestion
d. Swollen sores, ulcer, and carbuncles
e. Superficial visual obstruction and cataracts

2415. Fu Zi and Gan Jiang each are used to treat which of the patterns at right?

2416. Fu Zi and Lu Rong each are used to treat which of the patterns at right?

a. Extreme collapse of primordial energy, profuse respiration, and a minute or weak pulse
b. Devastated Yang disorders where the Yang Qi is extremely weak and there is abundant cold in the extremities
c. Delirium or coma, Wind stroke, convulsions, seizures
d. Deficient Kidney Yang, Interior Cold, cold extremities
e. Deficient Qi, fatigue, spontaneous sweating

2417. Which two herbs each are used to treat palpitations accompanied by a slow or weak pulse that sometimes comes at irregular intervals?

2418. Which two herbs each are used to treat focal distention with pain and fullness in the chest and epigastrium?

a. Zhi Gan Cao and Gui Zhi
b. Jie Geng and Xie Bai
c. Shan Yao and Wu Yao
d. Gua Lou and Zhi Shi
e. Shan Zha and Wu Zhu Yu

2419. Which two herbs each are used to treat wheezing due to rebellious Qi wheezing caused by Deficient Kidneys?

2420. Which two herbs each are used to treat chronic ulcerations or Yin-type boils that do not heal?

a. Chen Xiang and Bu Gu Zhi
b. Lu Rong and Rou Gui
c. Lu Rong and Huang Qi
d. Lu Rong and Gui Ban
e. Fu Zi and Rou Gui

2421. Which herb is known especially for treating recurring dysenteric disorders?

2422. Which herb would you select to treat malaria?

a. Huang Bai
b. Qing Pi
c. Bai Tou Weng
d. Ya Dan Zi
e. Ma Chi Xian

2423. Which treatment is indicated when there is Phlegm lurking above and below the diaphragm and excruciating pain in the thorax, neck and lower back?

2424. Which treatment is indicated for deep-rooted boils of the Yin type caused by Phlegm-Damp obstructing the meridians?

a. Bai Jie Zi with Gan Sui and Da Ji
b. Bai Jie Zi with Ma Huang and Xiong Ren
c. Bai Jie Zi with Su Zi and Lai Fu Zi
d. Bai Jie Zi with Rou Gui and Shu Di Huang
e. Bai Jie Zi applied topically in powder form

2425. Which herb would you select to treat wheezing due to Cold?

2426. Which herb would you select to treat wheezing due to Heat?

2427. Which herb would you select to treat wheezing due to Deficiency?

a. Ma Huang
b. Ge Jie
c. Ban Xia
d. Di Long
e. Tian Nan Xing

2428. Which herb treats Deficient Yang with constipation?

2429. Which herb treats Deficient Blood with constipation?

a. Da Fu Pi
b. Da Huang
c. Suo Yang
d. Dang Gui
e. Shang Lu

2430. Which treatment is indicated when there is vomiting and regurgitation of sour fluids from wheat-induced disharmony between the Liver and Stomach?

2431. Which treatment is indicated when there is vomiting due to Stomach Heat?

2432. Which treatment is indicated when there is vomiting due to Stomach Cold?

a. Ban Xia with Gan Jiang
b. Pi Pa Ye with Huang Lian
c. Wu Zhu Yu with Huang Lian
d. Xuan Fu Huan with Dai Zhe Shi
e. Zi Su Gang with Sha Ren

2433. Which herb treats flaming up of dominant Liver Fire with painful swollen red eyes?

2434. Which herb treats painful spasms in the abdomen caused by incoordination between the Liver and Spleen?

2435. Which herb treats irritability, restlessness, dizziness, and/or vertigo caused by Deficient Liver Yin with Deficient Yang transgressing upward?

a. Dai Zhe Shi
b. Long Gu
c. Ci Shi
d. Bai SHao
e. Jue Ming Zi

2436. Which herb would you select to treat distention and fullness in the chest and abdomen caused by Damp distresses?

2437. Which herb would you select to treat irregular menstruation caused by an inability to facilitate the flow of Liver Qi?

2438. Which herb would you select to treat rectal or uterine prolapse?

a. Zhi Shi
b. Fo Shou
c. Tan Xiang
d. Xiang Fu
e. Hou Po

2439. Which herb would you select to treat irritability and insomnia caused by Deficient Heart Yin and Deficient Liver Blood?

2440. Which herb would you select to treat irritability and insomnia caused by Excess-Heat disturbing the Heart?

a. Yuan Zhi
b. He Huan Pi
c. Zhu SHa
d. Suan Zao Ren
e. Fu Ling

2441. Which herb is incompatibile with San Leng?

2442. Which herb is incompatible with Yu Jin?

2443. Which herb is incompatible with Quan Niu Zi?

a. Liu Huang
b. Ba Dou
c. Ding Xiang
d. Mang Xiao
e. Rou Gui

2444. Which pattern at right indicates Yi Guan Jian?

2445. Which pattern at right indicates Yue Ju Wan?

2446. Which pattern at right indicates Si Ni San?

2447. Which pattern at right indicates Xiao Yao San?

2448. Which pattern at right indicates Chai Hu Shu Gan San?

a. The six constraints
b. Incoordination between the Liver and Spleen, Qi constraint in the Interior, pain and fullness in the chest and epigastrium, cold fingers and toes
c. Liver constraint with Deficient Blood, Deficient Spleen and Stomach energy disorder, hypochondriac pain, fatigue, reduced appetite, pale red tongue, wiry-rapid pulse
d. Constraint and clumping of Liver Qi, hypochondriac pain, fullness in the chest and hypochondria, alternating fever and chills
e. Pain in the chest and hypochondria, Deficient Yin of the Liver and Kidneys causing a parched dry throat, a concurrent case of Qi stagnation

---

2449. What function does Feng Feng perform in the Chuan Xiong Cha Tiao San?

2450. What function does Feng Feng perform in Xie Huang San?

2451. What function does Feng Feng perform in Tong Xie Yao Fang?

a. Relieve overcontrol of the Spleen by the Liver
b. Expel Wind, eliminate Damp, and alleviate pain
c. Disperse smoldering Fire in the Spleen and Stomach
d. Disperse Wind, release the Exterior, and alleviate pain
e. Disperse Wind, dissipate nodules, and reduce swelling

2452. Which pattern at right indicates Huang Qin Tang?

2453. Which pattern at right indicates Shao Yao Tang?

2454. Which pattern at right indicates Ge Gen Huang Qin Huang Lian Tang?

a. Dysentery caused by Damp-Heat evil, diarrhea with pus and blood, tenesmus, difficulty with defecation, burning sensation around the anus, darky scanty urine, greasy yellow tongue fur
b. Abdominal pain, dysenteric diarrhea, fever, bitter taste in the mouth, red tongue with yellow fur, rapid pulse
c. Heat dysentery due to postpartum, which has led to Deficient Blood
d. Fever, dysenteric diarrhea with foul-smelling stool, burning sensation around the anus, irritability and heat in the chest and epigastrium, thirst, wheezing, sweating, yellow tongue fur, rapid pulse
e. None of the above

2455. Which pattern indicates Xiao Chai Hu Tang?

2456. Which pattern indicates Da Chai Hu Tang?

2457. Which pattern indicates Hao Qin Qing Dan Tang?

a. Alternating fever and chills, fullness in the chest and hypochondria, bitter taste in the mouth, continuous vomiting, no bowel movement, yellow tongue fur, wiry-forceful pulse
b. Alternating fever and chills, generalized body aches, heavy sensation in the limbs, no appetite, soggy pulse
c. Alternating fever and chills, full sensation in the chest and hypochondria, heartburn, nausea and vomiting, reduced appetite, thin white tongue fur, wiry pulse
d. Alternating fever and chills, fullness and pain in the chest and hypochondria, headache in the lateral aspect of the forehead, vertigo, white tongue fur, wiry-slippery pulse
e. None of the above

2458. What function does Huang Qi perform in Yu Ping Feng San?

2459. What function does Huang Qi perform in Dang Gui Bu Xue Tang?

2460. What function does Huang Qi perform in Bu Zhong Yi Qi Tang?

2461. What function does Huang Qi perform in Bu Yang Huan Wu Tang?

a. Big dosage: strongly tonifies the Primordial Qi, impels the circulation of Blood, and eliminates Blood Stasis without injuring Vital Qi
b. Large dosage: strongly tonifies the Qi of the Spleen and Lungs, thereby reinforcing the source of Blood
c. Tonifies the Qi of the Middle Energizer, raises the sunken Yang, and stops perspiration
d. Tonifies the Qi, stabilizes the Exterior, and eliminates evils without injuring health
e. None of the above

2462. Which pattern indicates Jiao Ai Tang?

2463. Which pattern indicates Huang Tu Tang?

2464. Which pattern indicates Wen Jing Tang?

a. Injury and Deficiency of the Chong and Ren meridians, metrorrhagia caused by Deficient Blood but partial Cold
b. Deficiency and Cold of the Chong and Ren meridians, metrorrhagia caused by Blood Stasis
c. Deficient Spleen Yang, metrorrhagia caused by failure of the Spleen Qi to govern the Blood
d. Deficient Spleen Qi, metrorrhagia caused by instability of the Chong meridian
e. None of the above

2465. Which formula at right treats this pattern: headache, fever, hacking cough, dry throat and nose, irritability, thirst, dry tongue, big-deficient-rapid pulse?

2466. Which formula at right treats this pattern: slight headache, chills without sweating, cough with watery sputum, stuffy nose, dry throat, dry white tongue fur, wiry pulse?

2467. Which formula at right treats this pattern: slight fever, cough, slight thirst, thin white tongue fur, floating-rapid pulse?

a. Sang Ju Yin
b. Cang Chi Tang
c. Sang Xing Tang
d. Xing Su San
e. Qing Zao Jiu Fei Tang

2468. What is the main formula for treating coughs caused by Deficient Yin of the Lungs and Kidneys?

2469. What is the main formula for treating coughing and wheezing due to Deficient Yin that has caused consumptive Lung disease?

2470. What is the main formula for treating hacking coughs caused by Dry-Heat attacking the Lungs?

a. Bai He Gu Jin Tang
b. Qing Zao Jiu Fei Tang
c. Sha Shen Mai Men Dong
d. Mai Men Dong Tang
e. Yang Yin Qing Fei Tang

2471. How does Bu Dai Wan treat cases of roundworms?

2472. How does Fei Er Wan treat cases of roundworms?

2473. How does Wu Mei Wan treat cases of roundworms?

a. Tonify the Spleen and Stomach, eliminate evils, and restore healthy energy
b. Tonify Spleen Qi, reduce accumulation, and clear Heat
c. Reduce food stagnation, dry Damp, and clear the Liver
d. Warm Cold in the lower body and clear Heat in the upper body
e. None of the above

2474. Which patterns indicates Huang Lian Jie Du Tang?

2475. Which pattern indicates Xian Fang Huo Ming Yin?

2476. Which pattern indicates Wu Wei Xiao Du Yin?

2477. Which pattern indicates Si Miao Yang An Tang?

a. Boils and carbuncles with localized erythema and swelling, which are hot and painful with deep-rooted hard lesions that resemble nail heads or chestnuts, red tongue, rapid pulse
b. Localized, dark-red erythema that is very painful and accompanied by slight swelling and heat, fever, thirst, red tongue, rapid pulse
c. Carbuncles with skin lesions that are swollen, red, hot, and painful, fever, slight aversion to cold, thin white or slightly yellow tongue fur, rapid-forceful pulse
d. Carbuncles and other toxic swellings, high fever, irritability, dry mouth and throat, red tongue, yellow tongue fur, rapid-forceful pulse
e. None of the above

2478. Tian Hua Fen performs which of the functions at right in Fu Yuan Huo Xue Tang?

2479. Hua Fen performs which of the functions at right in Yu Ye Tang?

2480. Tian Hua Fen performs which of the functions at right in Xian Fang Huo Ming Yin?

a. Treat thirst by enriching the Yin and moistening Dry
b. Clear heat and resolve lumps
c. Disperse the Blood Stasis caused by traumatic physical injury
d. Promote urination and disperse accumulation
e. None of the above

2481. What is the method of administration for tonic medicine?

2482. What is the method of administration for medicine in cases of acute disease?

2483. What is the method of administration for medicine that irritates the Stomach and Intestines?

a. Should be taken before meals
b. Should be taken after meals
c. Should be taken on an empty stomach
d. Should be taken at regular intervals
e. Should be administered immediately

2484. Liang Ge San and Tao He Cheng Qi Tang each contain which of the following ingredients?

2485. Ma Zi Ren Wan and Huang Long Tang each contain which of the following ingredients?

a. Da Huang, Hou Po, and Zhi Shi
b. Da Huang, Mang Xiao, and Gan Cao
c. Da Huang, Mang Xiao, Hou Po, and Fu Zi
d. Da Huang and Ren Shen
e. Da Huang and Gan Jiang

2486. Which pattern indicates Zhu Ye Shi Gao Tang?

2487. Which pattern indicates Qing Shu Yi Qi Tang?

a. Fever, profuse sweating, irritability, thirst, desire to curl up in a fetal position, shortness of breath, apathy, deficient-rapid pulse
b. Fever, profuse sweating, irritability, thirst, insomnia, red tongue with little fur, deficient-rapid pulse
c. High fever, profuse sweating, thirst, irritability, slippery-rapid pulse
d. Fever, disturbed hidrosis, thirst, cough, tongue is red at the tip, floating-rapid pulse
e. Fever, profuse sweating, general sensation of heaviness, greasy red tongue

---

2488. Which formula at right treats this pattern: epigastric pain, a stifling sensation in the chest, and hypochondriac pain caused by stagnant Liver Qi and Cold congealing in the Stomach?

2489. Which formula at right treats this pattern: epigastric pain, vomiting, and acid regurgitation caused by Cold due to Deficient Stomach?

a. Li Zhong Wan
b. Wu Zhu Yu Tang
c. Liang Fu Wan
d. Hou Po Wen Zhang Tang
e. Ding Xian Shi Di Tang

2490. Xu Duan performs which of the functions at right?

2491. Sang Ji Sheng performs which of the functions at right?

a. Tonify the Liver and Kidneys, strengthen the sinews and bones, and treat hypertension
b. Tonify the Liver and Kidneys, strengthen the sinews and bones, expel Damp
c. Tonify the Liver and Kidneys, strengthen the sinews and bones, and promote movement of Blood
d. Tonify the Liver and Kidneys, strengthen the sinews and bones, aid the smooth flow of Qi and Blood
e. Tonify the Liver and Kidneys, benefit the Essence, moisten the Lungs, and enrich the Yin

---

2492. Shan Yao performs which of the functions at right?

2493. Bai Zhu performs which of the functions at right?

2494. Gan Cao performs which of the functions at right?

a. Tonify the Spleen, augment the Qi, expel Phlegm, stop coughing, moderate spasms, and alleviate pain
b. Tonify the Spleen, augment the Qi, nourish the Blood, calm the Spirit, moderate and harmonize the harsh properties of other herbs
c. Tonify the Spleen, augment the Qi, eliminate Damp, induce diuresis, stop sweating, prevent abortion
d. Tonify and augment the Spleen and Stomach, nourish the Lungs and strengthen the Kidneys to arrest spermatorrhea
e. Tonify the Spleen, augment the Qi, and generate fluids

2495. Sang Zhi performs which of the functions at right?

2496. Luo Shi Teng performs which of the functions at right?

2497. Hai Feng Teng performs which of the functions at right?

a. Dispel Wind-Damp, unblock the meridians, cool the Blood, and reduce swelling
b. Dispel Wind-Damp, unblock the meridians, dispers Cold, and alleviate pain
c. Dispel Wind-Damp, unblock the meridians, and relax the sinews
d. Dispel Wind-Damp, unblock the meridians, and expel pathogenic Wind from the sinews or skin
e. Dispel Wind-Damp, unblock the meridians, benefit the joints, and induce enuresis to alleviate edema

---

2498. Bai Jiang Can performs which of the functions at right?

2499. Chuan Xiong performs which of the functions at right?

2500. Bai Zhi performs which of the functions at right?

a. Release Wind, alleviate pain, reduce swelling, and expel pus
b. Release Wind, alleviate pain, warm the Lungs, and transform Phlegm
c. Release Wind, alleviate pain, and promote Blood circulation and the flow of Qi
d. Release Wind, alleviate pain, remove Damp, and disperse Cold
e. Release Wind, alleviate pain, transform Phlegm, and dissipate nodules

C. In the next section (questions 2501–3500), the questions come in sets of to two to five. To the right of each set of questions, you will find four possible answers. Use these to answer all of the questions in that set. *Each question has only one correct answer.*

2501. Which answers at right describe two herbs of similar nature increasing each other's effect?

2502. Which answers at right describe the relationship between Huang Bai and Zhi Mu?

2503. Which answers at right describe one herb inhibiting the toxic effect of another herb?

a. One herb enhances another herb's effect (*xiang shi*)
b. Mutual promotion (*xiang xu*)
c. Both of the above
d. None of the above

2504. Which answers at right describe what happens when one herb is used to counteract the negative effect of another herb?

2505. Which answers at right describe the relationship between Ren Shen and Wu Ling Zhi?

2506. Which answers at right describe the relationship between Gan Cao and Ba Dou?

a. One herb decreases another herb's toxicity (*xiang sha*)
b. Mutual antagonism (*shi jiu wei*)
c. Both of the above
d. None of the above

2507. Which answers at right describe what happens when two herbs inhibit or check each other, weakening or even canceling their original efficacy?

2508. Which answers at right describe what happens when two herbs combine to create toxic side effects?

2509. Which answers at right describe the relationship between Ren Shen and Sha Shen?

a. Incompatibility (mutual addition: *xiang fan*)
b. Mutual inhibition (*xiang wu*)
c. Both of the above
d. None of the above

2510. Which herbs are prohibited during pregnancy?

2511. Which herbs should be used with exceeding caution during pregnancy?

a. Herbs that are poisonous or drastic
b. Herbs that remove Blood Stasis to restore menstruation, herbs that relieve stagnation of Qi, herbs that have hot properties and pungent flavor, or herbs that have a lowering and sinking effect
c. Both of the above
d. None of the above

2512. Which statements at right are true of how flavors are assigned to herbs in materia medicas?

a. They refer to the actual tastes of the herbs
b. They are organized according to the effect of each herb rather than its actual taste
c. Both of the above
d. None of the above

2513. What is the reason for baking Yan Hu Suo in vinegar?

2514. What is the reason for carbonizing Da Huang?

2515. What is the reason for refining Zhen Shu to a powder with water?

a. To increase its efficacy
b. To change its character and function so as to meet particular therapeutic needs
c. Both of the above
d. None of the above

2516. What food is to be avoided in cases where a patient has a suppurative infection on the surface of the body and cutaneous pruritis?

2517. What food is to be avoided in cases where a patient has indigestion caused by Deficient Spleen and Stomach?

2518. What food is to be avoided in cases where a patient is suffering from a Cold syndrome?

a. Fish, shrimp, crabs, and other irritating fish-related food
b. Fried, greasy, and sticky food
c. Both of the above
d. None of the above

2519. Refining an herbal powder in water is done in which type of processing?

2520. Simmering is done in which type of processing?

2521. Roasting in ashes is done in which type of processing?

a. Water processing
b. Fire processing
c. Both of the above
d. None of the above

2522. Meridian tropism is based on which theories at right?

a. Theory of the viscera
b. Theory of the meridians and their collaterals
c. Both of the above
d. None of the above

2523. Fan Xie Ye is suitable for use after being prepared in which of the ways at right?

2524. Xuan Fu Hua is suitable for use after being prepared in which of the ways at right?

2525. Fu Ling is suitable for use after being prepared in which of the ways at right?

2526. Che Qian Ze is suitable for use after being prepared in which of the ways at right?

a. Decocted in a packet (*bao jian*)
b. Soaked in hot water
c. Both of the above
d. None of the above

2527. In what form is Zhi Bao Dan prescribed?

2528. In what form is Zi Xue Dan prescribed?

2529. In what form is Hui Chun Dan prescribed?

2530. In what form is An Gong Niu Huang Wan prescribed?

a. Pill
b. Powder
c. Both of the above
d. None of the above

2531. What role does the "assistant" perform in a formula?

2532. What role does the "chief" perform in a formula?

2533. What role does the "guide" perform in a formula?

a. Help to strengthen the effect of the principal herb
b. Produce the leading effect in the treatment of symptoms
c. Both of the above
d. None of the above

2534. What role does the "assistant" perform in a formula?

2535. What role does the "guide" perform in a formula?

a. Reduce or negate the toxicity of the principal and assistant herbs to prevent toxic side effects
b. Coordinate the effects of a formula's ingredients
c. Both of the above
d. None of the above

2536. What type of modification is made to Si Ni Tang to produce Tong Mai Si Ni Tang?

2537. What type of modification is made to Zeng Ye Tang to produce Zeng Ye Cheng Qi Tang?

a. Modification of dosages
b. Modification of ingredients
c. Both of the above
d. None of the above

2538. Ma Huang is used to treat which syndromes at right?

2539. Gui Zhi is used to treat which syndromes at right?

a. Exterior-Excess syndrome caused by exopathogenic Wind-Cold
b. Exterior-Deficiency syndrome caused by exopathogenic Wind-Cold
c. Both of the above
d. None of the above

2540. Which herbs at right can be used to clear Heat?

2541. Which herbs at right can be used to nourish fluids?

a. Chai Hu
b. Ge Gen
c. Both of the above
d. None of the above

2542. Jing Jie treats which ailments at right?

2543. Zi Su Ye treats which ailments at right?

a. Exterior patterns of Wind-Cold
b. Blood in the stool or uterine bleeding
c. Both of the above
d. None of the above

2544. Bo He is indicated for what kind of skin trouble?

2545. Niu Bang Zi is indicated for what kind of skin trouble?

a. Early stages of measles when there is incomplete expression of the rash
b. Red swellings, carbuncles, erythema, mumps
c. Both of the above
d. None of the above

2546. Sang Ye is indicated for which patterns at right?

2547. Ju Hua is indicated for which patterns at right?

2548. Dan Dou Chi is indicated for which patterns at right?

  a. Dry Lungs, coughing, and a dry mouth
  b. Dry, red, painful eyes caused by Wind-Heat in the Liver meridian
  c. Both of the above
  d. None of the above

2549. Which herbs at right treat Deficiency patterns of Exterior-Wind-Cold where there is sweating?

2550. Which herbs at right treat Excess patterns of Exterior-Wind-Cold where there is no sweating?

  a. Ma Huang
  b. Gui Zhi
  c. Both of the above
  d. None of the above

2551. Chai Hu performs which functions at right?

2552. Sheng Ma performs which functions at right?

2553. Ge Gen performs which functions at right?

  a. Raise the Yang Qi
  b. Clear Heat
  c. Both of the above
  d. None of the above

2554. Which meridians at right does Ju Hua enter?

2555. Which meridians at right does Sang Ye enter?

2556. Which meridians at right does Ge Gen enter?

  a. Liver
  b. Lung
  c. Both of the above
  d. None of the above

2557. Sheng Ma performs which functions at right?

2558. Chai Hu performs which functions at right?

2559. Man Jing Zi performs which functions at right?

  a. Raise the Yang Qi
  b. Spread Liver Qi, relieve constraint
  c. Both of the above
  d. None of the above

2560. Fu Ping performs which functions at right?

2561. Ge Gen performs which functions at right?

2562. Mu Zei performs which functions at right?

  a. Release the Exterior, vent rashes
  b. Remove water, reduce swelling
  c. Both of the above
  d. None of the above

2563. Which patterns at right does Jing Jie treat?

2564. Which patterns at right does Bo He treat?

  a. Exterior patterns of Wind-Cold
  b. Exterior patterns of Wind-Heat
  c. Both of the above
  d. None of the above

2565. After taking Gui Zhi Tang, what should a patient do?

2566. After taking Ma Huang Tang, what should a patient do?

2567. After taking Xiao Qing Long Tang, what should a patient do?

  a. Drink a small quantity of hot water or hot porridge
  b. Lie in a warm bed to induce sweating
  c. Both of the above
  d. None of the above

2568. Gui Zhi Tang contains which herbs at right?
2569. Ma Huang Tang contains which herbs at right?
2570. Xiao Qing Long Tang contains which herbs at right?

a. Gui Zhi and Zhi Gan Cao
b. Ma Huang and Bai Shao
c. Both of the above
d. None of the above

2571. Xiao Qing Long Tang performs which functions at right?
2572. Cong Chi Tang performs which functions at right?
2573. Ling Gan Wu Wei Jiang Xin Tang performs which functions at right?

a. Release the Exterior and expel Cold
b. Warm the Lungs and transform congested fluids
c. Both of the above
d. None of the above

2574. Ren Shen Bai Du San is indicated for which patterns at right?
2575. Chai Ge Jie Ji Tang is indicated for which patterns at right?

a. Fever and chills (chills predominant), no sweating, headache, generalized body aches, thin white tongue fur, floating-tight pulse
b. Increasing fever and decreasing chills, headache, stiffness of the extremities, orbital and eye pain, dry nasal passages, irritability, insomnia, thin yellow tongue fur, floating pulse
c. Both of the above
d. None of the above

2576. Zai Zao San performs which functions at right?
2577. Ren Shen Bai Du San performs which functions at right?
2578. Jiu Wei Qiang Huo Tang performs which functions at right?

a. Release the Exterior, expel Wind and Damp, and augment Qi
b. Release the Exterior, tonify Yang, induce sweating, and augment Qi
c. Both of the above
d. None of the above

2579. Ma Huang performs which functions at right in Ma Huang Xi Xin Fu Zi Tang?
2580. Ma Huang performs which functions at right in Ding Chuan Tang?
2581. Ma Huang performs which functions at right in Ma Huang Tang?
2582. Ma Huang performs which functions at right in Yang He Tang?

a. Release the Exterior
b. Arrest wheezing
c. Both of the above
d. None of the above

2583. Yin Qiao San contains which herbs at right?
2584. Sang Ju Yin contains which herbs at right?
2585. Cong Bai Jie Geng Tang contains which herbs at right?

a. Lian Qiao and Jie Geng
b. Gan Cao and Bo He
c. Both of the above
d. None of the above

2586. Yin Qiao San performs which functions at right?
2587. Sang Ju Yin performs which functions at right?

a. Disperse Wind-Heat
b. Clear Heat and relieve toxicity
c. Both of the above
d. None of the above

2588. Xuan Shen performs which functions at right?
2589. Sheng Di Huang performs which functions at right?
2590. Lu Gen performs which functions at right?

a. Clear Heat and nourish Yin
b. Cool the Blood and stop bleeding
c. Both of the above
d. None of the above

2591. Huang Qin performs which functions at right?
2592. Di Gu Pi performs which functions at right?
2593. Mu Dan Pi performs which functions at right?

a. Clear Lung Heat
b. Clear Deficiency Fire
c. Both of the above
d. None of the above

2594. Hong Teng treats which type of abscesses?
2595. Yu Xing Cao treats which type of abscesses?
2596. She Gan treats which type of abscesses?

a. Lung abscesses
b. Intestinal abscesses
c. Both of the above
d. None of the above

2597. Hu Huang Lian treats which disorders at right?
2598. Huang Lian treats which disorders at right?
2599. Huang Bai treats which disorders at right?

a. Damp-Heat dysenteric disorders
b. Hectic or tidal fever caused by Deficient Yin
c. Both of the above
d. None of the above

2600. Xuan Shen treats which disorders at right?
2601. Niu Bang Zi treats which disorders at right?
2602. Pang Da Hai treats which disorders at right?

a. Throat pain caused by Deficient Yin
b. Throat pain caused by Heat toxicity
c. Both of the above
d. None of the above

2603. Huang Lian and Wu Zhu Yu combined treat which disorders at right?
2604. Huang Lian and Mu Xiang combined treat which disorders at right?

a. Dysenteric disorders caused by Damp-Heat
b. Epigastric and abdominal pain with acid regurgitation caused by Liver Fire or Stomach Heat
c. Both of the above
d. None of the above

2605. Ban Bian Lian treats which disorders at right?
2606. Ban Zhi Lian treats which disorders at right?
2607. Ma Chi Xian treats which disorders at right?

a. Snake bites
b. Edema
c. Both of the above
d. None of the above

2608. Dan Zhu Ye treats which disorders at right?

2609. Deng Xin Cao treats which disorders at right?

2610. Lian Xin treats which disorders at right?

a. Heat patterns involving irritability
b. Heat stranguria
c. Both of the above
d. None of the above

2611. Huang Lian is considered the best treatment to clear which disorders at right?

2612. Huang Bai is considered the best treatment to clear which disorders at right?

2613. Huang Qin is considered the best treatment to clear which disorders at right?

a. Prime Minster Fire
b. Monarch Fire
c. Both of the above
d. None of the above

2614. Tian Hua Fen performs which functions at right?

2615. Zhi Mu performs which functions at right?

2616. Zi Cao treats which functions at right?

a. Generate fluids and stop thirst
b. Relieve toxicity and expel pus
c. Both of the above
d. None of the above

2617. Which herbs at right check malarial disorders?

2618. Which herbs at right clear Deficiency fevers?

2619. Which herbs at right clear Summer Heat?

a. Yin Chai Hu
b. Qing Hao
c. Both of the above
d. None of the above

2620. Huang Qin treats which disorders at right?

2621. Huang Bai treats which disorders at right?

2622. Chuan Xin Lian treats which disorders at right?

a. Fever caused by Deficient Yin
b. Damp-Heat in the Stomach and Intestines
c. Both of the above
d. None of the above

2623. Lian Qiao treats which disorders at right?

2624. Jin Yin Hua treats which disorders at right?

2625. Bai Tou Weng treats which disorders at right?

a. Diarrhea and dysentery with purulent, bloody stool
b. Suppurative infections or scrofula and tubercular adenitis caused by accumulation of noxious Heat
c. Both of the above
d. None of the above

2626. Yin Chai Hu treats which disorders at right?

2627. Chai Hu treats which disorders at right?

a. Fire from Deficient Yin with steaming bone syndrome, or from any Deficient Yin fever
b. Shao-Yang syndrome
c. Both of the above
d. None of the above

2628. Which herbs at right treat blood in the urine and vomiting of blood?

2629. Which herbs at right treat amenorrhea, abdominal masses, and lumps or bruises?

2630. Which herbs at right treat irritability associated with childhood nutritional impairment?

a. Mu Dan Pi
b. Di Gu Pi
c. Both of the above
d. None of the above

2631. Which herbs at right treat caoughing caused by Lung Heat?

2632. Which herbs at right treat vomiting caused by Stomach Heat?

2633. Which herbs at right treat steaming bone disorder with night sweats caused by Kidney Fire?

a. Huang Qin
b. Huang Lian
c. Both of the above
d. None of the above

2634. Which herbs at right treat dysenteric disorders caused by Damp-Heat?

2635. Which herbs at right treat carbuncles and abscesses caused by excessive Heat with toxicity?

2636. Which herbs at right treat malarial disorders?

a. Huang Lian
b. Bai Tou Weng
c. Both of the above
d. None of the above

2637. Which herbs at right treat coughing and wheezing caused by Lung Heat?

2638. Which herbs at right treat Deficient Yin and Lung Dry?

2639. Which herbs at right treat erythema, nosebleeds, and vomiting of blood?

a. Zhi Mu
b. Shi Gao
c. Both of the above
d. None of the above

2640. Which herbs at right treat cases where Heat has entered the nutritive or Blood level and there is vomiting of blood and nosebleeds?

2641. Which herbs at right treat cases where Heat has entered the Wei level and there is fever, chills, and headache?

2642. Which herbs at right treat cases where Heat has entered the Qi level and there is high fever without chills and irritability?

a. Xi Jiao
b. Shi Gao
c. Both of the above
d. None of the above

2643. Sheng Di Huang treats which patterns at right?

2644. Xuan Shen treats which patterns at right?

2645. Tu Niu Xi treats which patterns at right?

a. Warm febrile diseases where Heat enters the nutritive or Blood level and there is high fever, thirst, and a scarlet tongue
b. Deficient Yin with Heat signs, sore throat, and neck lumps due to Phlegm-Fire
c. Both of the above
d. None of the above

2646. Huang Lian performs which functions at right?
2647. Zhi Mu performs which functions at right?
2648. Jin Yin Hua performs which functions at right?

a. Release exogenous Heat
b. Clear Interior Heat
c. Both of the above
d. None of the above

2649. Qin Jiao performs which functions at right?
2650. Huang Bai performs which functions at right?
2651. Huang Lian performs which functions at right?

a. Clear Heat and dry Damp
b. Clear Deficiency-Fire
c. Both of the above
d. None of the above

2652. Shi Gao performs which functions at right?
2653. Di Gu Pi performs which functions at right?
2654. Ling Yang Jiao performs which functions at right?

a. Clear Deficiency-Fire
b. Clear Lung Heat
c. Both of the above
d. None of the above

2655. At what level does Mu Dan Pi act?
2656. At what level does Zi Cao act?
2657. At what level does Lu Gen act?

a. Qifen
b. Xuefen
c. Both of the above
d. None of the above

2658. Chai Hu is especially effective at performing which functions at right?
2659. Yin Chai Hu is especially effective at performing which functions at right?
2660. Qing Hao is especially effective at treating which functions at right?

a. Clear Deficiency-Heat
b. Treat alternating chills and fever
c. Both of the above
d. None of the above

2661. Zhi Mu performs which functions at right?
2662. Shi Gao performs which functions at right?
2663. Mu Dan Pi performs which functions at right?

a. Clear Lung Heat
b. Moisten Lung Dry
c. Both of the above
d. None of the above

2664. Huang Qin performs which functions at right?
2665. Di Gu Pi performs which functions at right?
2666. Ting Li Zi performs which functions at right?

a. Clear Lung Heat
b. Clear Lung Excess
c. Both of the above
d. None of the above

2667. Huang Lian enters which levels at right?
2668. Xi Jiao enters which levels at right?
2669. Sang Ye enters which levels at right?

a. Qifen
b. Xuefen
c. Both of the above
d. None of the above

2670. Jin Yin Hua treats which patterns at right?

2671. Huang Lian treats which patterns at right?

2672. Shi Gao treats which patterns at right?

a. Qifen high fever that may have slightly injured the body fluids
b. Qifen high fever that has severely injured the body fluids, mouth and tongue are dry
c. Both of the above
d. None of the above

2673. Lu Gen performs which functions at right?

2674. Bai Mao Gen performs which functions at right?

2675. Ban Lan Gen performs which functions at right?

a. Clear Heat and generate body fluids
b. Cool the Blood and stop bleeding
c. Both of the above
d. None of the above

2676. Qing Hao performs which functions at right?

2677. Hua Shi performs which functions at right?

2678. Xi Gua performs which functions at right?

a. Release Summer Heat and promote urination
b. Release Summer Heat and Deficiency-Heat
c. Both of the above
d. None of the above

2679. Shan Dou Gen performs which functions at right?

2680. She Gan performs which functions at right?

2681. Tu Niu Xi performs which functions at right?

a. Relieve Fire toxicity and improve the throat
b. Relieve Fire toxicity and transform Phlegm
c. Both of the above
d. None of the above

2682. Lian Qiao performs which functions at right?

2683. Lian Xin performs which functions at right?

2684. Mu Tong performs which functions at right?

a. Drain Heart Fire
b. Promote urination
c. Both of the above
d. None of the above

2685. Huang Lian combined with Bai Tou Weng treats which disorders at right?

2686. Huang Lian combined with Che Qian Zi treats which disorders at right?

2687. Huang Lian combined with Xi Xin treats which disorders at right?

a. Dysenteric disorders caused by epidemic toxins
b. Diarrhea caused by Damp-Heat
c. Both of the above
d. None of the above

2688. Bai He Gu Jin Tang and Yang Yin Qing Fei Tang each contain which of the herbs at right?

2689. Qing Ying Tang and Yang Yin Qing Fei Tang each contain which of the herbs at right?

2690. Qing Ying Tang and Tian Wang Bu Xin Dang each contain which of the herbs at right?

a. Sheng Di Huang, Xuan Shen, and Mai Men Dong
b. Bai Shao, Bai Mu, and Gan Cao
c. Both of the above
d. None of the above

2691. Dao Chi San treats which patterns at right?

2692. Long Dan Xie Gan Tang treats which patterns at right?

2693. Zuo Jin Wan treats which patterns at right?

2694. Xiao Yao San treats which patterns at right?

a. Hypochondrial pain and a bitter taste in the mouth
b. Epigastric distention, vomiting, and acid regurgitation caused by Liver Heat attacking the Stomach
c. Both of the above
d. None of the above

2695. Huang Lian performs which functions at right in Zuo Jin Wan?

2696. Huang Lian performs which functions at right in Qing Wei San?

2697. Huang Lian performs which functions at right in Huang Lian Jie Du Tang?

2698. Huang Lian performs which functions at right in Xiang Liang Wan?

a. Clear Heat and Middle Energizer Fire
b. Clear Heat and Dry Damp
c. Both of the above
d. None of the above

2699. Xie Qing Wan is indicated for which pathogeneses at right?

2700. Long Dan Xie Gan Tang is indicated for which pathogeneses at right?

2701. Dang Gui Long Hui Wan is indicated for which pathogeneses?

a. Flaming up of Liver and Gallbladder Excess-Fire
b. Damp-Heat evil attacking the Lower Energizer of the Liver and Gallbladder
c. Both of the above
d. None of the above

2702. Di Gu Pi performs which functions at right in Xie Bai San?

2703. Di Gu Pi performs which functions at right in Qing Gu San?

2704. Di Gu Pi performs which functions at right in Qin Jiao Bie Jia San?

a. Drain Heat from the Lungs
b. Nourish the Yin
c. Both of the above
d. None of the above

2705. Sheng Di Huang is the chief (monarch or *jun*) component in which formulas at right?

2706. Dang Gui is the chief (monarch or *jun*) component in which formulas at right?

2707. Shu Di Huang is the chief (monarch or *jun*) component in which formulas at right?

a. Dang Gui Liu Huang Tang
b. Tian Wang Bu Xin Dan
c. Both of the above
d. None of the above

2708. Liang Ge San contains which herbs at right?

2709. Da Huang Mu Dan Tang contains which herbs at right?

2710. Huang Lian Jie Du Tang contains which herbs at right?

a. Da Huang and Mang Xiao
b. Huang Qin and Zhi Zi
c. Both of the above
d. None of the above

2711. Which formulas at right treat this pattern: fever, sweating, thirst, shortness of breath, scanty and dark urine, deficient-rapid pulse?

2712. Which formulas at right treat this pattern: vomiting, parched mouth, lips and throat, choking cough, stifling sensation in the chest?

2713. Which formulas at right treat this pattern: high fever, profuse sweating, severe thirst and irritability?

a. Qing Shu Yi Qi Tang
b. Zhu Ye Shi Gao Tang
c. Both of the above
d. None of the above

2714. Xiang Ru San is indicated for which syndromes at right?

2715. Huo Xiang Zheng Qi San is indicated for which syndromes at right?

2716. Qing Luo Yin is indicated for which syndromes at right?

a. Vomiting and diarrhea caused by Exterior-Cold with Interior-Damp
b. Mild Summer Heat injuring the Qi level of the Lungs meridian
c. Both of the above
d. None of the above

2717. Bai Hu Tang treats which syndromes at right?

2718. Qing Shu Yi Qi Tang treats which syndromes at right?

2719. Liu Yi San treats which syndromes at right?

a. Exogenous Cold evil that enters the Interior and is transformed into Heat syndrome
b. Excess Heat caused by Heat evil entering the Qifen where it becomes hyperactive
c. Both of the above
d. None of the above

2720. Yu Nu Jian contains which herbs at right?

2721. Qing Shu Yi Qi Tang contains which herbs at right?

2722. Qing Hao Bie Jia Tang contains which herbs at right?

a. Xi Yang Shen and Huang Lian
b. Mai Men Dong and Zhi Mu
c. Both of the above
d. None of the above

2723. Gua Lou Ren treats which disorders at right?

2724. Xing Ren treats which disorders at right?

2725. Bai Jie Zi treats which disorders at right?

a. A stifling or distended sensation in the chest, with constriction pain or diaphragmatic pressure, caused by Phlegm accumulation in the chest
b. Constipation caused by Dry
c. Both of the above
d. None of the above

2726. Da Ji performs which functions at right?
2727. Gan Sui performs which functions at right?
2728. Yuan Hua performs which functions at right?

a. Drain water downward and drive out congested fluids
b. Reduce swelling and dissipate nodules
c. Both of the above
d. None of the above

2729. Yu Li Ren is indicated for which disorders at right?
2730. Huo Ma Ren is indicated for which disorders at right?
2731. Qian Niu Zi is indicated for which disorders at right?

a. Constipation and difficult urination
b. Roundworms or tapeworms
c. Both of the above
d. None of the above

2732. Huo Ma Ren performs which functions at right?
2733. Tian Men Dong performs which functions at right?
2734. Man Jing Zi performs which functions at right?

a. Moisten the Intestines and unblock the bowels
b. Nourish the Yin
c. Both of the above
d. None of the above

2735. Xiao Cheng Qi Tang treats which disorders at right?
2736. Da Cheng Qi Tang treats which disorders at right?
2737. Tiao Wei Qi Tang treats which disorders at right?

a. Yangming Yang organ syndrome
b. Retention of Heat evil causing watery diarrhea
c. Both of the above
d. None of the above

2738. Ma Zi Ren Wan contains which herbs at right?
2739. Ji Chuan Jian contains which herbs at right?
2740. Wen Pi Tang contains which herbs at right?

a. Da Huang, Hou Po, and Zhi Shi
b. Xing Ren and Shao Yao
c. Both of the above
d. None of the above

2741. Da Huang Fu Zi Tang treats which disorders at right?
2742. Ji Chuan Jian treats which disorders at right?
2743. Ma Zi Ren Wan treats which disorders at right?

a. Constipation with hard stool caused by depletion of fluids and slight Heat in the Interior
b. Constipation caused by Deficient Yang and Qi of the Kidneys
c. Both of the above
d. None of the above

2744. Run Chang Wan treats which disorders at right?
2745. San Wu Bei Ji Wan treats which disorders at right?
2746. Ji Chuan Jian treats which disorders at right?

a. Constipation caused by Deficient Spleen and Dry-Heat of the Stomach and Intestines
b. Abdominal pain and constipation caused by Cold accumulation in the Interior
c. Both of the above
d. None of the above

2747. Da Huang performs which functions at right in Tao He Cheng Qi Tang?

2748. Da Huang performs which functions at right in Da Cheng Qi Tang?

2749. Da Huang performs which functions at right in Da Xian Xiong Tang?

a. Attack and purge Blood Stasis
b. Cleanse pathogenic Heat
c. Both of the above
d. None of the above

2750. Tiao Wei Cheng Qi Tang contains which herbs at right?

2751. Da Cheng Qi Tang treats which disorders at right?

2752. Ma Zi Ren Wan contains which herbs at right?

2753. Xiao Cheng Qi Tang contains which herbs at right?

a. Da Huang and Mang Xiao
b. Zhi Shi and Hou Po
c. Both of the above
d. None of the above

2754. Jin Qian Cao performs which functions at right?

2755. Hai Jin Sha performs which functions at right?

2756. Yin Chen Hao performs which functions at right?

a. Relieve stranguria through diuresis
b. Clear Damp-Heat and expel jaundice
c. Both of the above
d. None of the above

2757. Tong Cao performs which functions at right?

2758. Mu Tong performs which functions at right?

2759. Wang Bu Liu Xing performs which functions at right?

a. Promote urination
b. Promote lactation
c. Both of the above
d. None of the above

2760. Dang Gua Ren treats which disorders at right?

2761. Yi Yi Ren treats which disorders at right?

2762. Fu Ling treats which disorders at right?

a. Diarrhea
b. Abscesses of the Lungs or Intestines
c. Both of the above
d. None of the above

2763. Jin Sha Teng treats which disorders at right?

2764. Chi Xiao Dou treats which disorders at right?

2765. Jin Qian Cao treats which disorders at right?

a. Urinary stones
b. Jaundice
c. Both of the above
d. None of the above

2766. Fu Ling treats which disorders at right?

2767. Hou Po treats which disorders at right?

2768. Yi Yi Ren treats which disorders at right?

a. Damp stagnated in the Middle Energizer
b. Edema, Deficient Spleen, and lassitude
c. Both of the above
d. None of the above

2769. Fu Ling treats which disorders at right?
2770. Che Qian Zi treats which disroders at right?
2771. Huang Qi treats which disorders at right?

a. Edema in Excess syndromes
b. Edema in Deficiency syndromes
c. Both of the above
d. None of the above

2772. Shi Wei treats which disorders at right?
2773. Jin Qian Cao treats which disorders at right?
2774. Dong Gua Pi treats which disorders at right?

a. Stranguria complicated by hematuria
b. Stranguria caused by urinary stones
c. Both of the above
d. None of the above

2775. Bei Xie treats which disorders at right?
2776. Hua Shi treats which disorders at right?
2777. Shan Yao treats which disorders at right?

a. Cloudy urine
b. Stranguria induced by overstrain
c. Both of the above
d. None of the above

2778. Qu Mai performs which functions at right?
2779. Di Fu Zi performs which functions at right?
2780. Bian Xu performs which functions at right?

a. Expel Damp and stop itching
b. Unblock the bowels
c. Both of the above
d. None of the above

2781. Which formulas at right treat diseases of the Taiyang meridian and Yang organs involving retention of congested fluids in the Lower Energizer and urinary difficulty?
2782. Which formulas at right treat urinary difficulty caused by clumping of Damp-Heat that injures the Yin?
2783. Which formulas at right treat urinary difficulty resulting from a weakened Wei Qi that allows an invasion of Wind and Damp, accompanied by symptoms of superficial edema, sweating, and an aversion to Wind?

a. Wu Ling San
b. Zhu Ling Tang
c. Both of the above
d. None of the above

2784. Gui Zhi performs which functions at right in Wu Ling San?
2785. Gui Zhi performs which functions at right in Ling Gui Zhu Gan Tang?
2786. Gui Zhi performs which functions at right in Xiao Qing Long Tang?
2787. Gui Zhi performs which functions at right in Wu Mei Wan?

a. Release the Exterior and disperse Cold
b. Warm the Yang and transform the Qi
c. Both of the above
d. None of the above

2788. Which formulas at right warm and transform Phlegm?
2789. Which formulas at right warm the Yang to eliminate Damp and transform and separate the turbid from the clear?
2790. Which formulas at right warm the Yang to promote diuresis?

a. Zhen Wu Tang
b. Bei Xie Fen Qing Yin
c. Both of the above
d. None of the above

2791. Which formulas at right treat adverse rising of fluids syndrome?

2792. Which formulas at right treat water retention syndrome?

2793. Which formulas at right treat fluid retention syndrome?

a. Ling Gui Zhu Gan Tang
b. Wu Ling San
c. Both of the above
d. None of the above

2794. Ba Zheng San treats which disorders at right?

2795. Bei Xie Fen Qing Yin treats which disorders at right?

2796. Xiao Ji Yin Zi treats which disorders at right?

a. Stranguria caused by static Heat accumulating in the Lower Energizer where it injures the Blood collaterala
b. Stranguria caused by clumping of Damp-Heat in the Lower Energizer
c. Both of the above
d. None of the above

2797. Bai Shao performs which functions at right in Shao Yao Tang?

2798. Bai Shao performs which functions at right in Zhan Wu Tang?

2799. Bai Shao performs which functions at right in Si Wu Tang?

a. Preserve Yin and alleviate pain
b. Alleviate abdominal pain and tenesmus caused by dysentery
c. Both of the above
d. None of the above

2800. Shi Pi Yin contains which herbs at right?

2801. Zhen Wu Tang contains which herbs at right?

2802. Hui Yang Jiu Ji Tang contains which herbs at right?

a. Fu Zi, Fu Ling, and Bai Zhu
b. Hou Po, Gan Jiang, and Gan Cao
c. Both of the above
d. None of the above

2803. Wu Ling San contains which herbs at right?

2804. Zhu Ling Tang contains which herbs at right?

2805. Wei Ling Tang contains which herbs at right?

a. Fu Ling and Zhu Ling
b. Ze Xie and Bai Zhu
c. Both of the above
d. None of the above

2806. Cang Zhu performs which functions at right?

2807. Bai Zhu performs which functions at right?

2808. Bai Dou Kou performs which functions at right?

a. Dry Damp and tonify the Spleen
b. Augment the Qi and promote urination
c. Both of the above
d. None of the above

2809. Bai Dou Kou performs which functions at right?

2810. Rou Dou Kou performs which functions at right?

2811. Cao Dou Kou performs which functions at right?

a. Treat Damp and warm the Middle Energizer
b. Bind up the Intestines and stop diarrhea
c. Both of the above
d. None of the above

2812. Sha Ren treats which disorders at right?
2813. Huo Xiang treats which disorders at right?
2814. Sang ji Sheng treats which disorders at right?

a. Morning sickness
b. Restless fetus
c. Both of the above
d. None of the above

2815. Sha Ren treats which disorders at right?
2816. Chen Pi trets which disorders at right?
2817. Cao Guo treats which disorders at right?

a. Damp obstructing the Middle Energizer
b. Phlegm-Damp coughs and wheezing
c. Both of the above
d. None of the above

2818. Cang Zhu treats which disorders at right?
2819. Bai Zhu treats which disorders at right?
2820. Hou Po treats which disorders at right?

a. Restless fetus
b. Poor appetite and abdominal distention
c. Both of the above
d. None of the above

2821. Pei Lan performs which functions at right?
2822. Huo Xiang performs which functions at right?
2823. Bai Dou Kou performs which functions at right?

a. Transform Damp and release Summer Heat
b. Stop vomiting
c. Both of the above
d. None of the above

2824. Ping Wei San is indicated for which pathogeneses at right?
2825. Lian Po Yin is indicated for which pathogeneses at right?
2826. San Miao Wan is indicated for which pathogeneses at right?

a. Damp-Cold stagnating in the Spleen and Stomach
b. Damp-Heat stagnating in the Spleen and Stomach
c. Both of the above
d. None of the above

2827. Ba Zheng San is indicated for which pathogeneses at right?
2828. Xuan Bi Teng is indicated for which pathogeneses at right?
2829. Gan Lu Xiao Du Dan is indicated for which pathogeneses at right?

a. Damp-Heat stagnating in the meridians
b. Damp-Heat stagnating in the Lower Energizer?
c. Both of the above
d. None of the above

2830. Ping Wei San contains which herbs at right?
2831. Huo Xiang Zheng Qi San contains which herbs at right?
2832. Bu Huan Jin Zheng Qi San contains which herbs at right?

a. Chen Pi and Hou Po
b. Huo Xiang and Ban Xia
c. Both of the above
d. None of the above

2833. Which statements at right apply to Ping Wei San?

2834. Which statements at right apply to Huo Xiang Zheng Qi San?

a. Add Sheng Jiang and Da Zao before preparing
b. Do not use to treat Fire caused by Deficient Yin
c. Both of the above
d. None of the above

2835. Hai Feng Teng performs which functions at right?

2836. Luo Shi Teng performs which functions at right?

2837. Hai Tong Pi performs which functions at right?

a. Dispel Wind-Damp and unblock the meridians
b. Promote urination and reduce edema
c. Both of the above
d. None of the above

2838. Qin Jiao performs which functions at right?

2839. Du Huo performs which functions at right?

2840. Qiang Huo performs which functions at right?

a. Disperse Wind-Cold-Damp painful obstruction, especially in the upper back and arms
b. Disperse Wind-Cold-Damp painful obstruction, especially in the lower back and legs
c. Both of the above
d. None of the above

2841. Fang Ji performs which functions at right?

2842. Bei Xie performs which functions at right?

2843. Wei Ling Xian performs which functions at right?

a. Expel Wind-Damp and alleviate pain
b. Expel Wind-Damp and promote urination
c. Both of the above
d. None of the above

2844. Wu Jia Pi treats which disorders at right?

2845. Song Jie treats which disorders at right?

2846. Xi Xian Cao treats which disorders at right?

a. Wind-Cold-Damp painful obstruction
b. Generation of weak or soft sinews and bone
c. Both of the above
d. None of the above

2847. Sang Zhi treats which disorders at right?

2848. Xi Xian Cao treats which disorders at right?

2849. Du Huo treats which disorders at right?

a. Wind-Heat-Damp painful obstruction
b. Irritability, insomnia, and forgetfulness
c. Both of the above
d. None of the above

2850. Hai Tong Pi treats which disorders at right?
2851. Qiang Huo treats which disorders at right?
2852. Sang Zhi treats which disorders at right?

a. Wind-Damp painful obstruction, especially in the lower back and knees
b. Wind-Heat-Damp painful obstruction, especially in the upper back and arms
c. Both of the above
d. None of the above

2853. Ren Dong Teng treats which disorders at right?
2854. Xi Xin treats which disorders at right?
2855. Wei Ling Xian treats which disorders at right?

a. Wind-Cold painful obstruction
b. Damp-Heat painful obstruction
c. Both of the above
d. None of the above

2856. Juan Bi Tang (from Bai Yi Xuan Feng) treats which disorders at right?
2857. Du Huo Ji Sheng Tang treats which disorders at right?
2858. Gui Zhi Shao Yao Zhi Mu Tang treats which disorders at right?

a. Wind-Cold-Damp evils obstructing the sinews and bones, injured Kidneys and Liver, Deficient Qi and Blood
b. Deficient energy of the Yingfen and Weifen, Wind-Cold-Damp evils causing pain
c. Both of the above
d. None of the above

2859. Qing Huo Sheng Shi Tang is indicated for which pathogeneses at right?
2860. Ji Ming San is indicated for which pathogeneses at right?
2861. San Bi Tang is indicated for which pathogeneses at right?

a. Damp-Cold settling in the legs and feet
b. Wind-Damp in the superficial aspects of the body and the muscles
c. Both of the above
d. None of the above

2862. Du Huo Ji Sheng Tang contains which herbs at right?
2863. Qing Huo Sheng Shi Tang contains which herbs at right?
2864. San Bi Tang contains which herbs at right?

a. Fang Feng and Du Huo
b. Ren Shen and Dang Gui
c. Both of the above
d. None of the above

2865. Fu Hai Shi performs which functions at right?
2866. Hai Ge Ke performs which functions at right?
2867. Tian Hua Fen performs which functions at right?

a. Soften hardness and dissipate nodules
b. Clear the Lungs and transform Phlegm
c. Both of the above
d. None of the above

2868. Tian Hua Fen performs which functions at right?
2869. Bai Zhi performs which functions at right?
2870. Jie Geng performs which functions at right?

a. Clear Heat and generate fluids
b. Transform Phlegm and expel pus
c. Both of the above
d. None of the above

2871. Ting Li Zi performs which functions at right?

2872. Sang Bai Pi performs which functions at right?

2873. Jie Geng performs which functions at right?

a. Clear Lung Heat
b. Drain Lung Excess
c. Both of the above
d. None of the above

2874. Bai Fu Zi performs which functions at right?

2875. Tian Nan Xing performs which functions at right?

2876. Ban Xia performs which functions at right?

a. Disperse Damp-Phlegm from the Spleen and Stomach
b. Disperse Wind-Phlegm from the Spleen and Stomach
c. Both of the above
d. None of the above

2877. Bai Bu treats which disorders at right?

2878. Bai Ji treats which disorders at right?

2879. Sha Shen treats which disorders at right?

a. Acute and chronic cough
b. Coughing due to Deficient Yin
c. Both of the above
d. None of the above

2880. Zhe Bai Mu treats which disorders at right?

2881. Bai Qian treats which disorders at right?

2882. Gua Lou treats which disorders at right?

a. Coughing due to Lung Heat
b. Coughing due to Deficient Yin
c. Both of the above
d. None of the above

2883. Which herbs at right stop coughing and calm wheezing?

2884. Which herbs at right treat chronic coughing caused by Deficient Lungs?

2885. Which herbs at right treat externally contracted Dry cough?

a. Zi Wan
b. Xing Ren
c. Both of the above
d. None of the above

2886. Which herbs at right treat coughing caused by Phlegm-Heat?

2887. Which herbs at right treat chronic coughing caused by Deficient Yin?

2888. Which herbs at right treat lung or breast abscesses?

a. Chuan Bei Mu
b. Zhi Bei Mu
c. Both of the above
d. None of the above

2889. Which herbs at right treat wheezing or coughing involving copious sputum and a gurgling sound in the throat?

2890. Which herbs at right treat coughing and wheezing caused by Lung Heat and involving thick yellow sputum?

a. Sang Bai Pi
b. Ting Li Zi
c. Both of the above
d. None of the above

2891. Xiao Qing Long Tang performs which functions at right?
2892. Ling Gui Zhu Gan Tang performs which functions at right?
2893. Bei Mu Gua Lou San performs which functions at right?

a. Warm the Lungs and transform Phlegm
b. Release the Exterior and disperse Cold
c. Both of the above
d. None of the above

2894. Which role does Ban Xia play in Er Chen Tang?
2895. Which role does Ban Xia play in Qing Qi Hua Tan Wan
2896. Which role does Ban Xia play in Mai Men Dong Tang?

a. Chief (monarch or *jun*) component
b. Deputy (minister or *chen*) component
c. Both of the above
d. None of the above

2897. Ling Gui Zhu Gan Tang performs which functions at right?
2898. Ling Gan Wu Wei Jiang Xin Tang performs which functions at right?
2899. Wu Pi San performs which functions at right?

a. Warm and transform Phlegm
b. Strengthen the Spleen and resolve Damp
c. Both of the above
d. None of the above

2900. Xiao Qing Long Tang is indicated for which pathogeneses at right?
2901. Ling Gan Wu Wei Jiang Xin Tang is indicated for which pathogeneses at right?
2902. San Zi Yang Qin Tang is indicated for which pathogeneses at right?

a. Cold fluids congested in the Interior
b. Exogenous Wind-Cold evils
c. Both of the above
d. None of the above

2903. Qing Zao Jiu Fei Tang is indicated for which pathogeneses at right?
2904. Zhi Sou San is indicated for which pathogeneses at right?

a. Dry-Heat attacking the Lungs
b. Wind evil
c. Both of the above
d. None of the above

2905. Mai Men Dong Tang is indicated for which pathogeneses at right?
2906. Yang Yin Qing Fei Tang is indicated for which pathogeneses at right?

a. Deficient Yin of the Lungs
b. Deficient Yin of the Stomach
c. Both of the above
d. None of the above

2907. Wen Dan Tang contains which herbs at right?
2908. Ding Xian Wan contains which herbs at right?
2909. Zhi Sou San contains which herbs at right?

a. Ban Xia and Chen Pi
b. Fu Ling and Gan Cao
c. Both of the above
d. None of the above

2910. Qing Qi Hua Tan Wan contains which herbs at right?

2911. Xing Su San contains which herbs at right?

2912. Wen Dan Tang contains which herbs at right?

a. Ban Xia, Chen Pi, Fu Ling, and Xing Ren
b. Huang Qin, Zhi Shi, Gua Lou Ren, and Dan Nan Xing
c. Both of the above
d. None of the above

2913. Xing Su San performs which functions at right?

2914. Qing Qi Hua Tan Wan performs which functions at right?

2915. Sang Xing Tang performs which functions at right?

a. Clears and disperses Warm-Dry
b. Gently disperses Cool-Dry
c. Both of the above
d. None of the above

2916. Qing Qi Hua Tan Wan is indicated for which patterns at right?

2917. Sang Xing Tang is indicated for which patterns at right?

2918. Bei Mu Gua Lou San is indicated for which patterns at right?

a. Moderate fever, dry hacking cough, dry mouth and throat, thirst, floating-rapid pulse at the right position
b. Coughing that produces viscous yellow sputum with difficulty, a feeling of distention and fullness in the chest and diaphragm, oliguria with reddish urine, red tongue with yellow fur, slippery-rapid pulse
c. Both of the above
d. None of the above

2919. Which formulas at right contain Xuan Shen, Sheng Di Huang, and Mai Men Dong?

2920. Which formulas at right contain Dang Gui, Shu Di Huang, and Jie Geng?

2921. Which formulas at right contain Ren Shen, Ban Xia, and E Jiao?

2922. Which formulas at right contain Bei Mu, Shao Yao, and Gan Cao?

a. Bai He Gu Jin Tang
b. Yang Yin Qing Fei Tang
c. Both of the above
d. None of the above

2923. Qing Zao Jiu Fei Tang performs which functions at right?

2924. Sang Xing Tang performs which functions at right?

2925. Xiang Su San performs which functions at right?

a. Strengthen, clear Heat, and nourish; used in cases where Warm-Dry has injured the Lungs
b. Clear small amount of Heat; used in mild cases of Warm-Dry
c. Both of the above
d. None of the above

2926. Mai Ya performs which functions at right?

2927. Gu Ya performs which functions at right?

2928. Shan Zha performs which functions at right?

a. Transform Blood Stasis and stop diarrhea
b. Reduce food stagnation and inhibit lactation
c. Both of the above
d. None of the above

2929. Mai Ya performs which functions at right?
2930. Ji Nei Jin performs which functions at right?
2931. Lai Fu Zi performs which functions at right?

a. Reduce food stagnation
b. Strengthen the Spleen
c. Both of the above
d. None of the above

2932. Lai Fu Zi performs which functions at right?
2933. Xiang Fu performs which functions at right?
2934. Qing Pi performs which functions at right?

a. Move the Qi
b. Transform accumulation
c. Both of the above
d. None of the above

2935. Which herbs at right treat constrained Liver Qi accompanied by distention and pain in the chest or breasts?
2936. Which herbs at right treat stagnation of Qi in the Spleen or Stomach accompanied by distention and pain in the epigastric or abdominal regions?
2937. Which herbs at right dry Damp and transform Phlegm?

a. Chen Pi
b. Qing Pi
c. Both of the above
d. None of the above

2938. Which herbs at right activate the Qi and soothe chest disorders, particularly in cases where a patient suffers from Deficient Qi?
2939. Which herbs at right break up stagnant Qi and reduce accumulation?
2940. Which herbs at right transform Phlegm and expel focal distention?

a. Zhi Shi
b. Zhi Ke
c. Both of the above
d. None of the above

2941. Fo Shou treats which disorders at right?
2942. Xiang Fu treats which disorders at right?
2943. Qing Pi treats which disorders at right?

a. Constrained Liver Qi
b. Stagnation of Qi in the Stomach
c. Both of the above
d. None of the above

2944. Xiang Fu performs which functions at right?
2945. Bai Ji Li performs which functions at right?
2946. Wu Yao performs which functions at right?

a. Facilitate the smooth flow of Liver Qi
b. Calm the Liver and anchor the Yang
c. Both of the above
d. None of the above

2947. Chen Pi performs which functions at right?
2948. Fo Shou performs which functions at right?
2949. Zhi Shi performs which functions at right?

a. Spread and regulate the Liver Qi and transform Phlegm
b. Strengthen the Spleen and adjust the Middle Energizer
c. Both of the above
d. None of the above

2950. Sang Bai Pi performs which functions at right?

2951. Da Fu Pi performs which functions at right?

2952. Ju Hong performs which functions at right?

a. Promote urination and reduce edema
b. Drain Heat from the Lungs and stop wheezing
c. Both of the above
d. None of the above

2953. Jiang Huang performs which functions at right?

2954. Mei Gui Hua performs which functions at right?

2955. Mu Xiang performs which functions at right?

a. Promote the movement of Qi
b. Promote Blood circulation
c. Both of the above
d. None of the above

2956. Su Zi Jiang Qi Tang performs which functions at right?

2957. Ju Pi Zhu Ru Tang performs which functions at right?

2958. Si Mo Tang performs which functions at right?

a. Direct rebellious Lung Qi down
b. Direct rebellious Stomach Qi down
c. Both of the above
d. None of the above

2959. Jin Ling Zi San treats which disorders at right?

2960. Hou Po Wen Zhong Tang treats which disorders at right?

2961. Gua Lou Xie Bai Bai Jiu Tang treats which disorders at right?

a. Stagnation of Liver Qi
b. Stagnation of Spleen and Stomach Qi
c. Both of the above
d. None of the above

2962. Liang Fu Wan treats epigastric pain associated with which causes at right?

2963. Dan Shen Yin treats epigastric pain associated with which causes at right?

2964. Jin Ling Zi San treats epigastric pain associated with which causes at right?

a. Stagnation of Qi and congealed Cold
b. Stagnation of Qi and Blood Stasis
c. Both of the above
d. None of the above

2965. Dang Gui performs which functions in Su Zi Jiang Tang?

2966. Dang Gui performs which functions in Fu Yuan Huo Xue Tang?

2967. Dang Gui performs which functions in Yi Guan Jian?

a. Treat cough from rebellious Qi
b. Nourish the Blood and moisten Dry
c. Both of the above
d. None of the above

2968. Xiao Qing Long Tang is indicated for which pathogeneses at right?

2969. Ding Chuan Tang is indicated for which pathogeneses at right?

2970. Zhi Sou San is indicated for which pathogeneses at right?

a. Wind-Cold constraining the Exterior and Phlegm-Heat smoldering in the Interior
b. Wind-Cold constraining the Exterior with congested fluids, which together cause the pores to close
c. Both of the above
d. None of the above

2971. Qian Cao Gen performs which functions at right?

2972. Bai Mao Gen performs which functions at right?

2973. Hua Rui Shi performs which functions at right?

a. Cool the Blood and stop bleeding
b. Dispel Blood Stasis and stop bleeding
c. Both of the above
d. None of the above

2974. Qian Cao Gen performs which functions at right?

2975. Ce Bai Ye performs which functions at right?

2976. Yu Jin performs which functions at right?

a. Invigorate the Blood, break up Blood Stasis, cool the Blood and reduce jaundice
b. Invigorate the Blood, break up Blood Stasis, cool the Blood, and stop bleeding
c. Both of the above
d. None of the above

2977. Xue Yu Tan performs which functions at right?

2978. Bai Ji performs which functions at right?

2979. Fu Ping performs which functions at right?

2980. Xian He Cao performs which functions at right?

a. Restrain leakage of Blood and stop bleeding
b. Reduce swelling and generate flesh
c. Both of the above
d. None of the above

2981. Huai Hua performs which functions at right?

2982. Ce Bai Ye performs which functions at right?

2983. Pu Huang performs which functions at right?

a. Cool the Blood and stop bleeding
b. Expel Phlegm and stop coughing
c. Both of the above
d. None of the above

2984. Di Yu performs which functions at right?

2985. Da Ji (Japanese thistle) performs which functions at right?

2986. San Qi performs which functions at right?

a. Cool the Blood and stop bleeding
b. Promote the generation of new flesh
c. Both of the above
d. None of the above

2987. E Jiao treats which disorders at right?

2988. Zong Lu Pi treats which disorders at right?

2989. Jiang Xiang treats which disorders at right?

a. Bleeding caused by Deficient Blood
b. Bleeding caused by Blood Stasis
c. Both of the above
d. None of the above

2990. Tu Bie Chong performs which functions at right?

2991. Shui Zhi performs which functions at right?

a. Break up and drive out Blood Stasis
b. Renew sinews and join bones
c. Both of the above
d. None of the above

2992. Yu Jin performs which functions at right?

2993. Zhi Zi performs which functions at right?

a. Invigorate the Blood and alleviate pain
b. Benefit the Gallbladder and reduce jaundice
c. Both of the above
d. None of the above

2994. Xing Ren performs which functions at right?

2995. Tao Ren performs which functions at right?

a. Break up Blood Stasis
b. Moisten the Intestines and unblock the bowels
c. Both of the above
d. None of the above

2996. Bai Shao performs which functions at right?

2997. Chi Shao performs which functions at right?

a. Clear Heat and Cool the Blood
b. Calm and curb the Liver Yang and alleviate pain
c. Both of the above
d. None of the above

2998. Ji Xue Teng performs which functions at right?

2999. Dang Gui performs which functions at right?

a. Tonify the Blood
b. Promote the movement of Blood
c. Both of the above
d. None of the above

3000. Da Huang treats which disorders at right?

3001. Hu Zhang treats which disorders at right?

a. Damp-Heat jaundice and traumatic injury
b. Wind-Damp painful obstruction and cough caused by Lung Heat
c. Both of the above
d. None of the above

3002. Yan Hu Suo is indicated for which disorders at right?

3003. Chuan Xiong is indicated for which disorders at right?

a. Stagnant Qi and Blood Stasis with abdominal pain
b. Headaches caused by Wind, Cold, Heat, or Deficient Blood
c. Both of the above
d. None of the above

3004. Chuan Xiong is indicated for which disorders at right?

3005. Niu Xi is indicated for which disorders at right?

a. Headaches caused by Wind, Cold, Heat, or Deficient Blood
b. Abdominal pain caused by Blood Stasis
c. Both of the above
d. None of the above

3006. Niu Xi is indicated for which disorders at right?

3007. Du Zhong is indicated for which disorders at right?

a. Soreness and pain in the lower back and knees caused by Deficient Liver and Kidneys
b. Pain in the lower back and knees caused by Damp-Heat painful obstruction
c. Both of the above
d. None of the above

3008. Which herbs at right promote the movement of Blood and Qi?

3009. Which herbs at right benefit the Gallbladder and reduce jaundice?

a. Yu Jin
b. Jiang Huang
c. Both of the above
d. None of the above

3010. Which herbs at right treat edema caused by Damp-Heat and accompanied by dysuria?

3011. Which herbs at right treat postpartum abdominal pain?

a. Yi Mu Cao
b. Shan Zha
c. Both of the above
d. None of the above

3012. Bu Yang Huan Wu Tang treats which disorders at right?

3013. Shi Xiao San treats which disorders at right?

3014. Qi Li San treats which disorders at right?

a. Bruising, swelling, pain, and/or bleeding associated with traumatic injuries
b. Pain caused by Blood Stasis that obstructs the vessels
c. Both of the above
d. None of the above

3015. Fu Yuan Huo Xue Tang contains which herbs at right?

3016. Sheng Hua Tang contains which herbs at right?

3017. Xue Fu Zhu Yu Tang contains which herbs at right?

a. Hong Hua and Chai Hu
b. Tao Ren and Dang Gui
c. Both of the above
d. None of the above

3018. Jiao Ai Tang performs which functions at right?

3019. Si Wu Tang performs which functions at right?

a. Warm and tonify to stop bleeding
b. Nourish the Blood and regulate menstruation
c. Both of the above
d. None of the above

3020. Huang Tu Tang is indicated for which disorders at right?

3021. Jiao Ai Tang is indicated for which disorders at right?

a. Deficiency-Cold patterns where there is blood in the stool
b. Deficiency-Cold patterns where there is abnormal uterine bleeding
c. Both of the above
d. None of the above

3022. Tao He Cheng Qi Tang is indicated for which disorders at right?

3023. Di Dang Tang is indicated for which disorders at right?

a. Accumulation of stagnant Blood in the Lower Energizer
b. Amenorrhea caused by Blood Stasis
c. Both of the above
d. None of the above

3024. Fu Zi treats which disorders at right?

3025. Rou Gui treats which disorders at right?

a. Yang exhaustion syndrome
b. Deficient Yang syndrome
c. Both of the above
d. None of the above

3026. Which herbs at right treat Shaoyin headaches?

3027. Which herbs at right treat parietal headaches?

a. Xi Xin and Du Huo
b. Gao Ben and Wu Zhu Yu
c. Both of the above
d. None of the above

3028. Which herbs at right treat vomiting caused by Stomach Cold?

3029. Which of the herbs at right treat exhausted Yang?

a. Ban Xia
b. Gan Jiang
c. Both of the above
d. None of the above

3030. Which herbs at right treat vomiting caused by Stomach Cold?

a. Ding Xiang
b. Bai Dou Kou
c. Both of the above
d. None of the above

3031. Which herbs at right treat Lung Cold that involves expectoration of thin watery or white sputum?

3032. Which herbs at right treat exhausted Yang where the extremities are cold?

a. Gan Jiang
b. Fu Zi
c. Both of the above
d. None of the above

3033. Which herbs at right disperse Cold and alleviate pain?

3034. Which herbs at right restore the devastated Yang and assist the Deficient Yang?

a. Chuan Wu
b. Fu Zi
c. Both of the above
d. None of the above

3035. Which formulas at right treat bleeding caused by Deficient Yang?

3036. Which formulas at right treat metrorrhagia caused by impairment of the Chong and Ren meridians?

a. Li Zhong Wan
b. Huang Tu Tang
c. Both of the above
d. None of the above

3037. Li Zhong Wan is indicated for which pathogeneses at right?

3038. Wu Zhu Yu Tang is indicated for which pathogeneses at right?

a. Deficient Cold Spleen and Stomach
b. Liver Cold attacking the Stomach
c. Both of the above
d. None of the above

3039. Sheng Jiang performs which functions at right in Gui Zhi Tang?

3040. Sheng Jiang performs which functions at right in Wu Zhu Yu Tang?

3041. Sheng Jiang performs which functions at right in Zhen Wu Tang?

a. Release the Exterior and expel Cold evils
b. Warm the Middle Energizer and direct rebellious Qi downward
c. Both of the above
d. None of the above

3042. Zhen Ren Yang Zang Tang performs which functions at right?

3043. Fu Zi Li Zhong Wan performs which functions at right?

a. Augment the Qi and strengthen the Spleen
b. Restrain leakage from the Intestines and stop diarrhea
c. Both of the above
d. None of the above

3044. What is the relationship between the chief (monarch or *jun*) and the deputy (minister or *chen*) herbs in Si Ni Tang?

3045. What is the relationship between the chief (monarch or *jun*) and the deputy (minister or *chen*) herbs in Zuo Jin Wan?

a. Mutual promotion
b. Corrigent method
c. Both of the above
d. None of the above

3046. Shen Fu Tang is indicated for which patterns at right?

3047. Si Ni Tang is indicated for which patterns at right?

a. Extremely cold extremities, lethargy, constant desire to sleep, vomiting, diarrhea, abdominal pain, deep-thin or submerged pulse
b. Cold extremities, hyperhidrosis, weak breathing, almost imperceptible pulse
c. Both of the above
d. None of the above

3048. Which formulas at right treat Excess in the upper body and Deficiency in the lower body where there is this pattern of symptoms: wheezing and gasping for breath, cold extremities, unremitting cold sweat, pale tongue with slippery white fur, faint pulse?

3049. Which formulas at right treat Excess in the upper body and Deficiency in the lower body where there is this pattern of symptoms: copious watery sputum, coughing and wheezing with shortness of breath, a stifling sensation in the chest and diaphragm, slippery or greasy white tongue fur?

a. Hei Xi Dan
b. Su Zi Jiang Qi Tang
c. Both of the above
d. None of the above

3050. What is the treatment principle by which Hei Xi Dan treats coughing and wheezing?

3051. What is the treatment principle by which Su Zi Jiang Qi Tang treats coughing and wheezing?

a. Direct rebellious Qi downward, stop coughing and wheezing and expel Phlegm, primarily treat the Excess in the upper body, warming the Kidneys and helping them to grasp Qi, secondarily treat the Deficiency in the lower body
b. Warm and strengthen the lower source and force the floating Yang downward
c. Both of the above
d. None of the above

3052. Sang Ji Sheng performs which functions at right?

3053. Wu Jia Pi performs which functions at right?

a. Dispel Wind-Damp, strengthen the sinews and bones, and promote urination
b. Tonify the Liver and Kidneys, strengthen the sinews, and calm the womb
c. Both of the above
d. None of the above

3054. Gou Qi Zi performs which functions at right?

3055. Nu Zhen Zi performs which functions at right?

a. Augment the Liver and Kidneys
b. Clear Heat from Deficiency and improve vision
c. Both of the above
d. None of the above

3056. Ji Xue Teng performs which functions at right?

3057. Dang Gui performs which functions at right?

a. Tonify the Blood and promote the movement of Blood
b. Invigorate the meridians and relax the sinews
c. Both of the above
d. None of the above

3058. Dang Shen performs which functions at right?

3059. Hai Er Shen performs which functions at right?

a. Tonify the Spleen and promote urination
b. Tonify the Kidneys and fortify the Yang
c. Both of the above
d. None of the above

3060. Which functions at right do Gui Ban and Bie Jia have in common?

3061. Which functions at right do Sang Shen Zi and Nu Zhen Zi have in common?

a. Nourish the Yin and anchor the Yang
b. Stabilize the Kidneys and retain the Essence
c. Both of the above
d. None of the above

3062. Gou Qi Zi performs which functions at right?

3063. Han Lian Cao performs which functions at right?

a. Tonify and nourish the Liver and Kidneys
b. Cool the Blood and stop bleeding
c. Both of the above
d. None of the above

3064. Xu Duan performs which functions at right?

3065. Gou Ji Performs which functions at right?

a. Tonify the Liver and Kidneys and strengthen the sinews and bones
b. Promote the movement of Blood and calm the fetus
c. Both of the above
d. None of the above

3066. Ji Xue Teng performs which functions at right?

3067. Dang Gui performs which functions at right?

a. Nourish the Blood
b. Promote the movement of Blood
c. Both of the above
d. None of the above

3068. Rou Gui performs which functions at right?

3069. Lu Rong performs which functions at right?

a. Warm the Kidneys and fortify the Yang
b. Disperse Cold and alleviate pain
c. Both of the above
d. None of the above

3070. Huang Qi performs which functions at right?

3071. Chai Hu performs which functions at right?

a. Strengthen Qi
b. Raise the Yang Qi
c. Both of the above
d. None of the above

3072. Huang Qi is indicated for which disorders at right?

3073. Bai Zhu is indicated for which disorders at right?

a. Deficiency with spontaneous sweating
b. A wound that is not healing and where pus has formed
c. Both of the above
d. None of the above

3074. Hu Tao Ren is indicated for which disorders at right?

3075. Ge Jie is indicated for which disorders at right?

a. Chronic coughing and wheezing resulting from Deficient Lungs and Kidneys
b. Constipation in the elderly or resulting from injured fluids after febrile illnesses
c. Both of the above
d. None of the above

3076. Bie Jia and Gui Ban are each contraindicated in which cases at right?

3077. Tian Men Dong and Mai Men Dong are each contraindicated in which cases at right?

a. During pregnancy
b. Cold resulting from Deficient Spleen and Stomach and involving diarrhea
c. Both of the above
d. None of the above

3078. Rou Cong Rong treats which disorders at right?

3079. Hu Tao Ren treats which disorders at right?

a. Constipation involving Dry Intestines
b. Deficient Yang of the Kidneys
c. Both of the above
d. None of the above

3080. Dong Chong Xia Cao treats which disorders at right?

3081. Bai He treats which disorders at right?

a. Chronic cough and wheezing resulting from Deficient Qi of the Lungs and Kidneys
b. Coughing and wheezing resulting from Deficient Yin of the Lungs
c. Both of the above
d. None of the above

3082. Lu Rong treats which disorders at right?

3083. Lu Jiao Jiao treats which disorders at right?

a. Deficiency-Cold bleeding
b. Deficient Yang of the Kidneys
c. Both of the above
d. None of the above

3084. Which herbs at right nourish the Yin and anchors the Yang?

3085. Which herbs at right benefit the Kidneys and strengthens the bones?

a. Gui Ban
b. Bie Jia
c. Both of the above
d. None of the above

3086. Which herbs at right tonify the Qi and raises the Yang?

3087. Which herbs at right generates body fluids?

a. Huang Qi
b. Tai Zi Shen
c. Both of the above
d. None of the above

3088. Rou Cong Rong performs which functions at right?

3089. Suo Yang performs which functions at right?

3090. Hu Tao Ren performs which functions at right?

a. Tonifies the Kidneys and strengthens the Yang
b. Warms the Lungs
c. Both of the above
d. None of the above

3091. Sheng Mai San performs which functions at right?

3092. Shen Ling Bai Zhu San performs which functions at right?

a. Strengthen the Spleen and augment the Qi
b. Regulate Stomach energy and leach out Damp
c. Both of the above
d. None of the above

3093. Huang Qi performs which functions at right in Bu Yang Huan Wu Tang?

3094. Huang Qi performs which functions at right in Dang Gui Bu Xue Tang?

a. Tonify the Qi and generate Blood
b. Tonify the Qi and impel the circulation of Blood
c. Both of the above
d. None of the above

3095. Si Jun Zi Tang performs which functions at right?

3096. Gui Pi Tang performs which functions at right?

3097. Dang Gui Bu Xue Tang performs which functions at right?

a. Tonify the Qi and strengthen the Spleen
b. Tonify the Qi and nourish Blood
c. Both of the above
d. None of the above

3098. Gan Cao Tang performs which functions at right?

3099. Ba Zhen Tang performs which functions at right?

3100. Yi Guan Jian performs which functions at right?

3101. Si Wu Tang performs which functions at right?

3102. Gui Pi Tang performs which functions at right?

a. Tonify the Qi
b. Tonify the Blood
c. Both of the above
d. None of the above

3103. Which formulas at right treat a pattern of hectic fever, night sweats, and red tongue with little fur, which has been caused by Deficient Yin of the Kidneys and Liver where there is flaming up of Deficiency-Fire?

3104. Which formulas at right treat a pattern of weakness in the lower back and knees, deterioration of the sinews and bones with accompanying reduction in function, difficulty in walking, and red tongue with little fur, which has been caused by Deficient Yin of the Kidneys and Liver?

a. Liu Wei Di Huang Wan
b. Da Bu Yin Wan
c. Both of the above
d. None of the above

3105. Jin Ling Zi San performs which functions at right?

3106. Hu Qian Wan performs which functions at right?

3107. Yi Quan Jian performs which functions at right?

3108. Zuo Gui Wan performs which functions at right?

3109. You Gui Wan performs which functions at right?

a. Nourish the Yin
b. Spread Liver Qi
c. Both of the above
d. None of the above

3110. Ma Huang Gen performs which functions at right?
3111. Wu Bei Zi performs which functions at right?
3112. Nuo Dao Gen performs which functions at right?

a. Stop sweating
b. Nourish the Yin
c. Both of the above
d. None of the above

3113. Rou Dou Kou performs which functions at right?
3114. Bai Dou Kou performs which functions at right?

a. Bind up the Intestines and stop diarrhea
b. Transform Damp and move Qi
c. Both of the above
d. None of the above

3115. Jin Ying Zi performs which functions at right?
3116. Sang Piao Xiao performs which functions at right?

a. Retain the Essence and restrain urine
b. Tonify the Kidneys and assist the Yang
c. Both of the above
d. None of the above

3117. Fu Xiao Mai performs which functions at right?
3118. He Zi performs which functions at right?

a. Bind up the Intestines and stop diarrhea
b. Contain the leakage of Lung Qi and improve the condition of the throat
c. Both of the above
d. None of the above

3119. Which functions at right do Wu Wei Zi and Ying Su Ke have in common?
3120. Which functions at right do Shu Di Huang and He Shou Wu have in common?

a. Contain the leakage of Lung Qi
b. Nourish the Kidney Yin
c. Both of the above
d. None of the above

3121. Wu Wei Zi performs which functions at right?
3122. Wu Mei performs which functions at right?

a. Contain the Leakage of Lung Qi and generate fluids
b. Bind up the Essence and quiet the Spirit
c. Both of the above
d. None of the above

3123. Qian Shi performs which functions at right?
3124. Lian Zi performs which functions at right?

a. Tonify the Kidneys and stabilize the Essence
b. Nourish the Heart and calm the Spirit
c. Both of the above
d. None of the above

3125. Yu Liang Shi performs which functions at right?	a. Astringe and stop bleeding
3126. Chi Shi Zhi performs which functions at right?	b. Bind up the Intestines and stop diarrhea
	c. Both of the above
	d. None of the above

3127. Jin Ying Zhi performs which functions at right?	a. Bind up the Intestines and stop diarrhea
3128. Fu Pen Zi performs which functions at right?	b. Stabilize the Kidneys and retain Essence
	c. Both of the above
	d. None of the above

3129. Ma Huang treats which disorders at right?	a. Wheezing resulting from Deficient Lungs and Kidneys
3130. Wu Wei Zi treats which disorders at right?	b. Chronic cough resulting from Deficient Lungs
	c. Both of the above
	d. None of the above

3131. Which herbs at right stabilize the Kidneys and retains the Essence and urine?	a. Jin Ying Zi
	b. Sang Piao Xiao
3132. Which herbs at right tonify the Kidneys and assists the Yang?	c. Both of the above
	d. None of the above

3133. Which herbs at right treat excessive leukorrhea?	a. Bai Guo
3134. Which herbs at right treat excessive sweating?	b. Qian Shi
	c. Both of the above
	d. None of the above

3135. Mu Li San is indicated for which pathogeneses at right?	a. The Weifen fails to protect the body
3136. Yu Ping Fen San is indicated for which pathogeneses at right?	b. The Heart Yang is not suppressed
	c. Both of the above
	d. None of the above

3137. Huang Qi performs which functions at right in Yu Ping Fen San?	a. Supplement the Qi and stabilize the Exterior
	b. Raise the Yang
3138. Huang Qi performs which functions at right in Dang Gui Bu Xue Tang?	c. Both of the above
	d. None of the above

3139. Which formulas at right treat this pattern: spontaneous sweating, aversion to drafts, liability to Wind pathogens, pale and shiny complexion, pale tongue with white fur, floating-deficient-soft pulse??

3140. Which formulas at right treat this pattern: fever, headache, sweating, aversion to wind, thin white tongue fur, floating-moderate pulse?

a. Yu Ping Fen San
b. Gui Zhi Tang
c. Both of the above
d. None of the above

3141. Which instructions at right apply to Si Shen Wan?

3142. Which instructions at right apply to Ji Ming San?

a. Take daily just before sunrise
b. After taking the decoction, drink a small quantity of porridge and then lie in a warm bed
c. Both of the above
d. None of the above

3143. Tao Hua Tang performs which functions at right?

3144. Si Shen Wan performs which functions at right?

a. Warm and tonify the Kidneys and Spleen
b. Bind up the Intestines and stop diarrhea
c. Both of the above
d. None of the above

3145. Shen Ling Bai Zhu San performs which functions at right?

3146. Zhen Ren Yang Zang Tang performs which functions at right?

a. Bind up the Intestines and stop diarrhea
b. Warm the Middle Energizer and tonify Deficiency
c. Both of the above
d. None of the above

3147. Bai Shao performs which functions at right in Zhen Ren Yang Zang Tang?

3148. Bai Shao performs which functions at right in Wan Dai Tang?

a. Nourish the Blood and regulate the Yin
b. Soften spasms and stop pain
c. Both of the above
d. None of the above

3149. Wu Wei Zi performs which functions at right in Sheng Mai San?

3150. Wu Wei Zi performs which functions at right in Si Shen Wan?

a. Bind up the Intestines and stop diarrhea
b. Bind up the Lungs and stop excessive sweating
c. Both of the above
d. None of the above

3151. Mu Li performs which functions at right?

3152. Long Gu performs which functions at right?

a. Calm the Liver, anchor and preserve the floating Yang, and prevent the leakage of fluids
b. Soften and dissolve hard masses
c. Both of the above
d. None of the above

3153. Wu Jia Pi performs which functions at right?

3154. He Huan Pi performs which functions at right?

a. Calm the Liver and relieve constraint
b. Invigorate the Blood and dissipate swelling
c. Both of the above
d. None of the above

3155. Qing Xiang Zi performs which functions at right?

3156. Zhen Zhu performs which functions at right?

a. Promote healing and generate flesh
b. Clear the Liver to treat eye disease
c. Both of the above
d. None of the above

3157. Ci Shi performs which functions at right?

3158. Mu LI performs which functions at right?

a. Calm the Liver and anchor the floating Yang
b. Grasp the Qi and alleviate asthma
c. Both of the above
d. None of the above

3159. Huang Qi is used by itself to treat which disorders at right?

3160. Calcined Long Gu treats which disorders at right?

a. Spontaneous perspiration resulting from Deficient Yang
b. Night sweats resulting from Deficient Yin
c. Both of the above
d. None of the above

3161. Ci Shi treats which disorders at right?

3162. Cang Zhu treats which disorders at right?

a. Night blindness
b. Blurred vision
c. Both of the above
d. None of the above

3163. Zhu Sha performs which functions at right?

3164. Yuan Zhi performs which functions at right?

a. Clear Heat and calm the Spirit
b. Nourish the Heart and calm the Spirit
c. Both of the above
d. None of the above

3165. Bie Jia is indicated for which disorders at right?

3166. Gui Ban is indicated for which disorders at right?

3167. Mu Li is indicated for which disorders at right?

a. Stirring of endopathic Wind of the Deficiency type with convulsions of the extremities resulting from the impairment of Yin by febrile diseases
b. Scrofula and subcutaneous nodules resulting from accumulation of Phlegm-Fire
c. Both of the above
d. None of the above

3168. Niu Huang performs which functions at right?

3169. Yuan Zhi performs which functions at right?

a. Vaporize Phlegm and open the orifices
b. Drain Heat and relieve Fire toxicity
c. Both of the above
d. None of the above

3170. Which herbs at right treat tetanic collapse, Phlegm collapse, and seizures?

3171. Which herbs at right treat abdominal masses and treat amenorrhea resulting from Blood Stasis?

a. Bing Pian
b. She Xiang
c. Both of the above
d. None of the above

3172. Xiong Huang performs which functions at right?

3173. Niu Huang performs which functions at right?

a. Clear Heat
b. Relieve toxicity
c. Both of the above
d. None of the above

3174. Ren Shen treats which disorders at right?

3175. She Xiang treats which disorders at right?

a. Coma resulting from Excess syndrome
b. Coma resulting from collapse of Qi syndrome
c. Both of the above
d. None of the above

3176. Which treatments at right are appropriate for Yangming Excess-Heat constipation involving impaired consciousness?

3177. Which treatments at right are appropriate for Damp-Cold syndromes where turbid Phlegm veils the sensory organs and impairs consciousness?

a. Open the orifices with herbs that are warm in nature
b. Open the orifices with herbs that are cool in nature
c. Both of the above
d. None of the above

3178. An Gong Niu Huang Wan is indicated for which disorders at right?

3179. Shen Fu Tang is indicated for which disorders at right?

a. Coma syndrome resulting from an acute attack of Heat evil
b. Coma syndrome resulting from an acute attack of Cold evil
c. Both of the above
d. None of the above

3180. Chan Tui performs which functions at right?

3181. Niu Bang Zi performs which functions at right?

3182. Shi Jue Ming performs which functions at right?

a. Extinguish Wind and stop convulsions
b. Improve vision and remove superficial visual obstruction
c. Both of the above
d. None of the above

3183. Quan Xie performs which functions at right?

3184. Di Long performs which functions at right?

a. Extinguish Wind and stop convulsions
b. Calm wheezing and promote urination
c. Both of the above
d. None of the above

3185. Quan Xie performs which functions at right?

3186. Jiang Can performs which functions at right?

a. Extinguish Wind and stop convulsions
b. Unblock the collaterals and stop pain
c. Both of the above
d. None of the above

3187. Tian Nan Xing performs which functions at right?

3188. Bai Fu Zi performs which functions at right?

3189. Wu Gong performs which functions at right?

a. Extinguish Wind and stop spasms
b. Dry Damp and expel Phlegm
c. Both of the above
d. None of the above

3190. Zhen Zhu Mu performs which functions at right?

3191. Ling Yang Xiao performs which functions at right?

3192. Long Gu performs which functions at right?

a. Calm the Liver and anchor the Yang
b. Extinguish Wind and stop spasms
c. Both of the above
d. None of the above

3193. Wu Gong performs which functions at right?

3194. Quan Xie performs which functions at right?

3195. Zhu Sha performs which functions at right?

a. Extinguish Wind, stop spasms, relieve toxins, and dissipate nodules
b. Unblock the collaterals and stop pain
c. Both of the above
d. None of the above

3196. Xiao Feng San contains which herbs at right?
3197. Chuan Xiong Cha Tiao San contains which herbs at right?
3198. Yu Zhen San contains which herbs at right?
3199. Da Qin Jia Tang contains which herbs at right?
3200. Jia Wei Xiang Su San contains which herbs at right?

a. Fang Feng
b. Jing Jie
c. Both of the above
d. None of the above

3201. Which formulas at right treat syndromes where Heat injures the Yin and Blood, stirring Deficiency-Wind inside?
3202. Which formulas at right treat syndromes where Wind-Heat-Damp causes weepy, itchy, red skin lesions?

a. Da Ding Feng Zgu
b. E Jiao Ji Zi Huang Tang
c. Both of the above
d. None of the above

3203. Which benefits at right are achieved by supplementing Di Huang Yin Zi with Wu Wei Zi?
3204. Which benefits at right are achieved by supplementing Xiao Qing Long Tang with Wu Wei Zi?
3205. Which benefits at right are achieved by supplementing Si Shen Wan with Wu Wei Zi?

a. Preserve the Yin and body fluids
b. Restrain the floating Yang
c. Both of the above
d. None of the above

3206. Dai Zhe Shi performs which functions at right in Zhen Gan Xi Feng Tang?
3207. Dai Zhe Shi performs which functions at right in Xuan Fu Dai Zhe Tang?

a. Calm the Liver and anchor the Yang
b. Directs Qi downward and controls rebelliousness thanks to its heavy nature
c. Both of the above
d. None of the above

3208. San Jia Fu Mai Tang contains which herbs at right?
3209. Zhen Gan Xi Feng Tang contains which herbs at right?
3210. Da Ding Feng Zhu contains which herbs at right?

a. Mu Li and Gui Ben
b. Bie Jia
c. Both of the above
d. None of the above

3211. Which herbs at right treat abdominal pain resulting from incoordination between the Liver and Stomach?
3212. Which herbs at right treat abdominal pain resulting from the accumulation of parasites?

a. Chuan Lian Zi
b. Ku Lian Gen Pi
c. Both of the above
d. None of the above

3213. Huang Bai uses which plant constituents at right?
3214. Ku Lian Pi uses which plant constituents at right?

a. Root bark
b. Tree bark
c. Both of the above
d. None of the above

3215. Lei Wan performs which functions at right?

3216. Guan Zhong performs which functions at right?

3217. Ku Lian Pi performs which functions at right?

a. Kill roundworms
b. Kill tapeworms
c. Both of the above
d. None of the above

3218. Wu Mei Wan and Da Jian Zhong Tang have which herbs at right in common?

3219. Wu Mei Wan and Dang Gui Si Ni Tang have which herbs at right in common?

a. Gui Zhi and Xi Xin
b. Chuan Jiao and Gan Jiang
c. Both of the above
d. None of the above

3220. Da Huang performs which functions at right in Da Huang Mu Dan Tang?

3221. Da Huang performs which functions at right in Tao He Cheng Qi Tang?

a. Drain Heat and break up Blood Stasis
b. Attack and purge Blood Stasis And Damp-Heat toxins
c. Both of the above
d. None of the above

3222. Da Huang Mu Dan Tang contains which herbs at right?

3223. Wei Jing Tang contains which herbs at right?

a. Tao Ren and Dong Gua Ren
b. Xing Ren and Huo Ma Ren
c. Both of the above
d. None of the above

3224. Shu Di Huang performs which functions at right in Yang He Tang?

3225. Shu Di Huang performs which functions at right in Liu Wei Di Huang Wan?

a. Nourish the Blood and tonify the Essence
b. Warm and Tonify the Blood
c. Both of the above
d. None of the above

3226. Ai Ye performs which functions at right?

3227. Pu Huang performs which functions at right?

3228. Ou Jie performs which functions at right?

a. Warm the womb and stop bleeding in cases resulting from Deficiency-Cold
b. Disperse Cold and alleviate menstrual pain in cases resulting from Deficiency-Cold
c. Both of the above
d. None of the above

3229. Fang Feng performs which functions at right?

3230. Jing Jie performs which functions at right?

3231. Mu Gua performs which functions at right?

a. Release the Exterior and expel Wind
b. Expel Wind-Damp and alleviate trembling
c. Both of the above
d. None of the above

3232. Nuo Dao Gen Xu performs which functions at right?

3233. He Zi performs which functions at right?

3234. Wu Bei Zi performs which functions at right?

a. Bind up the Intestines and stop diarrhea
b. Contain the leakage of Lung Qi and stop coughing
c. Both of the above
d. None of the above

3235. Gou Qi Zi performs which functions at right?

3236. Ba Ji Tian performs which functions at right?

3237. Bu Gu Zhi performs which functions at right?

a. Tonify the Kidneys and fortify the Yang
b. Disperse Wind and expel Damp
c. Both of the above
d. None of the above

3238. Zi Wan performs which functions at right?

3239. Zi Cao performs which functions at right?

3240. Zi Hua Di Ding performs which functions at right?

a. Clear Heat and relieve Fire toxicity
b. Invigorate the Blood and regulate the menses
c. Both of the above
d. None of the above

3241. Yi Mu Cao performs which functions at right?

3242. Xian He Cao performs which functions at right?

3243. Xi Xian Xao performs which functions at right?

a. Promote the movement of Blood and reduce masses
b. Restrain leakage of Blood and stop bleeding
c. Both of the above
d. None of the above

3244. Xi Xin performs which functions at right?

3245. Xin Yi Hua performs which functions at right?

3246. Hou Po performs which functions at right?

a. Disperse Wind-Cold and unblock the nasal orifices
b. Warm the Lungs and transform Phlegm
c. Both of the above
d. None of the above

3247. Li Lu is used in which of the ways at right?

3248. Gua Di is used in which of the ways at right?

3249. Chang Shan is used in which of the ways at right?

a. Taken orally to induce vomiting
b. Applied externally to fight scabies, lice, and ringworm
c. Both of the above
d. None of the above

3250. Duan (calcined) Long Gu performs which functions at right?

3251. Duan (calcined) Mu Li performs which functions at right?

3252. Chao (dry-fried) Suan Zao Ren performs which functions at right?

a. Stop nocturnal emissions with its astringent nature
b. Prevent abnormal sweating and quiet the Spirit
c. Both of the above
d. None of the above

3253. Qin Jiao is indicated for which disorders at right?
3254. Du Huo is indicated for which disorders at right?
3255. Ren Dong Tang is indicated for which disorders at right?

a. Damp-Heat painful obstruction
b. Wind-Cold-Damp painful obstruction
c. Both of the above
d. None of the above

3256. Wu Jia Pi performs which functions at right?
3257. Qian Nian Jian performs which functions at right?
3258. Sang Ji Sheng performs which functions at right?

a. Expel Wind-Damp
b. Strengthen the sinews and bones
c. Both of the above
d. None of the above

3259. Ren Shen and Dang Shen each treat which disorders at right?
3260. Ge Jie and Dong Xiong Xia Cao each treat which disorders at right?
3261. Fu Ling and Yi Yi Ren each treat which disorders at right?

a. Deficient Spleen syndrome
b. Deficient Lungs syndrome
c. Both of the above
d. None of the above

3262. Gan Jiang treats which disorders at right?
3263. Xi Xin treats which disorders at right?
3264. Qiang Huo treats which disorders at right?

a. Exterior-Cold syndrome
b. Interior-Cold syndrome
c. Both of the above
d. None of the above

3265. Chai Hu treats which disorders at right?
3266. Qing Pi treats which disorders at right?
3267. Yu Jin treats which disorders at right?

a. Constrained Liver Qi syndrome
b. Shao Yang syndrome
c. Both of the above
d. None of the above

3268. Mu Dan Pi treats which disorders at right?
3269. Qin Jiao treats which disorders at right?
3270. Bian Dou treats which disorders at right?

a. All types of pain syndromes
b. Steaming bone disorder
c. Both of the above
d. None of the above

3271. Sang Ji Sheng and Gou Ji each treat which disorders at right?
3272. Qiang Huo and Du Huo each treat which disorders at right?
3273. Ji Xue Teng and Hu Gu treat which disorders at right?

a. Deficient Kidney patterns that involve lumbago
b. Wind-Damp painful obstruction
c. Both of the above
d. None of the above

3274. Sha Ren treats which disorders at right?
3275. Ban Xia treats which disorders at right?
3276. Cao Guo treats which disorders at right?

a. Damp distress in the Middle Energizer
b. Restless fetus
c. Both of the above
d. None of the above

3277. Han Lian Cao performs which functions at right?

3278. Da Huang performs which functions at right?

a. Cool the Blood and stop bleeding
b. Promote healing of burns
c. Both of the above
d. None of the above

3279. Bai Zhu treats which disorders at right?

3280. Shan Yao treats which disorders at right?

3281. Zhu Ling treats which disorders at right?

a. Diabetes
b. Diarrhea resulting from Deficient Spleen
c. Both of the above
d. None of the above

3282. Bai Jiang Can performs which functions at right?

3283. She Tui performs which functions at right?

3284. She Chuang Zi performs which functions at right?

a. Extinguish Wind and stop spasms and convulsions
b. Expel Wind and stop itching
c. Both of the above
d. None of the above

3285. Wa Leng Zi treats which disorders at right?

3286. Wu Zei Gu treats which disorders at right?

3287. Shan Yao treats which disorders at right?

a. Stomach pain and acid regurgitation
b. Abdominal masses, scrofula, and goiters
c. Both of the above
d. None of the above

3288. Bo He treats which disorders at right?

3289. Bai Zhi treats which disorders at right?

3290. Yin Chai Hu treats which disorders at right?

a. Wind-Heat patterns with headache
b. Wind-Cold patterns with headache
c. Both of the above
d. None of the above

3291. Chuan Shan Jia treats which disorders at right?

3292. Wang Bu Liu Xing treats which disorders at right?

3293. Niu Xi treats which disorders at right?

a. Amenorrhea resulting from Blood Stasis
b. Insufficient lactation resulting from Blood Stasis
c. Both of the above
d. None of the above

3294. In which form is Gan Cao used when treating food poisoning or the poisonous effect of other herbs?

3295. In which form is Gan Cao used when treating painful spasms of the abdomen or legs resulting from injured Yin and Blood?

3296. In which form is Ma Huang used when treating Exterior disorders?

a. Raw
b. Honey-fried (zhi)
c. Both of the above
d. None of the above

3297. How is E Jiao prepared in order to arrest bleeding?

3298. How is E Jiao prepared in order to tonify the Blood and nourish the Yin?

3299. How is E Jiao prepared in order to moisten the Lungs?

a. Dissolved in wine
b. Dry fried *(chao)* with Hai Ge Fen
c. Both of the above
d. None of the above

3300. Long-term use of Gan Cao can lead to which of the disorders at right?

3301. Long-term use of Da Zao can lead to which of the disorders at right?

3302. Long-term use of Dang Shen can lead to which of the disorders at right?

a. Abdominal flatulence
b. Edema
c. Both of the above
d. None of the above

3303. Tian Nan Xing performs which functions at right?

3304. Ban Xia performs which functions at right?

3305. Jie Geng performs which functions at right?

a. Transform Phlegm resulting from Spleen Damp
b. Disperse Wind-Phlegm in the meridians
c. Both of the above
d. None of the above

3306. Che Qian Zi performs which functions at right?

3307. Hua Shi performs which functions at right?

3308. Jue Ming Zi performs which functions at right?

a. Clear Liver Fire to treat eye disease
b. Relieve stranguria through diuresis
c. Both of the above
d. None of the above

3309. Shi Wei is especially effective at treating which disorders at right?

3310. Jin Sha Teng is especially effective at treating which disorders at right?

3311. Yu Mi Xu is especially effective at treating which disorders at right?

a. Stones in the urine
b. Blood in the urine
c. Both of the above
d. None of the above

3312. Which statements at right are true of Su Zi?

3313. Which statements at right are true of Gua Lou?

3314. Which statements at right are true of Bai Fu Zi?

a. It is especially effective at transforming Phlegm resulting from Spleen Damp
b. It is especially effective at dispersing Wind-Phlegm in the meridians
c. Both of the above
d. None of the above

3315. Bai Zhi is very effective at treating which disorders at right?

3316. Gao Ben is very effective at treating which disorders at right?

3317. Wu Zhu Yu is very effective at treating which disorders at right?

a. Pain in the forehead
b. Parietal headache
c. Both of the above
d. None of the above

3318. Man Jing Zi is very effective at treating which disorders at right?

3319. Jing Jie is very effective at treating which disorders at right?

3320. Long Dan Cao is very effective at treating which disorders at right?

a. Headache resulting from Wind-Heat
b. Headache resulting from Liver Fire
c. Both of the above
d. None of the above

3321. Xin Yi Hua is very effective at treating which disorders at right?

3322. Xi Xin is very effective at treating which disorders at right?

3323. Bai Zhi is very effective at treating which disorders at right?

a. Headache resulting from sinusitis
b. Headache resulting from Wind-Cold
c. Both of the above
d. None of the above

3324. Fu Zi treats which disorders at right?

3325. Rou Gui treats which disorders at right?

3326. Gao Liang Jiang treats which disorders at right?

a. Devastated Yang syndrome
b. Deficient Yang of the Spleen and Kidneys syndrome
c. Both of the above
d. None of the above

3327. Yi Mu Cao performs which functions at right?

3328. Ze Lan performs which functions at right?

3329. Hong Hua performs which functions at right?

a. Invigorate the Blood and break up Blood Stasis
b. Promote urination and reduce edema
c. Both of the above
d. None of the above

3330. Tu Bie Chong performs which functions at right?

3331. Shui Zhi performs which functions at right?

3332. Zi Ran Tong performs which functions at right?

a. Break up and drive out Blood Stasis
b. Renew sinews and join bones
c. Both of the above
d. None of the above

3333. Da Zao performs which functions at right?

3334. Gan Cao performs which functions at right?

3335. Yi Tang performs which functions at right?

a. Tonify the Spleen and augment Qi
b. Alleviate abdominal pain
c. Both of the above
d. None of the above

3336. Yi Tang performs which functions at right?
3337. Gan Cao performs which functions at right?
3338. Bai He performs which functions at right?

a. Tonify the Middle Energizer and alleviate pain
b. Moisten the Lungs and stop coughs
c. Both of the above
d. None of the above

3339. Fu Xiao Mai performs which functions at right?
3340. Ma Huang Gen performs which functions at right?
3341. Nu Dao Gen Xu performs which functions at right?
3342. Hai Piao Xiao performs which functions at right?

a. Stop excessive sweating
b. Drain Fire resulting from Deficient Yin
c. Both of the above
d. None of the above

3343. Dong Gua Pi performs which functions at right?
3344. Chi Xiao Dou performs which functions at right?
3345. Dong Kui Zi performs which functions at right?

a. Clear Heat and promote urination
b. Reduce swelling and fire toxicity
c. Both of the above
d. None of the above

3346. Fu Zi performs which functions at right?
3347. Chuan Jiao performs which functions at right?
3348. Gui Zhi performs which functions at right?

a. Disperse Exterior-Cold
b. Disperse Interior-Cold
c. Both of the above
d. None of the above

3349. Rou Gui performs which functions at right?
3350. Fu Zi performs which functions at right?
3351. Xiao Hui Xiang performs which functions at right?

a. Supplement Fire and dispel Cold to relieve pain
b. Warm the Lungs and resolve Phlegm retention
c. Both of the above
d. None of the above

3352. Da Chai Hu Tang performs which functions at right?
3353. Xiao Chai Hu Tang performs which functions at right?
3354. Da Yuan Yin performs which functions at right?

a. Harmonize and release the Shao Yang
b. Drain internal clumping resulting from Heat
c. Both of the above
d. None of the above

3355. Si Ni San performs which functions at right?
3356. Xiao Yao San performs which functions at right?
3357. Tong Xie Yao Fang performs which functions at right?

a. Vent pathogenic influences and release constraint
b. Spread Liver Qi and tonify the Spleen
c. Both of the above
d. None of the above

3358. Si Ni San treats which disorders at right?

3359. Wu Zhu Yu Tang treats which disorders at right?

3360. Si Ni Tang treats which disorders at right?

a. Headache resulting from Jue Yin Deficiency-Cold and accompanied by retching and excessive salivation
b. Vomiting and diarrhea resulting from Shaoyin syndrome and accompanied by cold extremities and dysphoria
c. Both of the above
d. None of the above

3361. Hao Qin Qing Dan Tang performs which functions at right?

3362. Wen Dan Tang performs which functions at right?

3363. Du Chai Hu Tang performs which functions at right?

a. Clear the Gallbladder and harmonize the Stomach
b. Transform Phlegm
c. Both of the above
d. None of the above

3364. Chai Hu performs which functions at right in Xiao Chai Hu Tang?

3365. Chai Hu performs which functions at right in Si Ni San?

3366. Chai Hu performs which functions at right in Bu Zhong Yi Qi Tang?

a. Spread the Liver Qi to relieve Liver constraint
b. Dispel the pathogenic factor located halfway in the Exterior by driving it out
c. Both of the above
d. None of the above

3367. In cases of hypochondriac pain, Xiao Yao San is indicated for which pathogeneses at right?

3368. In cases of abdominal pain, Tong Xie Yao Feng is indicated for which pathogeneses at right?

3369. In cases of hypochondriac and chest pain, Yi Guan Jian is indicated for which pathogeneses at right?

a. Liver constraint with Deficient Blood
b. Incoordination between the Liver and Spleen
c. Both of the above
d. None of the above

3370. Which statements at right are true of Wu Mei Wan?

3371. Which statements at right are true of Ban Xia Xie Xin Tang?

a. It combines cooling and warming properties
b. It supports healthy energy to eliminate evils
c. Both of the above
d. None of the above

3372. Which herbs at right comprise the chief (monarch or *jun*) component of Si Ni San?

3373. Which herbs at right comprise the chief (monarch or *jun*) component of Xiao Chai Hu Tang

3374. Which herbs at right comprise the chief (monarch or *jun*) component of Da Chai Hu Tang?

a. Chai Hu
b. Dang Gui
c. Both of the above
d. None of the above

3375. Xiao Yao San contains which herbs at right?

3376. Hao Qin Qing Dan Tang contains which herbs at right?

3377. Tong Xie Yao Fang contains which herbs at right?

a. Bai Shao and Bai Zhu
b. Fu Ling and Gan Cao
c. Both of the above
d. None of the above

3378. Dang Gui Long Hui Wan treats which disorders at right?

3379. Long Dan Xie Gan Tang treats which disorders at right?

3380. Zuo Jin Wan treats which disorders at right?

a. Upward attack of Excessive Fire in the Liver, manifested as headache, conjunctival congestion, hypochondriac pain, a bitter taste in the mouth, deafness, pain and bulging in the ears
b. Downward flow of Damp-Heat from the Liver meridian, manifested as pruritis and swelling of the vulva, impotence, polyhidrosis around the external genitals, stranguria with turbid urine, and Damp-Heat leukorrhea
c. Both of the above
d. None of the above

3381. Gui Zhi Tang performs which functions at right?

3382. Xiang Ru San performs which functions at right?

a. Expel pathogenic factors from the muscles and skin
b. Regulate the Ying and Wei to relieve Exterior syndromes
c. Both of the above
d. None of the above

3383. Bai Shao performs which functions at right in Xiao Jian Zhong Tang?

3384. Bai Shao performs which functions at right in Dang Gui Si Ni Tang?

3385. Bai Shao performs which functions at right in Da Chai Hu Tang?

a. Replenish the Yin and Blood
b. Relieve spasms and pain
c. Both of the above
d. None of the above

3386. Which formulas at right harmonize and release the Shao Yang?

3387. Which formulas at right drain internal clumping resulting from Heat?

3388. Which formulas at right clear Gallbladder Heat and transforms Phlegm?

a. Da Chai Hu Tang
b. Xiao Chai Hu Tang
c. Both of the above
d. None of the above

3389. Gui Zhi Tang contains which herbs at right?

3390. Xiao Jian Zhong Tang contains which herbs at right?

3391. Zhi Gan Cao Tang contains which herbs at right?

a. Bai Shao and Gui Zhi
b. Sheng Jiang, Gan Cao, and Da Zao
c. Both of the above
d. None of the above

3392. Huo Xiang Zheng Qi San is indicated for which disorders at right?

3393. Ge Gen Huang Lian Huang Qin Tang is indicated for which disorders at right?

3394. Shao Yao Tang is indicated for which disorders at right?

a. Dysenteric diarrhea
b. A burning sensation around the anus
c. Both of the above
d. None of the above

3395. Gui Zhi performs which functions at right in Zhi Gan Cao Tang?

3396. Gui Zhi performs which functions at right in Zhi Shi Gua Lou Gui Zhi Tang?

a. Activate the Yang
b. Restore the pulse
c. Both of the above
d. None of the above

3397. Ci Zhu Wan performs which functions at right?

3398. Suan Zao Ren Tang performs which functions at right?

3399. Tian Wang Bu Xin Dan performs which functions at right?

a. Tranquilize the mind
b. Improve eyesight
c. Both of the above
d. None of the above

3400. Zhu Suan An Shen Wan contains which herbs at right?

3401. Tian Wang Bu Xin Dan contains which herbs at right?

3402. Suan Zao Ren Tang contains which herbs at right?

a. Zhu Sha and Huang Lian
b. Dang Gui and Sheng Di Huang
c. Both of the above
d. None of the above

3403. Jiao Ai Tang is indicated for which disorders at right?

3404. Huang Tu Tang is indicated for which disorders at right?

3405. Xiao Yi Yin Zi is indicated for which disorders at right?

a. Hemorrhage in Deficiency-Cold syndromes
b. Metrorrhagia and metrostaxis resulting from impaired and Deficient Chong and Ren meridians
c. Both of the above
d. None of the above

3406. Sheng Hua Tang is indicated for which disorders at right?

3407. Gui Zhi Fu Ling Tang is indicated for which disorders at right?

3408. Wen Jing Tang is indicated for which disorders at right?

a. Persistent uterine bleeding during pregnancy with immobile masses in the lower abdomen
b. Retention of lochia after childbirth with accompanying pain
c. Both of the above
d. None of the above

3409. Mai Ya, Yin Chen Hao, and Chuan Lian Zi perform which functions at right in Zhen Gan Xi Feng Tang?

3410. Mai Ya, Shan Zha, and Shen Qu perform which functions at right in Jian Pi Wan?

a. Clear the Liver Yang
b. Regulate the Liver Qi
c. Both of the above
d. None of the above

3411. Which formulas at right treat diabetes resulting from Deficient Kidneys and Stomach Dry?

3412. Which formulas at right treat atrophied Lungs (*fei wei*) caused by Heat resulting from Deficient Lungs and Stomach?

a. Mai Men Dong Tang
b. Yu Ye Tang
c. Both of the above
d. None of the above

3413. Zeng Ye Tang is indicated for which pathogeneses at right?

3414. Zeng Ye Cheng Qi Tang is indicated for which pathogeneses at right?

a. Retention of Heat evil
b. Depleted fluids
c. Both of the above
d. None of the above

3415. Lian Po Yin is indicated for which pathogeneses at right?

3416. Xuan Bi Tang is indicated for which pathogeneses at right?

3417. Ping Wei San is indicated for which pathogeneses at right?

a. Contained Damp-Heat in the meridians
b. Contained Damp-Heat in the Spleen and Stomach
c. Both of the above
d. None of the above

3418. Juan Bi Tang treats which disorders at right?

3419. Du Huo Ji Sheng Tang treats which disorders at right?

3420. Qiang Huo Sheng Shi Tang treats which disorders at right?

a. Wind-Cold-Damp evil obstructing the muscles and joints, leading to persistent arthralgia syndrome with Deficient Liver and Kidneys, and Deficient Qi and Blood
b. Deficient Qi of the Ying and Wei, leading to Wind-Cold-Damp obstruction that changes position and relatively early-stage pain (*bi*) syndrome
c. Both of the above
d. None of the above

3421. Zhi Shi Xiao Pi Wan contains which herbs at right?

3422. Jian Pi Wan contains which herbs at right?

a. All of the herbs in Si Jun Zi Tang
b. Huang Lian and Chen Pi
c. Both of the above
d. None of the above

3423. Zhi Shi Xiao Pi Wan performs which functions at right?

3424. Mu Xiang Bing Lang Wan performs which functions at right?

3425. Zhi Zhu Wan performs which functions at right?

a. Strengthen the Spleen
b. Reduce focal distention and eliminate fullness
c. Both of the above
d. None of the above

3426. Gui Pi Tang performs which functions at right?

3427. Xiao Yao San performs which functions at right?

3428. Jian Pi Wan performs which functions at right?

a. Strengthen the Spleen and nourish the Blood
b. Spread the Liver Qi
c. Both of the above
d. None of the above

3429. An Gong Niu Huang Wan is indicated for which disorders at right?

3430. Zi Xue Dan is indicated for which disorders at right?

3431. Huang Lian Jie Du Tang is indicated for which disorders at right?

a. High fever, irritability, and restlessness
b. Impaired consciousness and delirious speech
c. Both of the above
d. None of the above

3432. Zhen Zhu Mu Wan performs which functions at right?

3433. Suan Zao Ren Tang performs which functions at right?

3434. Ci Zhu Wan performs which functions at right?

a. Nourish the Blood and calm the Spirit
b. Clear Heat and eliminate irritability
c. Both of the above
d. None of the above

3435. Da Qin Jiao Tang contains which herbs at right?

3436. Chuan Xiong Cha Tiao San contains which herbs at right?

3437. Yin Qiao San contains which herbs at right?

a. Fang Feng and Jing Jie
b. Qiang Huo and Bai Zhi
c. Both of the above
d. None of the above

3438. Bu Yang Huan Wu Tang is indicated for which pathogeneses at right?

3439. Dan Shen Yin is indicated for which pathogeneses at right?

3440. Yu Ping Feng San is indicated for which pathogeneses at right?

a. Deficient Qi
b. Blood Stasis
c. Both of the above
d. None of the above

3441. Bu Zhong Yi Qi Tang contains which herbs at right?

3442. Shen Ling Bai Zhu San contains which herbs at right?

3443. Gui Pi Tang contains which herbs at right?

a. Ren Shen, Bai Zhu, Fu Ling, and Zhi Gan Cao
b. Dang Gui, Chen Pi, Sheng Ma, and Chai Hu
c. Both of the above
d. None of the above

3444. Bai He Gu Jin Tang contains which herbs at right?

3445. Tian Wang Bu Xin Dan contains which herbs at right?

3446. Yang Yin Qing Fei Tang contains which herbs at right?

a. Xuan Shen, Sheng Di Huang, and Mai Men Dong
b. Bai Shao, Dang Gui, and Bei Mu
c. Both of the above
d. None of the above

3447. Which formulas at right use a large dosage of Tao Ren?
3448. Which formulas at right use a large dosage of Dang Gui?
3449. Which formulas at right use a large dosage of Mai Men Dong?

a. Sheng Hua Tang
b. Bu Yang Huan Wu Tang
c. Both of the above
d. None of the above

3450. Chai Hu performs which functions at right in Da Chai Hu Tang?
3451. Chai Hu performs which functions at right in Bu Zhong Yi Qi Tang?
3452. Chai Hu performs which functions at right in Xiao Yao San?

a. Soothe the Liver and regulate the circulation of Qi
b. Focus the actions of the other herbs on the Liver and Gallbladder meridians
c. Both of the above
d. None of the above

3453. Qui Pi Tang contains which herbs at right?
3454. Du Huo Ji Sheng Tang contains which herbs at right?
3455. Bai He Gu Jin Tang contains which herbs at right?

a. Dang Gui and Ren Shen
b. Sheng Di Huang and Bai Shao
c. Both of the above
d. None of the above

3456. Da Ding Fen Zhu contains which herbs at right?
3457. E Jiao Ji Zi Huang Tang contains which herbs at right?
3458. San Jia Fu Mai Tang contains which herbs at right?

a. Ji Zi Huang, E Jiao, and Bai Shao
b. Gui Ban, Bie Jia, and Mu Li
c. Both of the above
d. None of the above

3459. Xue Fi Zhu Yu Tang contains which herbs at right?
3460. Sheng Hua Tang contains which herbs at right?
3461. Bu Yang Hua Wu Tang contains which herbs at right?

a. Hong Hua and Tao Ren
b. Dang Gui and Chuan Xiong
c. Both of the above
d. None of the above

3462. Su Zi Jiang Qi Tang contains which herbs at right?
3463. Ju PI Zhu Ru Tang contains which herbs at right?
3464. Ding Xiang Su Di Tang contains which herbs at right?

a. Ban Xia and Hou Po
b. Sheng Jiang and Ren Shen
c. Both of the above
d. None of the above

3465. Bai Dou Kou is indicated for which pathogeneses at right?
3466. Cang Zhu is indicated for which pathogeneses at right?
3467. Yi Yi Ren is indicated for which pathogeneses at right?

a. Disturbance of the Middle Energizer due to accumulation of Damp
b. Wind-Cold-Damp arthralgia
c. Both of the above
d. None of the above

3468. Which functions at right do Bu Gu Zhi and Suo Yang have in common?

3469. Which functions at right do Yin Yang Huo and Ba Ji Tian have in common?

3470. Which functions at right do Guang Fang Ji and Xi Xian Cao have in common?

a. Tonify the Kidneys and strengthen the Yang
b. Dispel Wind and eliminate Damp
c. Both of the above
d. None of the above

3471. Wu Zhu Yu is indicated for which disorders at right?

3472. Bu Gu Zhi is indicated for which disorders at right?

3473. Rou Dou Kou is indicated for which disorders at right?

a. Impotence, premature ejaculation, and enuresis resulting from Deficient Kidney Yang
b. Diarrhea occurring before dawn resulting from Deficient Yang of the Spleen and Kidneys
c. Both of the above
d. None of the above

3474. Hai Zao performs which functions at right?

3475. Fu Hai Shi performs which functions at right?

3476. Tian Zhu Huang performs which functions at right?

a. Clear Heat from the Lungs and expel Phlegm Heat
b. Soften hardness and dissipate Phlegm nodules
c. Both of the above
d. None of the above

3477. Huang Bai is indicated for which disorders at right?

3478. Shi Gao is indicated for which disorders at right?

3479. Zhi Mu is indicated for which disorders at right?

a. Epidemic febrile diseases with high fever and dire thirst
b. Hyperactivity of Fire marked by night sweats and hectic fever resulting from Deficient Yin
c. Both of the above
d. None of the above

3480. Tong Cao performs which functions at right?

3481. Yin Chen Hao performs which functions at right?

3482. Dong Kui Zi performs which functions at right?

a. Benefit the breasts
b. Promote urination
c. Both of the above
d. None of the above

3483. Which functions at right do Pu Gong Yin and Zi Hua Di Ding have in common?

3484. Which functions at right do Tian Ma and Gou Teng have in common?

3485. Which functions at right do Ling Yang Jiao and Niu Huang have in common?

a. Clear away Heat and toxins
b. Check endogenous Wind to relieve convulsions
c. Both of the above
d. None of the above

3486. Which functions at right do Yi Mu Cao and Ze Lan have in common?

3487. Which functions at right do Hong Hua and Niu Xi have in common?

3488. Which functions at right do Mu Tong and Ma Huang have in common?

a. Invigorate Blood cirulation to
b. remove Blood Stasis
c. Relieve edema by inducing enuresis
d. Both of the above
e. None of the above

3489. Ru Xiang and Mo Yao is indicated for which disorders at right?

3490. Bai Zhi and Zao Qiao Ci is indicated for which disorders at right?

3491. Qian Dan and Lu Gan Shi is indicated for which disorders at right?

a. Early-stage carbuncles where there is no pus
b. Carbuncles that are suppurated
c. Both of the above
d. None of the above

3492. Which functions at right do Dang Gui and Ji Xue Teng have in common?

3493. Which functions at right do Shu Di Huang and E Jiao have in common?

3494. Which functions at right do Gui Ban and Da Zao have in common?

a. Tonify the Blood and promote Blood circulation
b. Nourish the Blood and calm the Spirit
c. Both of the above
d. None of the above

3495. Which treatments at right do Sang Ji Sheng and Xu Duan have in common?

3496. Which treatmentss at right do Sha Ren and Huang Qin have in common?

3497. Which treatments at right do Chen Pi and Sheng Jiang have in common?

a. Treats pernicious vomiting
b. Treats threat of miscarriage
c. Both of the above
d. None of the above

3498. Shan Zhu Yu is indicated for which disorders at right

3499. Wu Wei Zi is indicated for which disorders at right?

3500. Lian Zi is indicated for which disorders at right?

a. Chronic cough and asthma resulting from Deficiency
b. Night sweats and nocturnal emissions
c. Both of the above
d. None of the above

Answers to the Questions

ANSWERS TO THE STOREHOUSE OF QUESTIONS

1. C	61. C	121. B	181. A	241. D	301. C	361. D
2. D	62. A	122. A	182. B	242. A	302. D	362. A
3. B	63. D	123. B	183. B	243. D	303. C	363. D
4. C	64. C	124. C	184. A	244. B	304. A	364. D
5. C	65. D	125. C	185. C	245. D	305. D	365. B
6. A	66. A	126. D	186. B	246. B	306. C	366. D
7. B	67. D	127. A	187. B	247. A	307. B	367. B
8. C	68. B	128. B	188. B	248. D	308. D	368. D
9. B	69. D	129. D	189. A	249. B	309. D	369. A
10. D	70. D	130. D	190. C	250. B	310. B	370. C
11. D	71. B	131. A	191. D	251. C	311. C	371. B
12. C	72. A	132. A	192. C	252. C	312. D	372. A
13. B	73. C	133. A	193. D	253. B	313. C	373. D
14. D	74. C	134. A	194. C	254. C	314. B	374. D
15. E	75. B	135. C	195. D	255. C	315. D	375. B
16. C	76. D	136. A	196. D	256. C	316. A	376. B
17. C	77. A	137. C	197. C	257. D	317. C	377. B
18. D	78. C	138. D	198. C	258. B	318. A	378. C
19. D	79. C	139. D	199. A	259. B	319. B	379. C
20. D	80. A	140. D	200. D	260. A	320. C	380. B
21. C	81. D	141. D	201. B	261. C	321. D	381. B
22. C	82. C	142. D	202. C	262. B	322. D	382. D
23. B	83. D	143. A	203. B	263. B	323. D	383. D
24. C	84. B	144. C	204. A	264. A	324. D	384. B
25. C	85. C	145. B	205. D	265. C	325. A	385. C
26. C	86. A	146. A	206. C	266. C	326. A	386. A
27. C	87. A	147. B	207. D	267. D	327. C	387. D
28. B	88. A	148. D	208. A	268. C	328. A	388. C
29. B	89. B	149. D	209. C	269. D	329. B	389. D
30. A	90. A	150. B	210. B	270. A	330. D	390. B
31. D	91. B	151. C	211. D	271. D	331. D	391. B
32. D	92. C	152. A	212. D	272. D	332. C	392. B
33. B	93. D	153. D	213. D	273. C	333. A	393. C
34. D	94. C	154. D	214. D	274. D	334. B	394. C
35. B	95. A	155. D	215. D	275. D	335. A	395. C
36. C	96. C	156. B	216. A	276. D	336. B	396. A
37. C	97. A	157. D	217. C	277. B	337. C	397. D
38. B	98. A	158. C	218. C	278. A	338. D	398. C
39. D	99. A	159. B	219. D	279. D	339. D	399. B
40. C	100. D	160. C	220. B	280. D	340. B	400. D
41. C	101. B	161. D	221. A	281. A	341. A	401. C
42. A	102. B	162. C	222. C	282. B	342. A	402. C
43. D	103. B	163. D	223. B	283. A	343. B	403. B
44. D	104. D	164. D	224. B	284. C	344. D	404. B
45. B	105. D	165. D	225. C	285. C	345. A	405. B
46. B	106. D	166. A	226. B	286. C	346. A	406. C
47. D	107. B	167. C	227. A	287. C	347. C	407. D
48. C	108. A	168. B	228. C	288. D	348. B	408. A
49. D	109. B	169. C	229. A	289. D	349. C	409. A
50. D	110. B	170. C	230. D	290. D	350. B	410. A
51. C	111. A	171. B	231. D	291. D	351. D	411. C
52. A	112. B	172. D	232. C	292. D	352. B	412. B
53. D	113. C	173. C	233. A	293. C	353. D	413. B
54. A	114. D	174. D	234. B	294. A	354. C	414. B
55. C	115. C	175. D	235. C	295. C	355. D	415. A
56. C	116. C	176. C	236. A	296. D	356. D	416. B
57. B	117. B	177. A	237. C	297. A	357. B	417. C
58. C	118. C	178. D	238. C	298. D	358. C	418. C
59. B	119. C	179. C	239. B	299. A	359. D	419. B
60. D	120. C	180. D	240. C	300. A	360. A	420. C

421. C	488. D	555. B	622. D	689. D	756. C	823. C
422. D	489. A	556. B	623. B	690. D	757. D	824. C
423. C	490. B	557. C	624. C	691. B	758. D	825. C
424. A	491. C	558. A	625. A	692. D	759. B	826. A
425. A	492. D	559. D	626. A	693. A	760. A	827. C
426. B	493. A	560. A	627. C	694. C	761. B	828. D
427. D	494. A	561. B	628. C	695. B	762. C	829. D
428. B	495. D	562. B	629. C	696. C	763. A	830. A
429. D	496. A	563. D	630. B	697. C	764. A	831. C
430. B	497. B	564. D	631. D	698. C	765. B	832. C
431. B	498. C	565. C	632. A	699. D	766. A	833. B
432. A	499. A	566. C	633. B	700. D	767. C	834. B
433. A	500. B	567. C	634. A	701. C	768. B	835. A
434. C	501. A	568. A	635. B	702. B	769. B	836. D
435. D	502. A	569. C	636. A	703. C	770. A	837. A
436. C	503. A	570. C	637. B	704. D	771. B	838. D
437. B	504. C	571. B	638. A	705. B	772. D	839. A
438. B	505. A	572. C	639. A	706. C	773. B	840. D
439. C	506. D	573. B	640. B	707. D	774. D	841. A
440. C	507. B	574. C	641. C	708. D	775. B	842. B
441. D	508. A	575. A	642. B	709. C	776. A	843. B
442. C	509. D	576. B	643. C	710. D	777. B	844. B
443. C	510. C	577. D	644. A	711. C	778. A	845. D
444. C	511. A	578. B	645. D	712. D	779. A	846. A
445. A	512. D	579. D	646. D	713. C	780. A	847. D
446. D	513. D	580. D	647. A	714. C	781. A	848. A
447. D	514. B	581. D	648. C	715. C	782. C	849. A
448. D	515. D	582. B	649. C	716. B	783. C	850. A
449. C	516. D	583. B	650. C	717. B	784. D	851. B
450. D	517. C	584. C	651. C	718. D	785. B	852. C
451. D	518. C	585. C	652. B	719. C	786. D	853. C
452. A	519. D	586. C	653. C	720. C	787. B	854. D
453. B	520. D	587. D	654. C	721. B	788. A	855. C
454. C	521. A	588. B	655. A	722. D	789. C	856. C
455. A	522. C	589. D	656. B	723. D	790. B	857. A
456. A	523. D	590. D	657. C	724. B	791. D	858. A
457. B	524. A	591. D	658. B	725. C	792. D	859. D
458. C	525. D	592. C	659. B	726. C	793. B	860. D
459. C	526. D	593. C	660. B	727. A	794. A	861. D
460. A	527. B	594. C	661. D	728. B	795. A	862. D
461. B	528. B	595. C	662. C	729. B	796. C	863. C
462. B	529. B	596. A	663. D	730. D	797. C	864. C
463. A	530. B	597. C	664. C	731. C	798. C	865. D
464. C	531. D	598. C	665. D	732. D	799. C	866. C
465. C	532. C	599. D	666. D	733. C	800. B	867. D
466. D	533. B	600. B	667. C	734. A	801. B	868. C
467. C	534. C	601. C	668. D	735. C	802. D	869. A
468. B	535. B	602. B	669. D	736. C	803. D	870. B
469. C	536. D	603. C	670. A	737. D	804. B	871. A
470. B	537. D	604. C	671. D	738. C	805. A	872. C
471. D	538. C	605. D	672. C	739. C	806. B	873. B
472. C	539. D	606. D	673. D	740. D	807. D	874. D
473. A	540. D	607. B	674. D	741. D	808. B	875. B
474. D	541. B	608. C	675. C	742. A	809. C	876. A
475. B	542. A	609. B	676. D	743. B	810. D	877. B
476. D	543. D	610. C	677. D	744. C	811. C	878. D
477. B	544. B	611. C	678. A	745. B	812. C	879. D
478. A	545. D	612. B	679. D	746. C	813. D	880. C
479. B	546. C	613. D	680. D	747. C	814. D	881. C
480. B	547. A	614. B	681. B	748. B	815. D	882. A
481. B	548. D	615. C	682. B	749. A	816. C	883. D
482. A	549. B	616. C	683. C	750. A	817. D	884. B
483. A	550. B	617. B	684. D	751. C	818. D	885. B
484. D	551. C	618. A	685. D	752. D	819. B	886. B
485. A	552. A	619. A	686. D	753. C	820. C	887. B
486. C	553. D	620. C	687. C	754. A	821. B	888. A
487. B	554. A	621. B	688. C	755. D	822. C	889. D

890. D	957. A	1024. C	1091. C	1158. B	1225. A	1292. C
891. D	958. D	1025. C	1092. D	1159. D	1226. D	1293. A
892. D	959. C	1026. A	1093. C	1160. D	1227. A	1294. B
893. D	960. A	1027. D	1094. D	1161. C	1228. C	1295. A
894. D	961. C	1028. C	1095. A	1162. D	1229. C	1296. B
895. C	962. D	1029. A	1096. D	1163. B	1230. D	1297. A
896. B	963. C	1030. D	1097. D	1164. A	1231. D	1298. C
897. A	964. B	1031. C	1098. C	1165. C	1232. C	1299. B
898. D	965. B	1032. B	1099. D	1166. D	1233. D	1300. D
899. A	966. B	1033. B	1100. D	1167. D	1234. B	1301. A
900. D	967. C	1034. B	1101. C	1168. A	1235. D	1302. B
901. B	968. B	1035. B	1102. C	1169. D	1236. D	1303. B
902. C	969. C	1036. A	1103. C	1170. A	1237. C	1304. A
903. C	970. D	1037. C	1104. C	1171. B	1238. B	1305. B
904. B	971. D	1038. A	1105. C	1172. D	1239. B	1306. D
905. C	972. D	1039. D	1106. D	1173. C	1240. D	1307. B
906. A	973. C	1040. A	1107. C	1174. D	1241. B	1308. B
907. C	974. B	1041. D	1108. D	1175. D	1242. B	1309. C
908. D	975. D	1042. A	1109. D	1176. C	1243. C	1310. D
909. D	976. D	1043. D	1110. B	1177. C	1244. D	1311. D
910. D	977. C	1044. D	1111. A	1178. D	1245. D	1312. C
911. C	978. C	1045. A	1112. A	1179. C	1246. A	1313. B
912. A	979. B	1046. A	1113. A	1180. B	1247. D	1314. B
913. B	980. A	1047. D	1114. D	1181. C	1248. C	1315. A
914. A	981. D	1048. C	1115. D	1182. D	1249. C	1316. A
915. B	982. A	1049. D	1116. C	1183. D	1250. B	1317. C
916. B	983. A	1050. A	1117. C	1184. D	1251. C	1318. B
917. A	984. D	1051. A	1118. C	1185. A	1252. D	1319. C
918. C	985. C	1052. A	1119. A	1186. D	1253. A	1320. C
919. B	986. C	1053. D	1120. D	1187. B	1254. A	1321. B
920. D	987. A	1054. A	1121. D	1188. C	1255. A	1322. C
921. D	988. D	1055. C	1122. B	1189. D	1256. B	1323. A
922. A	989. B	1056. B	1123. C	1190. A	1257. D	1324. B
923. A	990. D	1057. D	1124. B	1191. D	1258. D	1325. C
924. A	991. D	1058. C	1125. B	1192. C	1259. A	1326. B
925. B	992. D	1059. D	1126. A	1193. D	1260. B	1327. B
926. A	993. A	1060. B	1127. D	1194. C	1261. C	1328. A
927. C	994. D	1061. C	1128. A	1195. C	1262. D	1329. A
928. D	995. D	1062. B	1129. D	1196. D	1263. B	1330. B
929. D	996. D	1063. C	1130. D	1197. C	1264. C	1331. D
930. D	997. D	1064. D	1131. C	1198. A	1265. C	1332. D
931. C	998. D	1065. C	1132. C	1199. D	1266. D	1333. D
932. C	999. B	1066. A	1133. C	1200. A	1267. D	1334. D
933. D	1000. C	1067. B	1134. D	1201. B	1268. D	1335. A
934. A	1001. D	1068. C	1135. C	1202. C	1269. B	1336. C
935. C	1002. D	1069. C	1136. C	1203. D	1270. C	1337. C
936. D	1003. C	1070. A	1137. D	1204. D	1271. C	1338. B
937. D	1004. C	1071. D	1138. A	1205. B	1272. C	1339. D
938. C	1005. D	1072. C	1139. B	1206. A	1273. C	1340. B
939. C	1006. D	1073. D	1140. D	1207. A	1274. B	1341. A
940. C	1007. B	1074. D	1141. A	1208. A	1275. A	1342. B
941. A	1008. C	1075. A	1142. B	1209. A	1276. B	1343. B
942. D	1009. C	1076. A	1143. D	1210. A	1277. A	1344. B
943. D	1010. C	1077. B	1144. D	1211. D	1278. C	1345. B
944. B	1011. D	1078. B	1145. C	1212. C	1279. B	1346. A
945. C	1012. D	1079. B	1146. D	1213. C	1280. B	1347. D
946. C	1013. C	1080. C	1147. D	1214. D	1281. D	1348. D
947. D	1014. C	1081. D	1148. A	1215. D	1282. D	1349. D
948. A	1015. B	1082. A	1149. B	1216. D	1283. A	1350. D
949. C	1016. D	1083. A	1150. B	1217. B	1284. C	1351. D
950. B	1017. A	1084. D	1151. B	1218. D	1285. C	1352. D
951. D	1018. A	1085. D	1152. B	1219. D	1286. C	1353. D
952. B	1019. D	1086. B	1153. C	1220. D	1287. B	1354. D
953. A	1020. D	1087. D	1154. A	1221. C	1288. A	1355. B
954. D	1021. D	1088. A	1155. D	1222. C	1289. A	1356. A
955. C	1022. D	1089. D	1156. B	1223. D	1290. C	1357. D
956. A	1023. D	1090. D	1157. C	1224. B	1291. B	1358. C

#	Ans	#	Ans	#	Ans	#	Ans	#	Ans	#	Ans	#	Ans
1359.	D	1426.	D	1493.	D	1560.	C	1627.	C	1694.	D	1761.	D
1360.	A	1427.	B	1494.	C	1561.	B	1628.	D	1695.	D	1762.	B
1361.	C	1428.	A	1495.	A	1562.	D	1629.	B	1696.	C	1763.	C
1362.	C	1429.	B	1496.	A	1563.	C	1630.	C	1697.	C	1764.	D
1363.	D	1430.	B	1497.	D	1564.	B	1631.	C	1698.	D	1765.	D
1364.	C	1431.	B	1498.	C	1565.	D	1632.	B	1699.	C	1766.	D
1365.	D	1432.	A	1499.	B	1566.	C	1633.	D	1700.	C	1767.	C
1366.	B	1433.	D	1500.	D	1567.	C	1634.	C	1701.	D	1768.	D
1367.	B	1434.	A	1501.	D	1568.	B	1635.	C	1702.	A	1769.	C
1368.	D	1435.	A	1502.	D	1569.	B	1636.	C	1703.	D	1770.	A
1369.	D	1436.	B	1503.	D	1570.	C	1637.	D	1704.	B	1771.	D
1370.	C	1437.	B	1504.	C	1571.	B	1638.	B	1705.	B	1772.	A
1371.	C	1438.	C	1505.	D	1572.	C	1639.	D	1706.	D	1773.	D
1372.	C	1439.	A	1506.	C	1573.	D	1640.	D	1707.	C	1774.	C
1373.	A	1440.	B	1507.	C	1574.	B	1641.	B	1708.	D	1775.	A
1374.	B	1441.	A	1508.	D	1575.	D	1642.	A	1709.	C	1776.	C
1375.	D	1442.	B	1509.	C	1576.	C	1643.	D	1710.	A	1777.	D
1376.	B	1443.	D	1510.	D	1577.	C	1644.	C	1711.	B	1778.	C
1377.	A	1444.	B	1511.	C	1578.	A	1645.	A	1712.	C	1779.	C
1378.	D	1445.	A	1512.	B	1579.	C	1646.	C	1713.	D	1780.	B
1379.	D	1446.	A	1513.	A	1580.	C	1647.	B	1714.	C	1781.	B
1380.	B	1447.	C	1514.	B	1581.	B	1648.	D	1715.	D	1782.	C
1381.	C	1448.	A	1515.	A	1582.	C	1649.	C	1716.	C	1783.	D
1382.	B	1449.	D	1516.	A	1583.	C	1650.	B	1717.	D	1784.	D
1383.	D	1450.	B	1517.	B	1584.	D	1651.	C	1718.	B	1785.	D
1384.	D	1451.	A	1518.	B	1585.	A	1652.	B	1719.	D	1786.	C
1385.	D	1452.	C	1519.	D	1586.	C	1653.	C	1720.	B	1787.	C
1386.	D	1453.	C	1520.	D	1587.	C	1654.	C	1721.	A	1788.	C
1387.	B	1454.	C	1521.	B	1588.	B	1655.	C	1722.	C	1789.	C
1388.	D	1455.	B	1522.	C	1589.	D	1656.	C	1723.	D	1790.	D
1389.	B	1456.	C	1523.	B	1590.	B	1657.	D	1724.	C	1791.	D
1390.	C	1457.	A	1524.	A	1591.	B	1658.	C	1725.	C	1792.	A
1391.	B	1458.	A	1525.	B	1592.	A	1659.	C	1726.	D	1793.	A
1392.	D	1459.	B	1526.	C	1593.	C	1660.	C	1727.	B	1794.	C
1393.	A	1460.	D	1527.	C	1594.	C	1661.	C	1728.	A	1795.	C
1394.	C	1461.	A	1528.	D	1595.	C	1662.	D	1729.	C	1796.	C
1395.	C	1462.	B	1529.	B	1596.	D	1663.	D	1730.	D	1797.	C
1396.	B	1463.	B	1530.	A	1597.	B	1664.	D	1731.	C	1798.	A
1397.	C	1464.	C	1531.	A	1598.	C	1665.	C	1732.	A	1799.	D
1398.	C	1465.	A	1532.	C	1599.	D	1666.	D	1733.	B	1800.	D
1399.	D	1466.	B	1533.	D	1600.	C	1667.	A	1734.	D	1801.	E
1400.	D	1467.	A	1534.	B	1601.	C	1668.	B	1735.	B	1802.	D
1401.	D	1468.	D	1535.	A	1602.	C	1669.	A	1736.	A	1803.	A
1402.	D	1469.	B	1536.	D	1603.	C	1670.	C	1737.	C	1804.	C
1403.	C	1470.	A	1537.	B	1604.	C	1671.	C	1738.	D	1805.	C
1404.	D	1471.	B	1538.	C	1605.	B	1672.	C	1739.	D	1806.	B
1405.	B	1472.	A	1539.	D	1606.	C	1673.	D	1740.	C	1807.	C
1406.	A	1473.	C	1540.	C	1607.	D	1674.	B	1741.	C	1808.	A
1407.	C	1474.	D	1541.	C	1608.	D	1675.	C	1742.	D	1809.	D
1408.	B	1475.	C	1542.	C	1609.	B	1676.	C	1743.	C	1810.	A
1409.	D	1476.	C	1543.	C	1610.	C	1677.	D	1744.	C	1811.	B
1410.	D	1477.	A	1544.	C	1611.	C	1678.	D	1745.	B	1812.	C
1411.	D	1478.	A	1545.	D	1612.	D	1679.	A	1746.	D	1813.	B
1412.	B	1479.	B	1546.	C	1613.	D	1680.	A	1747.	D	1814.	C
1413.	A	1480.	B	1547.	D	1614.	D	1681.	C	1748.	A	1815.	D
1414.	B	1481.	C	1548.	B	1615.	D	1682.	C	1749.	C	1816.	B
1415.	B	1482.	D	1549.	D	1616.	B	1683.	D	1750.	D	1817.	C
1416.	D	1483.	D	1550.	C	1617.	C	1684.	D	1751.	D	1818.	C
1417.	C	1484.	C	1551.	C	1618.	C	1685.	C	1752.	C	1819.	D
1418.	C	1485.	D	1552.	A	1619.	B	1686.	C	1753.	B	1820.	D
1419.	B	1486.	A	1553.	A	1620.	D	1687.	C	1754.	D	1821.	C
1420.	A	1487.	D	1554.	B	1621.	C	1688.	C	1755.	C	1822.	A
1421.	B	1488.	A	1555.	D	1622.	A	1689.	D	1756.	C	1823.	E
1422.	C	1489.	C	1556.	C	1623.	D	1690.	C	1757.	B	1824.	D
1423.	B	1490.	C	1557.	B	1624.	D	1691.	D	1758.	D	1825.	D
1424.	A	1491.	D	1558.	D	1625.	D	1692.	D	1759.	A	1826.	C
1425.	B	1492.	D	1559.	C	1626.	D	1693.	B	1760.	D	1827.	E

1828.	D	1895.	E	1962.	A	2029.	A	2096.	A	2163.	B	2230.	A
1829.	B	1896.	B	1963.	E	2030.	B	2097.	E	2164.	E	2231.	B
1830.	A	1897.	C	1964.	A	2031.	E	2098.	A	2165.	C	2232.	C
1831.	D	1898.	E	1965.	A	2032.	A	2099.	C	2166.	A	2233.	E
1832.	B	1899.	D	1966.	A	2033.	D	2100.	D	2167.	D	2234.	A
1833.	C	1900.	E	1967.	C	2034.	E	2101.	B	2168.	E	2235.	A
1834.	C	1901.	C	1968.	C	2035.	B	2102.	E	2169.	C	2236.	D
1835.	D	1902.	A	1969.	C	2036.	C	2103.	A	2170.	A	2237.	C
1836.	B	1903.	B	1970.	A	2037.	A	2104.	B	2171.	A	2238.	D
1837.	E	1904.	C	1971.	A	2038.	E	2105.	C	2172.	C	2239.	B
1838.	E	1905.	A	1972.	D	2039.	D	2106.	C	2173.	D	2240.	C
1839.	A	1906.	B	1973.	A	2040.	A	2107.	A	2174.	B	2241.	E
1840.	C	1907.	E	1974.	B	2041.	B	2108.	C	2175.	C	2242.	A
1841.	D	1908.	B	1975.	B	2042.	D	2109.	B	2176.	E	2243.	C
1842.	A	1909.	C	1976.	E	2043.	B	2110.	A	2177.	B	2244.	B
1843.	A	1910.	A	1977.	A	2044.	A	2111.	B	2178.	C	2245.	E
1844.	B	1911.	B	1978.	B	2045.	E	2112.	C	2179.	D	2246.	B
1845.	E	1912.	A	1979.	E	2046.	C	2113.	A	2180.	B	2247.	D
1846.	C	1913.	B	1980.	D	2047.	D	2114.	C	2181.	C	2248.	A
1847.	E	1914.	C	1981.	B	2048.	B	2115.	B	2182.	E	2249.	C
1848.	A	1915.	B	1982.	A	2049.	C	2116.	D	2183.	B	2250.	A
1849.	C	1916.	C	1983.	C	2050.	D	2117.	E	2184.	C	2251.	B
1850.	B	1917.	D	1984.	D	2051.	A	2118.	B	2185.	B	2252.	C
1851.	D	1918.	A	1985.	B	2052.	D	2119.	D	2186.	D	2253.	D
1852.	E	1919.	A	1986.	A	2053.	C	2120.	C	2187.	C	2254.	D
1853.	D	1920.	B	1987.	A	2054.	A	2121.	A	2188.	B	2255.	A
1854.	A	1921.	A	1988.	E	2055.	A	2122.	D	2189.	B	2256.	C
1855.	C	1922.	B	1989.	B	2056.	B	2123.	D	2190.	D	2257.	B
1856.	B	1923.	E	1990.	C	2057.	C	2124.	B	2191.	D	2258.	D
1857.	C	1924.	C	1991.	A	2058.	D	2125.	C	2192.	C	2259.	C
1858.	B	1925.	A	1992.	B	2059.	D	2126.	D	2193.	B	2260.	B
1859.	A	1926.	E	1993.	C	2060.	A	2127.	A	2194.	D	2261.	D
1860.	E	1927.	A	1994.	B	2061.	D	2128.	E	2195.	A	2262.	D
1861.	A	1928.	E	1995.	E	2062.	A	2129.	C	2196.	B	2263.	A
1862.	B	1929.	A	1996.	E	2063.	B	2130.	E	2197.	C	2264.	B
1863.	E	1930.	D	1997.	D	2064.	E	2131.	D	2198.	D	2265.	B
1864.	A	1931.	E	1998.	A	2065.	D	2132.	A	2199.	A	2266.	A
1865.	B	1932.	C	1999.	B	2066.	A	2133.	B	2200.	D	2267.	A
1866.	A	1933.	A	2000.	A	2067.	C	2134.	A	2201.	B	2268.	B
1867.	D	1934.	A	2001.	E	2068.	B	2135.	A	2202.	D	2269.	E
1868.	E	1935.	E	2002.	C	2069.	C	2136.	C	2203.	C	2270.	D
1869.	B	1936.	A	2003.	D	2070.	D	2137.	A	2204.	A	2271.	A
1870.	E	1937.	B	2004.	A	2071.	A	2138.	C	2205.	D	2272.	B
1871.	A	1938.	C	2005.	A	2072.	B	2139.	B	2206.	A	2273.	A
1872.	C	1939.	A	2006.	C	2073.	C	2140.	D	2207.	D	2274.	C
1873.	E	1940.	B	2007.	D	2074.	D	2141.	E	2208.	E	2275.	E
1874.	D	1941.	C	2008.	E	2075.	A	2142.	A	2209.	A	2276.	D
1875.	C	1942.	B	2009.	A	2076.	E	2143.	B	2210.	D	2277.	E
1876.	B	1943.	A	2010.	C	2077.	E	2144.	D	2211.	B	2278.	A
1877.	E	1944.	C	2011.	B	2078.	A	2145.	C	2212.	C	2279.	C
1878.	B	1945.	D	2012.	C	2079.	C	2146.	A	2213.	A	2280.	D
1879.	C	1946.	A	2013.	A	2080.	C	2147.	B	2214.	B	2281.	B
1880.	C	1947.	B	2014.	B	2081.	B	2148.	A	2215.	B	2282.	D
1881.	E	1948.	E	2015.	D	2082.	D	2149.	C	2216.	C	2283.	C
1882.	A	1949.	C	2016.	E	2083.	A	2150.	A	2217.	E	2284.	C
1883.	B	1950.	A	2017.	C	2084.	C	2151.	E	2218.	D	2285.	B
1884.	C	1951.	C	2018.	E	2085.	E	2152.	D	2219.	C	2286.	C
1885.	A	1952.	B	2019.	D	2086.	A	2153.	E	2220.	B	2287.	E
1886.	B	1953.	D	2020.	C	2087.	C	2154.	A	2221.	B	2288.	C
1887.	D	1954.	A	2021.	D	2088.	B	2155.	A	2222.	B	2289.	D
1888.	A	1955.	E	2022.	E	2089.	A	2156.	B	2223.	B	2290.	B
1889.	E	1956.	D	2023.	A	2090.	B	2157.	C	2224.	D	2291.	A
1890.	C	1957.	D	2024.	C	2091.	E	2158.	A	2225.	A	2292.	B
1891.	A	1958.	E	2025.	D	2092.	A	2159.	D	2226.	E	2293.	B
1892.	C	1959.	C	2026.	E	2093.	C	2160.	B	2227.	C	2294.	A
1893.	A	1960.	A	2027.	E	2094.	E	2161.	D	2228.	B	2295.	E
1894.	A	1961.	E	2028.	D	2095.	D	2162.	A	2229.	A	2296.	A

2297. C	2364. B	2431. B	2498. E	2565. C	2632. B	2699. A
2298. A	2365. C	2432. A	2499. C	2566. B	2633. D	2700. C
2299. D	2366. D	2433. E	2500. A	2567. D	2634. C	2701. A
2300. D	2367. E	2434. D	2501. B	2568. A	2635. A	2702. C
2301. C	2368. E	2435. B	2502. B	2569. A	2636. D	2703. B
2302. D	2369. C	2436. E	2503. D	2570. C	2637. C	2704. B
2303. B	2370. B	2437. D	2504. A	2571. C	2638. A	2705. C
2304. A	2371. C	2438. A	2505. B	2572. A	2639. D	2706. A
2305. D	2372. B	2439. D	2506. D	2573. B	2640. A	2707. A
2306. E	2373. D	2440. C	2507. B	2574. D	2641. D	2708. C
2307. C	2374. E	2441. D	2508. B	2575. B	2642. B	2709. A
2308. C	2375. A	2442. C	2509. D	2576. B	2643. A	2710. B
2309. D	2376. D	2443. B	2510. A	2577. A	2644. C	2711. A
2310. A	2377. D	2444. E	2511. B	2578. D	2645. D	2712. B
2311. E	2378. C	2445. A	2512. C	2579. A	2646. B	2713. D
2312. B	2379. B	2446. B	2513. A	2580. C	2647. B	2714. A
2313. C	2380. E	2447. C	2514. B	2581. C	2648. C	2715. C
2314. B	2381. A	2448. D	2515. D	2582. D	2649. B	2716. D
2315. A	2382. B	2449. D	2516. A	2583. C	2650. C	2717. C
2316. E	2383. B	2450. C	2517. B	2584. C	2651. A	2718. D
2317. C	2384. C	2451. A	2518. D	2585. C	2652. B	2719. D
2318. A	2385. A	2452. B	2519. A	2586. C	2653. C	2720. B
2319. A	2386. B	2453. A	2520. C	2587. A	2654. D	2721. C
2320. E	2387. E	2454. D	2521. B	2588. A	2655. B	2722. D
2321. D	2388. A	2455. C	2522. C	2589. C	2656. B	2723. C
2322. C	2389. E	2456. A	2523. B	2590. D	2657. A	2724. B
2323. C	2390. C	2457. E	2524. A	2591. A	2658. B	2725. A
2324. B	2391. D	2458. D	2525. D	2592. C	2659. A	2726. C
2325. D	2392. B	2459. B	2526. A	2593. B	2660. C	2727. C
2326. E	2393. A	2460. C	2527. A	2594. B	2661. C	2728. A
2327. D	2394. E	2461. A	2528. B	2595. A	2662. A	2729. A
2328. A	2395. A	2462. A	2529. A	2596. D	2663. D	2730. D
2329. C	2396. B	2463. C	2530. A	2597. C	2664. A	2731. C
2330. B	2397. D	2464. B	2531. C	2598. C	2665. A	2732. C
2331. A	2398. E	2465. E	2532. B	2599. C	2666. B	2733. C
2332. B	2399. A	2466. D	2533. D	2600. C	2667. A	2734. D
2333. E	2400. C	2467. A	2534. A	2601. B	2668. B	2735. A
2334. A	2401. C	2468. A	2535. B	2602. B	2669. D	2736. C
2335. A	2402. B	2469. D	2536. A	2603. B	2670. C	2737. A
2336. D	2403. A	2470. B	2537. B	2604. A	2671. A	2738. C
2337. B	2404. D	2471. A	2538. A	2605. C	2672. C	2739. D
2338. B	2405. B	2472. B	2539. C	2606. A	2673. A	2740. D
2339. E	2406. A	2473. D	2540. C	2607. A	2674. B	2741. D
2340. C	2407. E	2474. D	2541. B	2608. C	2675. D	2742. B
2341. B	2408. A	2475. C	2542. C	2609. C	2676. B	2743. A
2342. C	2409. C	2476. A	2543. A	2610. A	2677. A	2744. D
2343. A	2410. A	2477. B	2544. A	2611. B	2678. A	2745. B
2344. E	2411. C	2478. C	2545. C	2612. A	2679. A	2746. D
2345. C	2412. D	2479. A	2546. C	2613. D	2680. C	2747. C
2346. B	2413. C	2480. B	2547. B	2614. C	2681. A	2748. B
2347. D	2414. B	2481. A	2548. D	2615. A	2682. A	2749. B
2348. E	2415. B	2482. E	2549. B	2616. D	2683. A	2750. A
2349. B	2416. D	2483. B	2550. A	2617. B	2684. C	2751. C
2350. E	2417. A	2484. B	2551. A	2618. C	2685. C	2752. B
2351. D	2418. D	2485. A	2552. C	2619. B	2686. B	2753. B
2352. A	2419. A	2486. B	2553. B	2620. B	2687. D	2754. C
2353. E	2420. B	2487. A	2554. C	2621. A	2688. C	2755. C
2354. B	2421. D	2488. C	2555. C	2622. B	2689. A	2756. C
2355. D	2422. D	2489. B	2556. D	2623. B	2690. A	2757. C
2356. C	2423. A	2490. C	2557. A	2624. C	2691. D	2758. C
2357. D	2424. D	2491. A	2558. C	2625. A	2692. A	2759. B
2358. A	2425. A	2492. D	2559. D	2626. A	2693. C	2760. B
2359. E	2426. D	2493. C	2560. C	2627. B	2694. A	2761. C
2360. D	2427. B	2494. A	2561. A	2628. C	2695. A	2762. A
2361. B	2428. C	2495. E	2562. D	2629. A	2696. A	2763. A
2362. C	2429. D	2496. A	2563. C	2630. D	2697. A	2764. B
2363. D	2430. C	2497. B	2564. B	2631. A	2698. B	2765. C

2766. C	2833. C	2900. C	2967. B	3034. B	3101. B	3168. C
2767. A	2834. C	2901. A	2968. B	3035. C	3102. C	3169. A
2768. C	2835. A	2902. D	2969. A	3036. D	3103. C	3170. B
2769. C	2836. A	2903. A	2970. D	3037. A	3104. D	3171. B
2770. A	2837. C	2904. B	2971. C	3038. C	3105. B	3172. B
2771. B	2838. D	2905. C	2972. A	3039. C	3106. A	3173. C
2772. C	2839. B	2906. A	2973. B	3040. B	3107. C	3174. B
2773. B	2840. A	2907. A	2974. B	3041. D	3108. A	3175. A
2774. D	2841. C	2908. C	2975. D	3042. C	3109. D	3176. D
2775. A	2842. A	2909. D	2976. A	3043. A	3110. A	3177. A
2776. D	2843. A	2910. C	2977. A	3044. A	3111. A	3178. A
2777. C	2844. C	2911. A	2978. C	3045. B	3112. C	3179. D
2778. B	2845. A	2912. D	2979. D	3046. B	3113. A	3180. C
2779. A	2846. D	2913. B	2980. A	3047. A	3114. B	3181. D
2780. A	2847. A	2914. D	2981. A	3048. A	3115. A	3182. B
2781. A	2848. C	2915. A	2982. C	3049. B	3116. C	3183. A
2782. B	2849. D	2916. B	2983. D	3050. B	3117. D	3184. C
2783. D	2850. A	2917. A	2984. C	3051. A	3118. C	3185. C
2784. C	2851. D	2918. D	2985. C	3052. B	3119. A	3186. A
2785. B	2852. B	2919. C	2986. D	3053. A	3120. B	3187. C
2786. A	2853. B	2920. A	2987. A	3054. A	3121. C	3188. C
2787. D	2854. A	2921. D	2988. D	3055. C	3122. A	3189. A
2788. D	2855. A	2922. C	2989. B	3056. C	3123. A	3190. A
2789. C	2856. B	2923. A	2990. C	3057. A	3124. C	3191. C
2790. A	2857. A	2924. B	2991. A	3058. D	3125. C	3192. A
2791. B	2858. D	2925. D	2992. C	3059. D	3126. C	3193. C
2792. B	2859. B	2926. B	2993. B	3060. A	3127. C	3194. C
2793. C	2860. A	2927. D	2994. B	3061. D	3128. B	3195. D
2794. B	2861. D	2928. A	2995. C	3062. A	3129. D	3196. C
2795. D	2862. C	2929. C	2996. B	3063. C	3130. C	3197. C
2796. A	2863. A	2930. C	2997. A	3064. C	3131. C	3198. A
2797. B	2864. C	2931. A	2998. C	3065. A	3132. B	3199. A
2798. A	2865. C	2932. C	2999. C	3066. C	3133. C	3200. C
2799. D	2866. C	2933. A	3000. A	3067. C	3134. D	3201. C
2800. C	2867. B	2934. C	3001. C	3068. C	3135. C	3202. D
2801. A	2868. C	2935. B	3002. A	3069. A	3136. A	3203. C
2802. A	2869. D	2936. A	3003. C	3070. C	3137. A	3204. D
2803. C	2870. B	2937. C	3004. C	3071. B	3138. D	3205. D
2804. A	2871. C	2938. B	3005. B	3072. C	3139. A	3206. C
2805. C	2872. C	2939. C	3006. C	3073. A	3140. B	3207. B
2806. A	2873. B	2940. C	3007. A	3074. C	3141. D	3208. C
2807. C	2874. B	2941. C	3008. C	3075. A	3142. A	3209. A
2808. D	2875. B	2942. A	3009. A	3076. C	3143. B	3210. C
2809. A	2876. A	2943. C	3010. A	3077. B	3144. C	3211. A
2810. B	2877. C	2944. A	3011. C	3078. C	3145. D	3212. C
2811. A	2878. B	2945. C	3012. D	3079. C	3146. C	3213. B
2812. C	2879. B	2946. D	3013. B	3080. C	3147. C	3214. C
2813. A	2880. A	2947. B	3014. A	3081. B	3148. D	3215. C
2814. B	2881. D	2948. C	3015. C	3082. B	3149. B	3216. C
2815. A	2882. A	2949. D	3016. B	3083. C	3150. A	3217. A
2816. C	2883. C	2950. C	3017. C	3084. C	3151. C	3218. B
2817. A	2884. A	2951. A	3018. C	3085. A	3152. A	3219. A
2818. B	2885. B	2952. D	3019. B	3086. A	3153. D	3220. B
2819. C	2886. C	2953. C	3020. C	3087. B	3154. C	3221. A
2820. B	2887. A	2954. C	3021. B	3088. B	3155. B	3222. A
2821. A	2888. C	2955. A	3022. C	3089. A	3156. C	3223. A
2822. C	2889. B	2956. A	3023. C	3090. C	3157. C	3224. B
2823. B	2890. C	2957. B	3024. C	3091. D	3158. A	3225. A
2824. A	2891. C	2958. C	3025. B	3092. C	3159. A	3226. C
2825. B	2892. A	2959. A	3026. A	3093. B	3160. C	3227. D
2826. D	2893. D	2960. B	3027. B	3094. A	3161. B	3228. D
2827. B	2894. A	2961. D	3028. C	3095. A	3162. A	3229. C
2828. A	2895. D	2962. A	3029. B	3096. C	3163. A	3230. A
2829. D	2896. D	2963. B	3030. C	3097. B	3164. B	3231. B
2830. A	2897. C	2964. B	3031. A	3098. C	3165. C	3232. D
2831. C	2898. A	2965. C	3032. C	3099. C	3166. A	3233. C
2832. C	2899. B	2966. D	3033. C	3100. B	3167. C	3234. C

3235.	D	3273.	B	3311.	A	3349.	C	3387.	A	3425.	C	3463.	B
3236.	C	3274.	C	3312.	D	3350.	A	3388.	D	3426.	A	3464.	B
3237.	A	3275.	A	3313.	D	3351.	D	3389.	C	3427.	C	3465.	A
3238.	D	3276.	A	3314.	B	3352.	C	3390.	C	3428.	D	3466.	C
3239.	A	3277.	A	3315.	A	3353.	A	3391.	B	3429.	C	3467.	D
3240.	A	3278.	C	3316.	B	3354.	A	3392.	A	3430.	C	3468.	A
3241.	A	3279.	B	3317.	B	3355.	C	3393.	C	3431.	A	3469.	C
3242.	B	3280.	C	3318.	A	3356.	B	3394.	C	3432.	A	3470.	D
3243.	D	3281.	D	3319.	A	3357.	B	3395.	C	3433.	C	3471.	D
3244.	C	3282.	C	3320.	B	3358.	D	3396.	A	3434.	D	3472.	C
3245.	A	3283.	A	3321.	C	3359.	A	3397.	C	3435.	B	3473.	B
3246.	B	3284.	B	3322.	C	3360.	B	3398.	A	3436.	C	3474.	B
3247.	C	3285.	C	3323.	C	3361.	C	3399.	A	3437.	D	3475.	C
3248.	A	3286.	A	3324.	C	3362.	C	3400.	C	3438.	C	3476.	A
3249.	A	3287.	D	3325.	B	3363.	D	3401.	B	3439.	B	3477.	B
3250.	A	3288.	A	3326.	D	3364.	B	3402.	D	3440.	A	3478.	A
3251.	A	3289.	B	3327.	C	3365.	C	3403.	B	3441.	B	3479.	C
3252.	B	3290.	D	3328.	C	3366.	D	3404.	C	3442.	A	3480.	C
3253.	C	3291.	C	3329.	A	3367.	A	3405.	D	3443.	A	3481.	D
3254.	B	3292.	C	3330.	C	3368.	B	3406.	B	3444.	C	3482.	C
3255.	A	3293.	A	3331.	A	3369.	D	3407.	C	3445.	A	3483.	A
3256.	C	3294.	A	3332.	C	3370.	C	3408.	D	3446.	A	3484.	B
3257.	C	3295.	B	3333.	A	3371.	C	3409.	C	3447.	D	3485.	C
3258.	C	3296.	A	3334.	C	3372.	A	3410.	D	3448.	A	3486.	C
3259.	C	3297.	D	3335.	C	3373.	A	3411.	B	3449.	D	3487.	A
3260.	B	3298.	A	3336.	C	3374.	A	3412.	A	3450.	D	3488.	B
3261.	A	3299.	B	3337.	C	3375.	C	3413.	B	3451.	D	3489.	C
3262.	B	3300.	C	3338.	B	3376.	B	3414.	C	3452.	A	3490.	A
3263.	C	3301.	A	3339.	C	3377.	A	3415.	B	3453.	A	3491.	B
3264.	A	3302.	D	3340.	A	3378.	A	3416.	A	3454.	C	3492.	A
3265.	C	3303.	C	3341.	C	3379.	C	3417.	D	3455.	B	3493.	C
3266.	A	3304.	A	3342.	D	3380.	D	3418.	B	3456.	C	3494.	A
3267.	A	3305.	D	3343.	A	3381.	C	3419.	A	3457.	A	3495.	B
3268.	B	3306.	C	3344.	C	3382.	D	3420.	D	3458.	B	3496.	C
3269.	B	3307.	B	3345.	A	3383.	C	3421.	A	3459.	C	3497.	A
3270.	D	3308.	A	3346.	B	3384.	A	3422.	C	3460.	B	3498.	B
3271.	C	3309.	C	3347.	B	3385.	B	3423.	C	3461.	C	3499.	C
3272.	B	3310.	C	3348.	C	3386.	C	3424.	B	3462.	A	3500.	D